New Paradigms in Biomedical Engineering

New Paradigms in Biomedical Engineering

Edited by Eden Morrison

STATES
ACADEMIC PRESS
www.statesacademicpress.com

States Academic Press,
109 South 5th Street,
Brooklyn, NY 11249, USA

Visit us on the World Wide Web at:
www.statesacademicpress.com

ISBN: 978-1-63989-382-9

Cataloging-in-Publication Data

New paradigms in biomedical engineering / edited by Eden Morrison.
p. cm.
Includes bibliographical references and index.
ISBN 978-1-63989-382-9
1. Biomedical engineering. 2. Medicine. 3. Bioengineering. I. Morrison, Eden.
R856 .N49 2022
610.28--dc23

Table of Contents

Preface

Biomedical engineering is the branch of medical science that involves the application of engineering principles and concepts to biology and medicine for diagnostic and therapeutic purposes. It combines the biological sciences with the design and problem-solving skills of engineering for the advancement of healthcare treatment including monitoring, diagnosis and therapy. Biochemical engineering is a multidisciplinary field that draws concepts from mechanical engineering, chemical engineering, electrical engineering, materials science, computer science and biology. There are various applications of biomedical engineering such as design and development of active and passive medical devices, medical imaging, orthopedic implants, biomedical signal processing, and tissue and stem cell engineering. The ever growing need of advanced technology is the reason that has fueled the research in the field of biomedical engineering in recent times. This book is a compilation of chapters that discuss the most vital concepts and emerging trends in this field. As this field is emerging at a fast pace, it will help the readers to better understand the new paradigms in biomedical engineering.

Significant researches are present in this book. Intensive efforts have been employed by authors to make this book an outstanding discourse. This book contains the enlightening chapters which have been written on the basis of significant researches done by the experts.

Finally, I would also like to thank all the members involved in this book for being a team and meeting all the deadlines for the submission of their respective works. I would also like to thank my friends and family for being supportive in my efforts.

Editor

1

Image Processing Methods for Automatic Cell Counting In Vivo or In Situ Using 3D Confocal Microscopy

Manuel G. Forero[1] and Alicia Hidalgo[2]
[1]*Cardiff University,*
[2]*University of Birmingham,*
United Kingdom

1. Introduction

Image processing methods have opened the opportunity to extract quantitative information from confocal microscopy images of biological samples, dramatically increasing the range of questions that can be addressed experimentally in biology. Biologists aim to understand how cells behave and what genes do to build a normal animal, and what goes wrong in disease or upon injury. For this, they look at how alterations in gene function and application of drugs affect tissue, organ or whole body integrity, using confocal microscopy images of samples stained with cell specific markers. Image-processing methods have enormous potential to extract information from this kind of samples, but surprisingly, they are still relatively underexploited. One useful parameter to quantify is cell number. Cell number is the balance between cell division and cell death; it is controlled tightly during growth and it can be altered in disease, most notoriously neurodegeneration and cancer. Injury (e.g. spinal cord injury) results in an increase in cell death, plus a homeostatic regulation of cell proliferation. Thus to understand normal animal development, injury responses and disease, it is important to find out how many cells die or divide, or how many cells of a given type there are in an organ. Generally, cells are counted using automated methods after dissociating cells from a tissue (e.g. fluorescence-activated cell sorting, FACS, based), or when they are distributed in a dish in cell culture experiments, using image processing techniques in 2D (e.g. using Metamorph software). However, these approaches alter the normal cellular contexts and the procedures themselves can alter the relative numbers of cells. To maintain information relevant to how genes and cells behave in the organism, it is best to count cells in vivo (i.e. in the intact animal) or at least in an entire organ or tissue (i.e. in situ). Counting in vivo or in situ is generally carried out manually, or it consists of estimates of number of cells stained with a particular cell marker or inferences from anatomical alterations. These methods can be extremely time-consuming, estimates can be inaccurate, and the questions that can be addressed using these methods are limited. Manual counting can be experimentally cumbersome, tedious, labour intensive and error prone. The advent of confocal microscopy, which allows the capture of 3D images, has enabled the development of automatic and semi-automatic image processing methods to count cells in whole tissues or entire small animals. Whereas excellent automated methods can be purchased commercially and are widely used to count cells after dissociation or in cell culture, fewer methods have been developed to count cells in situ or in vivo. Such methods are challenging, as they require large stacks of images to capture the whole sample, and can encounter greater difficulty in distinguishing labelled cells from background signal. Some automatic techniques have been developed to segment cell nuclei from mammalian tissue sections or from whole Drosophila brains in 2D and 3D images (Lin et al., 2003; Shimada et al., 2005; Wählby 2003; Wählby et al., 2004), but they are not useful to analyse large sample sizes because the intensive computation slows down the process. Identifying all the nuclei is extremely challenging from the point of view of imaging because cells can be tightly packed. In any case, counting all nuclei is not always most informative, as it does not qualify on cell type (is the number of neurons or glia altered?) or cell state (do the changes affect dividing or dying cells?). Cell Profiler (Carpenter, 2006) enables combinations of image-processing methods that can be used to count cells, but it is not very user friendly for most biologists as it requires computation expertise.

We have developed a range of publicly available methods that can count the number of dividing or dying cells, neurons or glia, in intact specimens of fruit-fly Drosophila embryos (Forero et al, 2009, 2010, 2010a). Quantification is automatic, accurate, objective and fast, enabling reliable comparisons of multiple specimens of diverse genotypes. Additionally, results are reproducible: automatic programs perform consistently and always yield the same cell count for a given sample regardless of the number of times it is counted. Drosophila is a powerful model organism generally used to investigate gene function, developmental processes and model human diseases. Working in vivo or in situ with Drosophila is one of the main reasons behind using it as a model organism. Using Drosophila, researchers have investigated the number of dying cells, glial cells, and progeny cells in a neuroblast lineage, or the number of cells within mosaic cell clones (Maurange et al 2008; Bello et al, 2006, 2008; Rogulja-Ortmann et al. 2007; Franzdottir et al. 2009; Ho et al. 2009). Our methods can be used to automate these quantitative analyses. Although our image processing methods were developed from Drosophila images, these methods can be adapted to work on other sample types (i.e. mammalian tissues).

The identification and counting of cells is a difficult task both for the human eye and for image processing: i) Most often, cell visualisation with immunohistochemical markers results in background signal (i.e. spots) as well as the signal corresponding to the cells; ii) there is also natural variability within biological samples, as cell size and shape can vary; iii) if a marker detects abundant cells, they can be tightly packed and it can be difficult to determine the boundaries between adjacent cells; iv) and the properties of the detector, the fluorescence settings and the lasers can also introduce error (Dima et al., 2002). As a result, it can be difficult to decide what is a cell and what is not. Consequently, manual counting is extremely error prone. Image processing methods are ideal for objective quantifications, since once a good method has been established to identify the objects, all samples are treated in the same way thus eliminating error. When analysing cell counts in whole organisms (i.e. Drosophila embryos), tissues or organs, it is not appropriate to use projections of a stack of images into a single 2D image, since this will occlude cells and form tight clusters rendering it impossible to separate the individual cells. In vivo quantification requires object recognition in 3D, which is achievable using confocal microscopy.

In this chapter, we review the most relevant steps to be considered in the development of automatic methods to segment and count cells in 3D for in-situ or in vivo preparations. The principles described will enable researchers of multiple disciplines to apply the logic of image processing to modify the currently available programs making them applicable to their own samples and research questions, as well as help them make further developments. For two complementary reviews of image processing techniques and a description of some of the existing software employed to analyse biology samples, please see (Meijering & Cappellen, 2007) and (Peng, 2008).

2. Methodology

Counting cells in Drosophila is a complex task, due to variability in image quality resulting from different cell markers. Cells are segmented according to their characteristics. But cell shape changes with cell state (i.e. arrest, mitosis, or apoptosis). For instance, during mitosis the shape is irregular and it can be difficult to determine when a dividing cell can be considered as two daughter cells. Nuclei and glia cells have a more regular shape, between elliptical and circular. Apoptotic cells have initially a very irregular shape, later on very round, and can appear subdivided into different parts depending on the timing within apoptosis. Depending on the kind of cells or cell state to be visualised, a different cell marker (i.e. antibody) is employed. As a result, different image-processing methods must be developed to quantify cells of different qualities.

2.1 Visualisation of distinct cell types and states using immunohistochemistry

Cells to be counted in Drosophila embryos were visualised with immunohystochemistry methods, using antibodies as follows (Figure 1). (1) Dying (apoptotic) cells were stained with anti-cleaved-Caspase-3 (hereafter called Caspase) (Figure 1a), a widely used marker for apoptotic cells. The protein Caspase-3 is evolutionarily conserved. The commercially available antibodies that we have used (Caspase-3, Cell Signalling Technology) cross-react with a wide range of species, including Drosophila. Caspase is initially cytoplasmic and as apoptosis progresses it reveals intense, round, shrunken cells. Organisms stained with Caspase yield images with cells of irregular shape and size, low signal intensity and high intensity background. (2) Dividing (mitotic) cells were stained with anti-pHistone-H3 (hereafter called pH3, Figure 1b). pH3 labels the phosphorylated state of the evolutionarily conserved Histone-H3 characteristic of M-phase (mitosis) of the cell cycle. The commercially available antibodies we used (Upstate Biotechnology) work well in a wide range of species. The embryonic nuclei stained with pH3 are sparsely distributed and do not tend to overlap or form large clusters. As pH3 stains chromosomes, shape can be irregular. Nuclei can appear connected and must be separated. (3) Glial cell nuclei were stained with anti-Repo (hereafter called Repo) (Figure 1c). Repo (Developmental Studies Hybridoma Bank, Iowa) is the general nuclear marker for all glial cells, except the midline glia, in Drosophila. Nuclei stained with Repo tend to be rather regular. pH3 and Repo antibodies yield high signal intensity and low background, and stain nuclei that are relatively sparsely distributed in the organism. (4) Neuronal nuclei were stained with anti-HB9 (hereafter called HB9, gift of H. Brohier) in embryos (Figure 1d). Pan-neuronal anti-Elav does not consistently yield stainings of comparable quality and visualising all nuclei compromises resolution during object identification. Thus, a compromise solution is using HB9, which stains with strong signal and low background a large subset of interneurons and all motorneurons.

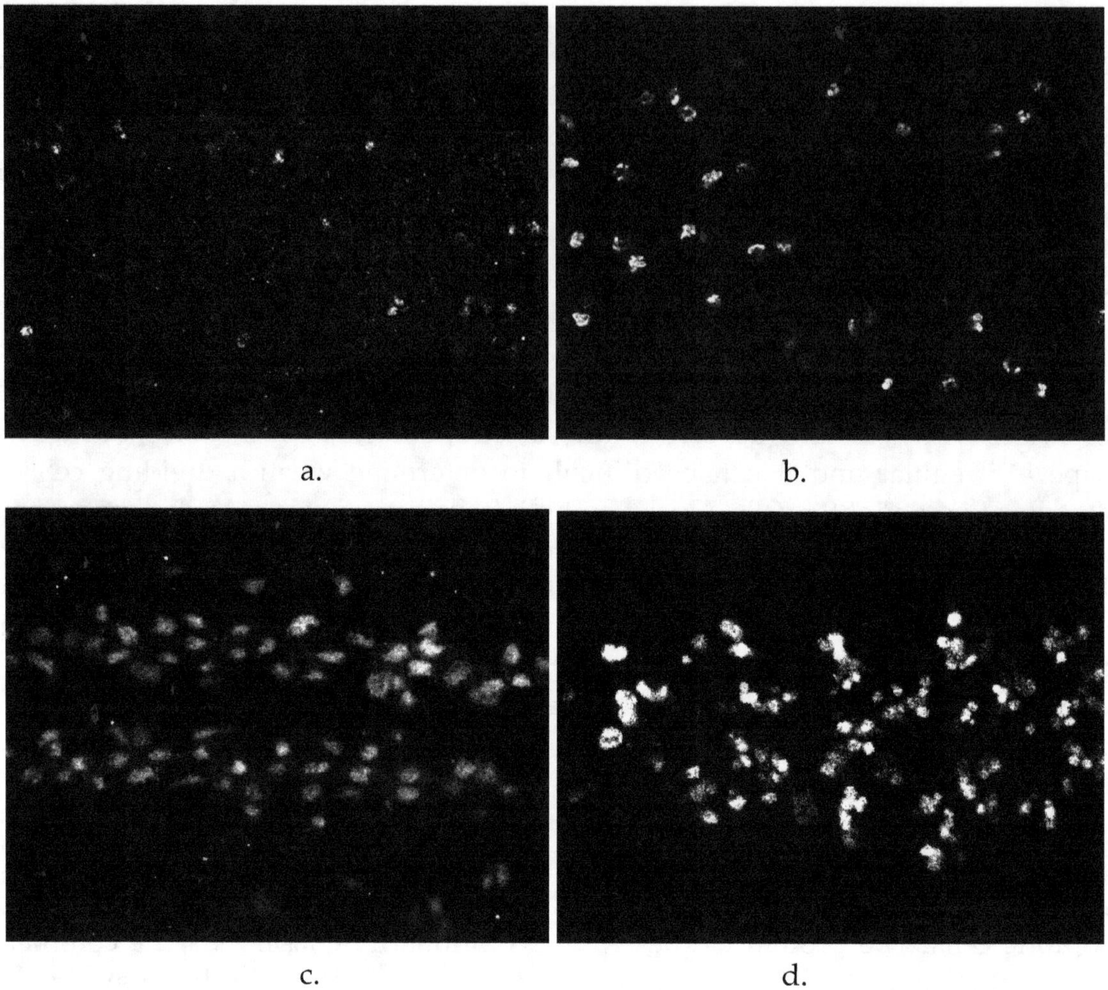

Fig. 1. Drosophila embryos labelled with: (a) Anti-cleaved-Caspase-3 to visualise apoptotic cells. (b) Anti-p-Histone-H3 to visualise mitotic cells. (c) Anti-Repo to visualise glial cells. (d) Anti-HB9 to visualise a subset of neuronal nuclei. A fraction of the ventral nerve cord is shown in each case; all images show single confocal optical sections.

Whole embryos were dechorionated in bleach, then fixed in 4% formaldehyde in phosphate buffer (PBS) for 20 minutes at room temperature, washed in PBS with 0.1% Triton-X100 (Sigma) and stained following standard protocols (Rothwell and Sullivan, 2000). Embryos were incubated in diluted primary antibodies overnight at 4°C and the following day in secondary antibodies for 2 hours at room temperature. Antibodies were diluted in PBS 0.1% Triton as follows: (1) Rabbit anti-cleaved-Caspase-3 1:50; (2) Guinea-pig HB9 1:1000; (3) Mouse anti-Repo at 1:100; (4) Rabbit-anti-phospho-Histone-H3 at 1:300. Secondary antibodies were directly conjugated to Alexa-488 and used at 1:250. Anti-Caspase had a tendency to yield high background, and different batches produced by Upstate Biotechnology had different staining qualities. Thus each new batch had to be optimised. To reduce background, embryos were first blocked in 1% Bovin Serum Albumin (BSA, Sigma) and incubated in very small volumes (10 microliters worth of embryos in a 50-100 microliter volume of diluted antibody), and the antibody was not reused. Signal amplification was not used (i.e. no avidin) since this raised the Caspase background considerably. All other antibodies were more robust and worked well using standard conditions, and antibody aliquots were reused multiple times. Samples were mounted in Vectashield (Vector Labs) or

70% glycerol. Mounted whole embryos were scanned using a BioRad Radiance 2000 or Leica TCS-SP2-AOBS laser scanning confocal microscopes. The settings at the confocal microscope were fixed for all samples and acquisition was set to ensure that the dynamic range of the histogram covered all grey values. The conditions for scanning were 60x lens, no zoom and 0.5μm slice step, acquisition resolution of 512 x 512 pixels, no averaging. Fixed iris (pinhole =1), laser intensity, gain and offset were maintained throughout all samples of the same experiment. Software algorithms were developed and evaluated using Java and ImageJ under an Ubuntu Linux platform in a PC Pentium 4 running at 3 GHz with 1.5 GB RAM.

2.1 Development

Most published techniques segment and count cells in two dimensions. With the appearance of confocal microscopes, which allow to visualise cells plane by plane in 3D, new techniques have been developed to count them in 3D.

In general, the automatic and semiautomatic techniques developed to count cells follow these steps:

- Acquisition.
- Filtering for noise reduction.
- Segmentation.
- Post processing, including morphological filtering and separation of cells.
- Classification.

2.2 Acquisition

The acquisition protocol is a very important step. If the quality of the images is poor or strongly changes from one stack to another, it renders the development of an automatic counting method challenging. For a given experiment were all samples are labelled with the same cell marker and fluorophore, there can be considerable variability in the quality of the images, and if of bad quality it can even become impossible for an experienced biologist to identify reliably the cells. Therefore, several parameters must be optimised experimentally, such as those relating to the treatment of samples (e.g. fixative, detergent, dilutions of antibodies, incubation period, etc.) and the acquisition (e.g. laser intensity, filters, gain and offset of the amplifiers, magnification, etc). Once the best quality of images is obtained, all of these parameters must be fixed, and samples that do not produce images of adequate quality should be rejected.

3D image processing techniques can be used to improve the quality of segmentation. This is important when the signal to noise ratio is low, given that some spots can be considered noise in a 2D image, but recognized as true particles in 3D (Gué, 2005). To work in 3D, other techniques should be considered before filtering. In fluorescence confocal microscopy signal intensity decreases with tissue thickness. Thus, frequently 3D techniques apply an intensity correction. One of the simplest techniques employs the maxima or the average of the foreground on each image to construct a function of the intensity attenuation and the inverse function is used to compensate the intensity loss (Adiga, 2000; Lin, 2003; Wählby, 2004). However, the result is not always satisfactory, especially when the background or the foreground changes abruptly or the background has some complexity, making it difficult to define the foreground automatically. This is a common issue in Drosophila samples. More complex techniques can also be used, although they are time-consuming (Conchello, 1995; Guan, 2008; Kervrann, 2004; Rodenacker, 2001; Roerdink, 1993; Wu, 2005) or require complex acquisition (Can, 2003).

Images are also degraded by out-of-focus blur, albeit to a lesser degree than with epi-fluorescence. The Z resolution is lower than in the X-Y plane, which affects the results of 3D segmentation techniques. De-blurring and restoration techniques, which both improve image definition and reduce noise should be considered before applying 3D segmentation techniques. Some of these methods are based on the knowledge of the Point Spread Function (PSF) or are blind when the PSF is unknown. The Richarson-Lucy (Richardson , 1972; Lucy, 1974) and the Tikhonov deconvolution methods are two of the best known methods. Others include maximum likelihood estimation, Wiener and wavelets (see review by Sarder & Nehorai, 2006). Deconvolution methods can achieve very good results, but at the expense of a very high computational cost. However, if a convenient segmentation technique is used to process each image based only in its properties, an intensity correction procedure can be avoided. Given such complexity and pitfalls, techniques have been developed to take the alternative route of avoiding these steps. Accordingly, images are filtered and segmented in 2D, and 3D techniques are only applied once the intensity of the cells is no longer relevant, i.e. after the images have been segmented, thus gaining speed in the process.

2.3 Filtering

3D restoration methods improve the quality of the images reducing noise. When these methods are not employed, other noise reduction techniques must be used. In confocal microscopy images, noise follows a Poisson distribution as image acquisition is based on photon emission. Given that the number of photons produced is very small, statistical variation in the number of detected photons is the most important source of noise. Although some researchers employ linear filters like the Gaussian operator to reduce noise in confocal microscopy (Wählby, 2004; Fernandez, 2010), they are not the most recommended to reduce Poisson noise, which is signal dependent. Additionally, the use of linear filters results in a lower definition of the cell borders, making it more difficult to distinguish cells, especially when they are tightly packed. In the Poisson distribution the mean and variance are not independent. Therefore, variance stabilising transformations (VST), like the Anscombe (Anscombe, 1948) and, the Freeman and Tukey (Freeman & Tukey, 1950) transforms, which approximately transform a random variable following a Poison distribution into a Gaussian, could be applied (Kervrann, 2004a) before the use of a linear filter.

Bar-Lev and Enis (Bar-Lev & Enis 1988) developed a method for obtaining a class of variance stabilizing transformations, which includes the Ascombe and, Freeman and Tukey transforms. In this case, images are transformed, then filtered by using a linear operator and then the inverse transform is applied before segmentation. However these transforms have an important limitation, as they are not useful when the number of counts or photons per pixel is lower than about 20 (Starck, 2002). Furthermore, bad results are also related to the inverse process (Makitalo & Foi, 2011). New efforts have been made to improve these two aspects (Foi, 2008, 2009; Makitalo & Foi, 2011, 2011a), but their developments have not been tested for cell counting in confocal microscopy samples. Other models based on the analysis of the acquisition system have been proposed (Calapez & Rosa, 2010).

Given the nature of the noise, non-linear filters are more appropriate. These filters in general reduce the noise and the significant intensity heterogeneity typical of confocal images, without strongly affecting the signal provided by the stained cells. The median filter is one of the simplest methods and we found it provides good results (Forero et al, 2009, 2010, 2010a). Many other median filter variations can also be employed, although they can require a more exhaustive and time-consuming calculation, and some parameters to be fixed (Mitra, 2001;

Forero & Delgado, 2003). Outlier filters can also serve to eliminate noise, while keeping the edges on the image. In this kind of filter the value of each pixel p is replaced by the mean or the median of the pixels included in a window centered in p, if the original value of p is further from the mean or the median than a threshold t defined by the user. Noise reduction techniques based on wavelets are also employed to filter confocal images. They can yield good results with an appropriate bank of filters. Other edge preserving methods like bilateral filters (Tomasi & Manduchi, 1998) can also be employed (Shen, 2009; Rodrigues, 2008). 3D filters have also been used, but the computational cost is higher and results can be affected by the difference in the resolution between the x-y plane and the z-axis. 2D restoration of the 3D methods mentioned above can also be employed, but unfortunately they are still time-consuming.
In addition to the Poisson noise filters, other filters may be required to eliminate noise specific to the kind of images being processed. For example, signal intensity is heterogeneous in HB9 labelled nuclei, and image background is characterised by extremely small spots or particles of very high intensity. To eliminate these small spots and render signal intensity uniform, a grey scale morphological opening with a circular structural element of radius r, higher than the typical radius of the spots, is applied to each slice of the stack. As a generalization, particles of any particular size can be eliminated by morphological granularimetry. In this way, granularimetry defined as:

$$G = \text{Open}\ (r_{min}) - \text{Open}\ (r_{max}) \tag{1}$$

is used to eliminate particles of radius between r_{max} and r_{min}.
Another morphological noise reduction technique, the alternating sequential filter (ASF) has also been used to reduce noise in confocal images (Fernandez, 2010). This filter removes particles starting from the smallest ones and moving toward the largest ones by doing an alternating succession of opening and closing morphological operations with structural elements of progressively larger size (Sternberg, 1986; Serra, 1988).

2.4 Segmentation

After filtering, segmentation is carried out. Segmentation is a procedure that subdivides the image in disjoint regions or classes in order to identify the structures or objects of interest appearing in the image. These structures can be basically identified by their similarity or discontinuity. On the one hand, the detection of the edges or contours of the objects of interest is given by searching the local discontinuities in the intensity of the grey levels of the image. On the other hand, the extraction of the objects can be found by searching the homogeneous areas in the grey level values. Thresholding techniques allow separating the pixels of the image between background and foreground. In the simplest case, bilevel or binarisation, the pixels take only two possible different grey levels. The objects in the foreground are considered to belong only to one class and are separated from the background by choosing an optimum threshold grey level t, in the interval $[0, L]$, where L is the maximum grey level in the image, based on certain criteria. Mathematically, binarisation is a process of transformation that converts an image represented by the function $q(x, y)$ into the image $r(x, y)$ given by:

$$r(x,y) = \begin{cases} 1 & \text{if} \quad q(x,y) > t \\ 0 & \text{if} \quad q(x,y) \le t \end{cases} \tag{2}$$

where (x, y) represent the position of each pixel in the image.

A third kind of method to segment cells in confocal microscopy consists on the use of active contour models. In their original description, snakes (Kass et al. 1988), the active contours were seen as a dynamic elastic band that was located outside or inside the objects to be segmented, and by contraction or expansion of the band the borders of the objects were obtained. The snakes look for the borders by minimizing the energy of the band, using the gradient of the image as one of the parameters to calculate the energy. This technique is very sensitive to noise and initiation (i.e. where the band is initially located), and several methods have been developed to overcome the limitations of finding a good initiation and of segmenting nuclei (Clocksin, 2003; Chan et al., 2000, Chan & Vese, 2001, Osher & Sethian, 1988), using level sets (Cheng, 2009).
As cell borders are fuzzy, we preferred thresholding to edge detection methods for segmentation. Depending on the intensity variation in the cells through each image, local or global thresholding can be employed. An alternative consists on using more than one global threshold (Long et al., 2007). Long et al. calculates a first threshold and cells detected over that threshold are segmented and counted. Then the regions where the cells have been counted are ignored and a new threshold is calculated. This second threshold is lower than the first one and allows detecting cells of lower intensity. Then these new cells are also processed and counted.
Due to fluorescence attenuation through the stack of images, cells are more clearly seen in the first slices and for this reason using only one threshold to binarise the whole stack is not appropriate. Instead, a threshold value is found for each image. The method chosen to find the threshold t is critical and varies with the marker employed to label the cells or nuclei and the characteristics of the resulting images. Thus a different binarisation method was developed for each cell marker.

2.4.1 Neuronal nuclei

The method employed to binarise images depends on the characteristics of the distribution of the intensities of the objects and background in the images, which can be studied trough the histogram. One of the most popular thresholding methods, Otsu, works especially well when the typical histogram of the images is bimodal, with a Gaussian distribution. It works also well in highly contrasted images, where there is a strong intensity difference between foreground and background. This was the case for nuclei labelled with HB9 antibodies, and therefore this was the method employed to binarise such images (Forero et al, 2010). A frequent case to be considered when working with stacks, is when no cells or nuclei but only background appear in some images. Whereas a very low threshold can be found, this would yield false nuclei. To solve this problem, low thresholds are not taken into account when the maximum intensity of an image is lower than a quarter of the maximum grey level or if the threshold is lower than 20, a value found empirically corresponding to the highest standard intensity of the background. In these cases, images are binarised using the last valid threshold obtained in a previous image of the stack. If a very low threshold is found in the first image of the stack, the threshold takes the value of the maximum grey level and the binarised image becomes black. The resulting binarised images are employed as masks and combined, using a logic AND operation, with the images resulting of the opening operation to produce images were the background becomes black (grey level 'zero') and the intensities of the foreground remain unmodified. For further details, see (Forero et al, 2010).

2.4.2 Apoptotic cells

The typical histogram $h(q)$, where q is the grey level intensity, of median-filtered Caspase images is composed of two modes, the first one corresponding to the background and the second one to the sample. There isn't a third mode that would belong to the apoptotic cells, due to the very small number of pixels belonging to them. In some Caspase images, the histogram becomes unimodal, when the background is so low as to disappear, and images only include the sample.

The following thresholding method was developed. The shape of the second mode, corresponding to the sample, can be roughly approximated to a Gaussian function $G(q)$, and the pixels belonging to the Caspase cells are considered outliers. The highest local maximum of the histogram serves to identify the sample mode. To identify the outliers, assuming the sample's pixel grey level intensities are normally distributed, the Gaussian function $G_b(q)$ that best fits the shape of the sample's mode is found. This is achieved by minimizing the square error between the histogram $h(q)$ in the interval corresponding to the mode and $G(q)$, that is

$$G_b(q) = \arg\left(\min_{q_{\min} < q_c < q_{\max}} error(q) \right) \tag{3}$$

where

$$error(q) = \sum_{q_c}^{q_{\max}} [G(q) - h(q)]^2 \tag{4}$$

and

$$G(q) = e^{-\frac{q-\mu(q)^2}{2\sigma(q)^2}} \tag{5}$$

$\mu(q)$ and $\sigma(q)$ are the mean and standard deviation of the mode respectively, calculated in the interval $[q, q_{\max}]$, given by

$$\mu(q) = \frac{\sum_{q=q_c}^{q_{\max}} h(q)q}{\sum_{q=q_c}^{q_{\max}} h(q)} \qquad \sigma(q) = \frac{\sum_{q=q_c}^{q_{\max}} h(q)(q-\mu)^2}{\sum_{q=q_c}^{q_{\max}} h(q)} \tag{6}$$

q_c is a cut-off value given by the global minimum between the first and the second modes, if the histogram is bimodal, or the first local minimum of the histogram, if it is unimodal, and $q_{\max}$ is the maximum grey level of the histogram. The threshold is obtained from the standard score (z-score), which rejects the outliers of the Gaussian function. The z-score is given by

$$z = \frac{(q - \mu_b)}{\sigma_b} \tag{7}$$

where μ_b and σ_b are the mean and standard deviation of the best Gaussian function respectively and q is pixel intensity. It is considered that a grey level is an outlier if $z \geq 3$, therefore the threshold t is given by

$$t = \mu_b + 3\sigma_b \tag{8}$$

2.4.3 Mitotic and glial cells

In images stained with either pH3 or Repo in Drosophila embryos, the mode corresponding to the cells is almost imperceptible due to the corresponding small number of pixels compared to the number of background pixels. Given the low number of foreground pixels the histogram can be considered unimodal. To binarise unimodal images, rather than using thresholding techniques, we assumed that the background follows a Gaussian distribution *G(q)* and considered the pH3 cells outliers. To identify the best Gaussian function, we minimised the square error in the histogram *h*(*q*) in the interval between the mode and threshold, given by

$$t = \mu_b + 3\sigma_b \tag{10}$$

following the same procedure employed to threshold apoptotic cells explained before.

2.5 Post-processing

After segmentation, or in parallel, other methods can also be developed to reduce remaining noise, to separate abutting cells and to recover the original shape of the objects before the classification. Which method is used will depend on the object to be discriminated.

2.5.1 Filtering

Some raw Caspase images have small spots of high intensity, which can be confused with cells in later steps of the process. To eliminate these spots without affecting the thresholding technique (if the spot filter is applied before thresholding the histogram is modified affecting the result), the raw images are filtered in parallel and the result is combined with the thresholding outcome. If a square window of side greater than the diameter of a typical spot, but smaller than the diameter of a cell, is centered in a cell, the mean of the pixel intensities inside the window should be close to the value of the central pixel. If the window is centered in a spot, the pixel mean should be considerably lower than the intensity of the central pixel. To eliminate the spots, a mobile window W is centered in each pixel. Let $p(x,y)$ and $s(x,y)$ be the original input image and the resulting filtered image respectively, and $m(x,y)$ the average of the intensities inside the window centered in (x,y). If $m(x,y)$ is lower than a certain proportion α with respect to the central pixel, it becomes black, otherwise it retains its intensity. That is

$$s(x,y) = \begin{cases} 0 & \text{if} \quad m(x,y) < \alpha p(x,y) \\ p(x,y) & \text{if} \quad m(x,y) \geq \alpha p(x,y) \end{cases} \tag{11}$$

where

$$m(x,y) = \sum_{x,y \in W} p(x,y) \tag{12}$$

After thresholding, cells and small spots appear white, while after spot filtering the spots appear black. The result from both images is combined using the following expression:

$$q(x,y) = \begin{cases} 0 & \text{if} \quad \min[t(x,y), s(x,y)] = 0 \\ 1 & \text{if} \quad \min[t(x,y), s(x,y)] > 0 \end{cases} \tag{13}$$

where $q(x, y)$ is the resulting image and $t(x, y)$ the image resulting form thresholding.

The combination of filtering and thresholding results in separating candidate objects (Caspase-positive cells) from background. The spot filter also separates cells that appear very close in the z-axis.

To render the Caspase-positive cells more similar in appearance to the original raw images, three-dimensional morphological operations are then performed throughout the whole stack. Firstly, morphological closing followed by opening are applied to further remove noise and to refine the candidate structures. Secondly, the objects containing holes are filled with foreground colour verifying that each hole is surrounded by foreground pixels.

2.5.2 Cell separation

Cells that appear connected must be separated. This is most challenging. Several automatic and semi-automatic methods deal with the problem of how to separate cells within clusters in order to recognise each cell. Initially some seeds or points identifying each cell are found. A seed is a small part of the cell, not connected to any other, that can be used to mark it. If more than one seed is found per cell, it will be subdivided (i.e. over-segmentation), but if no seed is found the cell will not be recognised. In some semiautomatic methods seeds are marked by hand. Several methods have been proposed to identify only one seed per cell avoiding over-segmentation. The simplest method consists of a seeding procedure developed during the preparation of the samples to avoid overlaps between nuclei (Yu et al., 2009). More practical approaches involve morphological filters (Vincent, 1993) or clustering methods (Clocksin, 2003; Svensson, 2007). Watershed based algorithms are frequently employed for contour detection and cell segmentation (Beucher & Lantuejoul, 1979; Vincent & Soille, 1991), some employing different distance functions to separate the objects (Lockett & Herman, 1994; Malpica, 1997). In this way, cells are separated by defining the watershed lines between them. Hodneland et al. (Hodneland, 2009) employed a topographical distance function and Svensson (Svensson, 2007) presented a method to decompose 3D fuzzy objects, were the seeds are detected as the peaks of the fuzzy distance transforms. These seeds are then used as references to initiate a watershed procedure. Level set functions have been combined with watershed in order to reduce over-segmentation and render the watershed lines more regular. In the method developed by Yu et al. (Yu et al., 2009) the dynamic watershed is constrained by the topological dependence in order to avoid merged and split cell segments. Hodneland et al. (Hodneland, 2009) also combine level set functions and watershed segmentation in order to segment cells, and the seeds are created by adaptive thresholding and iterative filling. Li et al. propose a different approach, based on gradient flow tracking (Li et al. 2007, 2008). These procedures can produce good results in 2D, although they are generally time consuming. They do not provide good results if the resolution of the images is low and the borders between the cells are imperceptible.

Watershed and h-domes are two morphological techniques commonly used to separate cells. These two techniques are better understood if 2D images or 3D stacks are seen as a topological relief. In the 2D case the height in each point is given by the intensity of the pixel in that position where the cells are viewed as light peaks or domes separated by dark valleys (Vincent, 1993). The basic idea behind watershed consists in imaging a flooding of the image, where the water starts to flow from the lower points of the image. The edges between the regions of the image tend to be placed on the watershed. Frequently, the watershed is applied to the gradient of the image, so the watershed is located in the crests, i.e. in the highest values. Watershed and domes techniques are also applied on distance images. In this way, each pixel or voxel of an object takes the value of the minimum distance to the background, and the highest distance will correspond to the furthest point from the borders. The cells are again localized at the domes of the mountains, while the watershed is used to find the lowest points in the valleys that are used to separate the mountains, i.e. the cells (Malpica et al., 1997). In this way, watershed can be used to divide joined objects, using the inverted of the distance transformation and flooding the mountains starting from the inverted domes that are used as seeds or points from where the flooding begins. The eroded points and the resulting points of a top-hat transformation can also be used as seeds in several watershed procedures.

2.5.2.1 Apoptotic cells

The solution to the cell separation problem depends on the shape of the cells and how close they are. Apoptotic cells, for example, do not appear very close, although it is possible to find some abutting one another. They can also have a very irregular shape and can appear subdivided. Therefore, we reached a compromise when trying to separate cells. When watershed was used in 3D many cells were subdivided resulting in a cell being counted as multiple cells, thus yielding false positives. On the other hand, if a technique to subdivide cells is not used, abutting cells can be counted only as one, yield false negatives. In general, if there are few abutting cells, the number of false negatives is low. A compromise solution was employed. Instead of using a 3D watershed, a 2D watershed starting from the last eroded points was used, thus separating objects in each plane. In this way, irregular cells that were abutting in one slice were separated, whilst they were kept connected in 3D. The number of false negatives was reduced without increasing the number of false positives. Although some cells can still be lost, this conservative solution was found to be the best compromise.

2.5.2.2 Mitotic and glial cells

Mitotic and glial cells in embryos were separated by defining the watershed lines between them. To this end, the first step consisted in marking each cell with a seed. In order to find the seeds a 3D distance transformation was applied. To mark the cells, we applied a 3D h-dome operator based on a morphological gray scale reconstruction (Vincent, 1993). We found $h = 7$ to be the standard minimum distance between the centre of a cell and the surrounding voxels. This marked all the cells, even if they were closely packed. To avoid a cell having more than one seed, we found the h-domes transform of an image $q(x,y)$. A morphological reconstruction of $q(x,y)$ was performed by subtracting from $q(x,y)-h$, where h is a positive scalar, the result of the reconstruction from the original image (Vincent, 1992, 1993), that is

$$D_h(q(x,y)) = q(x,y) - \rho(q(x,y) - h) \tag{14}$$

where the reconstruction

$$\rho(q(x,y) - h) \tag{15}$$

is also known as the h-maxima transform. The h extended-maxima, i.e. the regional maxima of the h-maxima transform, can be employed to mark the cells (Vincent, 1993; Wählby 2003, Wählby et al. 2004). However, we found that a more reliable identification of the cells that prevented losing cells, was achieved by the binarisation method of thresholding the h-domes images (Vincent, 1993). Given that each seed is formed of connected voxels, 3D domes could be identified and each seed labelled with 18-connectivity.

Due to the intensity variation of the cells, several seeds can be found in one cell, resulting in over-segmentation. To prevent over-segmentation after watershed, redundant seeds must be eliminated, to result in only one seed per cell. Wählby et al. (Wählby et al., 2004) have used the gradient among the seeds as a way to determine if two seeds belong to a single cell and then combine them. However, we found that for mitotic cells a simpler solution was successful at eliminating excess seeds. Multiple seeds can appear in one cell if there are irregularities in cell shape. The resulting extra peaks tend not to be very high and, when domes are found, they tend to occupy a very small number of voxels (maximum of 10). Instead, true seeds are formed of a minimum of 100 voxels. Consequently, rejecting seeds of less than 20 voxels eliminated most redundant seeds.

Recently, Cheng and Rajapakse (Cheng and Rajapakse, 2009) proposed an adaptive h transform in order to eliminate undesired regional minima, which can provide an alternative way of avoiding over-segmentation. Following seed identification, the 3D watershed employing the Image Foresting Transform (IFT) was applied (Lotufo & Falcao, 2000; Falcao et al., 2004), and watershed separated very close cells.

2.5.2.3 Neuronal nuclei

To identify the seeds in images of HB9 labelled cells, a 2D regional maxima detection was performed and following the method proposed by Vincent (Vincent, 1993), a h-dome operator based on a morphological gray scale reconstruction was applied to extract and mark the cells. The choice of h is not critical since a range of values can provide good results (Vincent, 1993). The minimum difference between the maximum grey level of the cells and the pixels surrounding the cells is 5. Thus, h=5 results in marking cells, while distinguishing cells within clusters. Images were binarised by thresholding the h-domes images.

Some nuclei were very close. As we did with the mitotic cells, a 3D watershed algorithm could be employed to separate them. However in our tests the results were not always good. We found better and more time-computing efficient results from employing both the intensity and the distance to the borders as parameters to separate nuclei. In this way, first a 2D watershed was applied to separate nuclei in 2D, based on the intensity of the particles. Subsequently, 3D erosion was used in order to increase their separation and a 3D distance transformation was applied. In this way each voxel of an object takes the value of the minimum distance to the background. Then the 3D domes were found and used as seeds to mark every cell. A fuzzy distance transform (Svensson, 2007), which combines the intensity of the voxels and the distance to the borders, was also tested. Whilst with our cells this did not work well, it might be an interesting alternative with different kinds of cells when working with other kinds of cells. The images were then binarised. Once the seeds were found, they were labelled employing 18-connectivity and from the seeds a 3D region growing was done to recover the original shape of each object, using as mask the stack resulting from the watershed (see Forero et al, 2010).

2.6 Classification

The final step is classification, whereby cells are identified and counted. This step is done according to the characteristics that allow to identify each cell type and reject other particles. A 3D labelling method (Lumia, 1983; Thurfjell, 1992; Hu, 2005) is first employed to identify each candidate object, which is then one by one either accepted or rejected according to the selected descriptors. To find the features that better describe the cells, a study of the best descriptors must be developed. Several methods are commonly employed to do this. Some methods consider that descriptors follow a Gaussian distribution, and use the Fisher discriminant to separate classes (Fisher, 1938; Duda et al., 2001). Other methods select the best descriptors after a Principal Components Analysis (Pearson, 1901; Duda, 2001). In this method, a vector of descriptors is obtained for each sample and then the principal components are obtained. The descriptors having the highest eigen values, that is, those having the highest dispersion, are selected as best descriptors. It must be noted that this method can result on the selection of bad descriptors when the two classes have a very high dispersion along a same principal component, but their distribution overlaps considerably. In this case the descriptor must be rejected.

In our case, we found that dying cells stained with Caspase and mitotic cells with pH3 are irregular in shape. Therefore, they cannot be identified by shape and users distinguish them from background spots of high intensity by their bigger size. Thus, apoptotic and mitotic cells were selected among the remaining candidate objects from the previous steps based only on their volume. The minimum volume can be set empirically or statistically making it higher than the volume occupied by objects produced by noise and spots of high intensity that can still remain. The remaining objects are identified as cells and counted. Using statistics, a sufficient number of cells and rejected particles can be obtained to establish their mean and standard deviation, thus finding the best values that allow to separate both classes using a method like the Fisher discriminator.

Nuclei have a very regular, almost spherical, shape. In this case more descriptors can be used to better describe cells and get a better identification of the objects. 2D and 3D descriptors can be employed to analyse the objects. Here we only present some 2D descriptors. For a more robust identification the representation of cells should preferably be translation, rotation and scale invariant. Compactness, eccentricity, statistical invariant moments and Fourier descriptors are compliant with this requirement. We did not use Fourier descriptors for our studies given the tiny size of the cells, which made obtaining cells' contours very sensitive to noise. Therefore, we only considered Hu's moments, compactness and eccentricity.

Compactness C is defined as

$$C = \frac{P^2}{A} \tag{16}$$

where A and P represent the area and perimeter of the object respectively. New 2D and 3D compactness descriptors to analyse cells have been introduced by Bribiesca (2008), but have not been tested yet.

Another descriptor corresponds to the flattening or eccentricity of the ellipse, whose moments of second order are equal to those of the object. In geometry texts the eccentricity of an ellipse is defined as the ratio between the foci length a and the major axis length D of its best fitting ellipse

$$E = \frac{a}{D} \tag{16}$$

Its value varies between 0 and 1, when the degenerate cases appear, being 0 if the ellipse is in fact a circumference and 1 if it is a line segment. The relationship between the focal length and the major and minor axes, D and d respectively, is given by the equation

$$D^2=d^2+a^2 \tag{17}$$

then,

$$E=\frac{\sqrt{D^2-d^2}}{D} \tag{18}$$

Nevertheless, some authors define the eccentricity of an object as the ratio between the length of the major and minor axes, also being named aspect ratio, and elongation because it quantifies the extension of the ellipse and is given by

$$e=\frac{d}{D}=\sqrt{1-E^2} \tag{19}$$

In this case, eccentricity also varies between 0 and 1, but being now 0 if the object is a line segment and 1 if it is a circumference.

The moment invariants are obtained from the binarised image of each cell; pixels inside the boundary contours are assigned to value 1 and pixels outside to value 0. The central moments are given by:

$$\mu_{rs}=\sum_{x=0}^{N-1}\sum_{y=0}^{M-1}(x-\overline{x})^r(y-\overline{y})^s f(x,y) \qquad \text{for } r, s = 0, 1, \ldots, \infty \tag{20}$$

where $f(x,y)$ represents a binary image, p and q are non-negative integers and $(\overline{x},\overline{y})$ is the barycentre or centre of gravity of the object and the order of the moment is given by $r + s$. From the central moments Hu (Hu, 1962) defined seven rotation, scale and translation invariant moments of second and third order

$$\begin{aligned}
&\phi_1=\eta_{20}+\eta_{02}\\
&\phi_2=(\eta_{20}-\eta_{02})^2+4\eta_{11}^2\\
&\phi_3=(\eta_{30}-3\eta_{12})^2+(3\eta_{21}-\eta_{03})^2\\
&\phi_4=(\eta_{30}+\eta_{12})^2+(\eta_{21}+\eta_{03})^2\\
&\phi_5=(\eta_{30}-3\eta_{12})(\eta_{30}+\eta_{12})\left[(\eta_{30}+\eta_{12})^2-3(\eta_{21}+\eta_{03})^2\right]+\\
&(3\eta_{21}-\eta_{03})(\eta_{21}+\eta_{03})\left[3(\eta_{30}+\eta_{12})^2-(\eta_{21}+\eta_{03})^2\right]\\
&\phi_6=(\eta_{20}-\eta_{02})\left[(\eta_{30}+\eta_{12})^2-(\eta_{21}+\eta_{03})^2\right]+4\eta_{11}(\eta_{30}+\eta_{12})(\eta_{21}+\eta_{03})\\
&\phi_7=(3\eta_{21}-\eta_{03})(\eta_{30}-\eta_{12})\left[(\eta_{30}+\eta_{12})^2-3(\eta_{21}+\eta_{03})^2\right]+\\
&(3\eta_{12}-\eta_{30})(\eta_{21}+\eta_{03})\left[3(\eta_{30}+\eta_{12})^2-(\eta_{21}+\eta_{03})^2\right]
\end{aligned} \tag{21}$$

Moments ϕ_1 to ϕ_6 are, in addition, invariant to object reflection, given that only the magnitude of ϕ_7 is constant, but its sign changes under this transformation. Therefore, ϕ_7 can be used to recognize reflected objects. As it can be seen from the equations, the first two moments are functions of the second order moments. ϕ_1 is function of μ_{20} and μ_{02}, the moments of inertia of the object with respect to the coordinate axes x and y, and therefore corresponds to the moment of inertia, measuring the dispersion of the pixels of the object

with respect to its centre of mass, in any direction. ϕ_2 indicates how isotropic or directional the dispersion is.
One of the most common errors in the literature consists of the use of the whole set of Hu's moments to characterise objects. They must not be used simultaneously since they are dependant (Flusser, 2000), given that

$$\phi_3 = \frac{\phi_5^2 + \phi_7^2}{\phi_4^3} \tag{22}$$

Since Hu's moments are not basis (meaning by a basis the smallest set of invariants by means of which all other invariants can be expressed) given that they are not independent and the system formed by them is incomplete, Flusser (2000) developed a general method to find bases of invariant moments of any order using complex moments. This method also allows to describe objects in 3D (Flusser et al, 2009).
As cells have a symmetrical shape, the third and higher odd order moments are close to zero. Therefore, the first three-order Hu's moment ϕ_3 is enough to recognize symmetrical objects, the others being redundant.
That is, eccentricity can be also derived from Hu's moments by:

$$e = \sqrt{\frac{\phi_1 - \sqrt{\phi_2}}{\phi_1 + \sqrt{\phi_2}}} \tag{23}$$

and, from Equation (19) it can be found that:

$$E = \sqrt{1 - e^2} = \frac{2\sqrt{\phi_2}}{\phi_1 + \sqrt{\phi_2}} \tag{24}$$

Therefore, eccentricity is not independent of the first two Hu's moments and it must not be employed simultaneously with these two moments for classification.

3. Conclusion

We have presented here an overview of image processing techniques that can be used to identify and count cells in 3D from stacks of confocal microscopy images. Contrary to methods that count automatically dissociated cells or cells in culture, these 3D methods enable cell counting in vivo (i.e. in intact animals, like Drosophila embryos) and in situ (i.e. in a tissue or organ). This enables to retain normal cellular context within an organism. To give practical examples, we have focused on cell recognition in images from fruit-fly (Drosophila) embryos labelled with a range of cell markers, for which we have developed several image-processing methods. These were developed to count apoptotic cells stained with Caspase, mitotic cells stained with pH3, neuronal nuclei stained with HB9 and glial nuclei-stained with Repo. These methods are powerful in Drosophila as they enable quantitative analyses of gene function in vivo across many genotypes and large sample sizes. They could be adapted to work with other markers, with stainings of comparable qualities used to visualise cells of comparable sizes (e.g. sparsely distributed nuclear labels like BrdU, nuclear-GFP, to count cells within a mosaic clone in the larva or adult fly).

Because automatic counting is objective, reliable and reproducible, comparison of cell number between specimens and between genotypes is considerably more accurate with automatic programs than with manual counting. While a user normally gets a different result in each measurement when counting manually, automatic programs obtain consistently a unique value. Thus, although some cells may be missed, since the same criterion is applied in all the stacks, there is no bias or error. Consistent and objective criteria are used to compare multiple genotypes and samples of unlimited size. Furthermore, automatic counting is considerably faster and much less labour intensive.

Following the logical steps explained in this review, the methods we describe could be adapted to work on a wide range of tissues and samples. They could also be extended and combined with other methods, for which we present an extended description, as well as with some other recent developments that we also review. This would enable automatic counting in vivo from mammalian samples (i.e. brain regions in the mouse), small vertebrates (e.g. zebra-fish) or invertebrate models (e.g. snails) to investigate brain structure, organism growth and development, and to model human disease.

4. References

Adiga, P.U. & Chaudhuri B. (2001). Some efficient methods to correct confocal images for easy interpretation. *Micron,* Vol. 32, No. 4, (June 2001), pp. 363-370, ISSN 09684328

Anscombe, F. J. (1948). The transformation of Poisson, Binomial and Negative-Binomial data. *Biometrika,* Vol. 35, No. 3/4, (December 1948), pp. 246-254, ISSN 00063444

Bar-Lev, S.K. & Enis, P. (1988). On the classical choice of variance stabilizing transformations and an application for a Poisson variate. *Biometrika,* 1988, Vol. 75, No. 4, (December 1988), pp. 803-804, ISSN 00063444

Bello B.C., Izergina N., Cussinus E. & Reichert H. (2008). Amplification of neural stem cell proliferation by intermediate progenitor cells in Drosophila brain development. *Neural Development,* Vol. 3, No. 1, (February 2008), pp. 5, ISSN 17498104

Bello B, Reichert H & Girth F. (2006). The brain tumor gene negatively regulates neural progenitor cell proliferation in the larval central brain complex of Drosophila. *Development,* Vol. 133, No. 14, (July 2006), pp. 2639-2648, ISSN 10116370

Beucher, S. & Lantuejoul, C. (1979). Use of watersheds in contour detection *International workshop on image processing: Real-time and motion detection/estimation. IRISA,* (September 1979), Vol. 132, pp. 2.1-2.12

Bribiesca, E. (2008). An easy measure of compactness for 2D and 3D shapes. *Pattern Recognition.* Vol. 41, No. 2, (February 2008), pp. 543-554, ISSN 0031-3203

Calapez, A. & Rosa, A. (2010). A statistical pixel intensity model for segmentation of confocal laser scanning microscopy images. *IEEE Transactions on Image Processing,* Vol. 19, No. 9, (September 2010), pp. 2408-2418, ISSN 10577149

Can, A. et al. (2003). Attenuation correction in confocal laser microscopes: A novel two-view approach. *Journal of Microscopy,* Vol. 211, No. 1, (July 2003), pp. 67-79, ISSN 00222720

Carpenter AE et al. (2006). CellProfiler: image analysis software for identifying and quantifying cell phenotypes *Genome Biology,* Vol. 7, No. 10, (October 2006), Article R1000, ISSN 14656906

Chan, T. F.; Sandberg, B. Y. & Vese, L. A. (2000). Active contours without edges for vector-valued images. *Journal of Visual Communication and Image Representation*. Vol. 11, No. 2, (February 2000), pp. 130-141, ISSN 10473203

Chan, T. & Vese, L. (2001). Active contours without edges. *IEEE Transactions on Image Processing*. Vol 10, No. 2, (February 2001), pp. 266-277, ISSN 10577149

Cheng, J. & Rajapakse, J. (2009). Segmentation of clustered nuclei with shape markers and marking function, *IEEE Transactions on Biomedical Engineering*, Vol. 56, No. 3, (March 2009), pp. 741-748, ISSN 00189294

Clocksin, W. (2003). Automatic segmentation of overlapping nuclei with high background variation using robust estimation and flexible contour models. *Proceedings 12th International Conference on Image Analysis and Processing*, pp. 682-687, ISBN 0769519482, Mantova, Italy, September 17-19, 2003

Conchello, J.A. (1995). Fluorescence photobleaching correction for expectation maximization algorithm. *Three-Dimensional microscopy: image acquisition and processing. Proceedings of the 1995 SPIE symposium on electronic imaging: Science and technology*. Wilson, T. & Cogswell C. J. (Eds.). Vol. 2412, pp. 138-146, ISBN 9780819417596, March 23, 1995

Dima, A.; Scholz, M. & Obermayer, K. (2002). Automatic segmentation and skeletonization of neurons from confocal microscopy images based on the 3-D wavelet transform. *IEEE Transactions on Image Processing*, 2002, *Vol.11*, No.7, (July 2002), pp. 790-801, ISSN 10577149

Duda, R.; Hart, P. & Stork, D. (2001). *Pattern classification*. John Wiley & sons, 2nd Ed. ISBN 9780471056690

Falcao, A.; Stolfi, J. & de Alencar Lotufo, R. (2004). The image foresting transform: theory, algorithms, and applications. *IEEE Transactions on Pattern Analysis and Machine Intelligence*. Vol. 26, No. 1 (January 2004), pp. 19-29, ISSN 01628828

Fernandez, R.; Das, P.; Mirabet, V.; Moscardi, E.; Traas, J.; Verdeil, J.L.; Malandain, G. & Godin, C. (2010). Imaging plant growth in 4D: robust tissue reconstruction and lineaging at cell resolution. *Nature Methods*, Vol. 7, No. 7, (July 2010), pp. 547-553, ISSN 15487091

Fisher, R. A. (1938). The use of multiple measurements in taxonomic problems. *Annals of Eugenics*. Vol. 7, pp. 179-188

Flusser, J. (2000). On the Independence of Rotation Moment Invariants. *Pattern Recognition.*, Vol. 33, No. 9, (September 2000), pp. 1405-1410, ISSN 0031-3203

Flusser, J.; Zitova, B. & Suk, T. (2009). *Moments and Moment Invariants in Pattern Recognition*. Wiley, ISBN 9780470699874

Foi, A. (2008). Direct optimization of nonparametric variance-stabilizing transformations. 8èmes Rencontres de Statistiques Mathématiques. CIRM, Luminy, December.

Foi, A. (2009). Optimization of variance-stabilizing transformations. Available from http://www.cs.tut.fi/~foi/, preprint.

Forero, M.G. & Delgado, L.J. (2003). Fuzzy filters for noise removal. In: *Fuzzy Filters for Image Processing*, Nachtegael M.; Van der Weken, D.; Van De Ville, D. & Etienne E.E, (Eds.), (July 2003), pp. 1–24, Springer, Berlin, Heidelberg, New York, ISBN 3540004653

Forero, M. G.; Pennack, J. A.; Learte, A. R. & Hidalgo, A. (2009). DeadEasy Caspase: Automatic counting of apoptotic cells in Drosophila. *PLoS ONE, Public Library of Science*, Vol.4, No.5, (May 2009), Article e5441, ISSN 19326203

Forero, M. G.; Pennack, J. A. & Hidalgo, A. (2010). DeadEasy neurons: Automatic counting of HB9 neuronal nuclei in Drosophila. *Cytometry A*, Vol.77, No.4, (April 2010), pp. 371-378, ISSN 15524922

Forero, M. G.; Learte, A. R.; Cartwright, S. & Hidalgo, A. (2010a). DeadEasy Mito-Glia: Automatic counting of mitotic cells and glial cells in Drosophila. *PLoS ONE, Public Library of Science*, Vol.5, No.5, (May 2010), Article e10557, ISSN 19326203

Franzdóttir S.R., Engelen D, Yuva-Aydemir Y, Schmidt I, Aho A, Klämbt C. (2009) Switch in FGF signalling initiates glial differentiation in the Drosophila eye. *Nature*, Vol. 460, No. 7256, (August 2009), pp. 758-761, ISSN 00280836

Freeman, M.F. & Tukey, J.W. (1950). Transformations related to the angular and the square root. *The Annals of Mathematical Statistics*, Vol. 21, No. 4, (December 1950), pp. 607-611, ISSN 00034851

Guan, Y.Q. et al. (2008). Adaptive correction technique for 3D reconstruction of fluorescence microscopy images. *Microscopy Research and Technique*, Vol. 71, No. 2, (February 2008), pp. 146-157, ISSN 1059910X

Gué, M.; Messaoudi, C.; Sun, J.S. & Boudier, T. (2005). Smart 3D-Fish: Automation of distance analysis in nuclei of interphase cells by image processing. *Cytometry A*, Vol. 67, No. 1, (September 2005), pp. 18-26, ISSN 15524922

Hodneland, E.; Tai, X.-C. & Gerde, H.-H. (2009). Four-color theorem and level set methods for watershed segmentation. *International Journal of Computer Vision*, Vol. 82, No. 3, (May 2009), pp. 264-283, ISSN: 09205691

Ho M.S., Chen M., Jacques C., Giangrande A., Chien C.Y. (2009). Gcm protein degradation suppresses proliferation of glial progenitors. *PNAS*, Vol. 106, No. 16, (April 2009), pp. 6778-6783, ISSN: 00278424

Hu, M. (1962).Visual pattern recognition by moment's invariant. *IRE Transaction on information theory*, Vol. 8, No. 2, (February 1962), pp. 179-187, ISSN 00961000

Hu, Q.; Qian, G. & Nowinski, W. L. (2005). Fast connected-component labelling in three-dimensional binary images based on iterative recursion. *Computer Vision and Image Understanding*, Vol. 89, No. 3, (September 2005) pp. 414-434, ISSN 10773142

Kass, M.; Witkin, A. & Terzopoulos, D. (1988). Snakes: Active contour models, *International Journal of Computer Vision*. Vol. 1, No. 4, (January 1988), pp. 321-331, ISSN 09205691

Kervrann, C.; Legland, D. & Pardini, L. (2004). Robust incremental compensation of the light attenuation with depth in 3D fluorescence microscopy. *Journal of Microscopy*. 214, (June 2004), pp. 297-314, ISSN 00222720

Kervrann, C. (2004a). An adaptive window approach for image smoothing and structures preserving, *Proceedings of the European Conforence on Computer Vision ECCV04*. Vol. 3023, pp. 132-144, ISBN 354021982X, Prague, Czech Republic, May 11-14, 2004

Li, G.; Liu, T.; Tarokh, A.; Nie, J.; Guo, L.; Mara, A.; Holley, S. & Wong, S. (2007). 3D cell nuclei segmentation based on gradient flow tracking. *BMC Cell Biology*, Vol. 8, No. 1, (September 2007), Article 40, ISSN 14712121

Li, G.; Liu, T.; Nie, J.; Guo, L.; Chen, J.; Zhu, J.; Xia, W.; Mara, A.; Holley, S. & Wong, S. (2008). Segmentation of touching cell nuclei using gradient flow tracking. *Journal of Microscopy*, Vol. 231, No. 1, (July 2008), pp. 47-58, ISSN 00222720

Lin, G.; Adiga, U.; Olson, K.; Guzowski, J.; Barnes, C. & Roysam, B. (2003). A hybrid 3D watershed algorithm incorporating gradient cues and object models for automatic segmentation of nuclei in confocal image stacks. *Cytometry A,* Vol.56, No.1, (November 2003), pp. 23-36, ISSN 15524922

Long, F.; Peng, H. & Myers, E. (2007). Automatic segmentation of nuclei in 3D microscopy images of C. Elegans. *Proceedings of the 4th IEEE International Symposium on Biomedical Imaging: From Nano to Macro,* pp. 536–539, ISBN 1424406722, Arlington, VA, USA, April 12-15, 2007

Lotufo, R. & Falcao, A. (2000). The ordered queue and the optimality of the watershed approaches, *in* Mathematical Morphology and its Applications to Image and Signal Processing, Kluwer Academic Publishers, (June 2000), pp. 341-350

Lucy, L. B. (1974). An iterative technique for the rectification of observed distributions. *Astronomical Journal.* Vol. 79, No. 6, (June 1974), pp. 745–754, ISSN 00046256

Lumia, R. (1983). A new three-dimensional connected components algorithm. *Computer Vision, Graphics, and Image Processing.* Vol. 22, No. 2, (August 1983), pp. 207-217, ISSN 0734189X

Makitalo, M. & Foi, A. (2011). Optimal inversion of the Anscombe transformation in low-count Poisson image denoising. *IEEE Transactions on Image Processing,* Vol. 20, No.1, (January 2011), pp. 99 -109, ISSN 10577149

Makitalo, M. & Foi, A. (2011a). A closed-form approximation of the exact unbiased inverse of the Anscombe variance-stabilizing transformation. *IEEE Transactions on Image Processing.* Accepted for publication, ISSN 10577149

Malpica, N.; de Solórzano, C. O.; Vaquero, J. J.; Santos, A.; Vallcorba, I.; Garcia-Sagredo, J. M. & del Pozo, F. (1997). Applying watershed algorithms to the segmentation of clustered nuclei. *Cytometry,* Vol. 28, No. 4, (August 1997), pp. 289-297, ISSN 01964763

Maurange, C, Cheng, L & Gould, A.P. (2008). Temporal transcription factors and their targets schedule the end of neural proliferation in Drosophila. *Cell.* Vol. 133, No. 5, (May 2008), pp. 591-902, ISSN 00928674

Meijering, E. & Cappellen, G. (2007). Quantitative biological image analysis. In: *Imaging Cellular and Molecular Biological Functions,* Shorte, S.L. & Frischknecht, F. (Eds.), pp. 45-70, Springer, ISBN 978-3-540-71331-9, Berlin Heidelberg

Mitra, S. K. & Sicuranza, G. L. (Eds.). (2001). *Nonlinear Image Processing,* Elsevier, ISBN 8131208443

Osher, S. & Sethian, J. A. (1988). Fronts propagating with curvature-dependent speed: Algorithms based on Hamilton-Jacobi formulations. *Journal of Computational Physics* Vol. 79, No. 1, (November 1988), pp. 12-49, ISSN 00219991

Pearson, K. (1901). On lines and planes of closest fit to systems of points in space. *Philosophical Magazine,* Vol. 2, No. 6, (July-December 1901), pp. 559–572, ISSN 14786435

Peng, H. (2008). Bioimage informatics: a new area of engineering biology. *Bioinformatics,* Vol. 24, No. 17, (September 2008), pp. 1827-1836, ISSN 13674803

Richardson, W. H. (1972). Bayesian-based iterative method of image restoration. *Journal of the Optical Society of America.* Vol. 62, No.1, (January 1972), pp. 55-59, ISSN 00303941

Rodenacker, K. et al. (2001). Depth intensity correction of biofilm volume data from confocal laser scanning microscopes. *Image Analysis and Stereology,* Vol. 20, No. Suppl. 1, (September 2001), pp. 556-560, ISSN 15803139

Rodrigues, I.; Sanches, J. & Bioucas-Dias, J. (2008). Denoising of medical images corrupted by Poisson noise. *15th IEEE International Conference on Image Processing, ICIP 2008,* pp. 1756-1759, ISBN 9781424417650, October 12-15, 2008

Roerdink, J.B.T.M. & Bakker, M. (1993). An FFT-based method for attenuation correction in fluorescence confocal microscopy. *Journal of Microscopy.* Vol. 169, No.1, (1993), pp. 3-14, ISSN 00222720

Rogulja-Ortmann, A; Lüer, K; Seibert, J; Rickert, C. & Technau, G.M. (2007). Programmed cell death in the embryonic central nervous system of Drosophila Melanogaster. *Development*, Vol. 134, No. 1, (January 2007), pp. 105-116, ISSN 1011-6370

Rothwell, W.F. & Sullivan, W. (2000) Fluorescent analysis of Drosophila embryos. In: *Drosophila protocols.* Ashburner, M.; Sullivan, W. & Hawley, R.S., (Eds.), Cold Spring Harbour Laboratory Press, pp. 141-158, ISBN 0879695862

Sarder, P. & Nehorai, A. (2006). Deconvolution methods for 3-D fluorescence microscopy images. *IEEE Signal Processing Magazine,* Vol. 23, No.3, (May 2006), pp.32-45, ISSN 10535888

Serra, J. (1988), *Image Analysis and Mathematical Morphology Vol. II: Theoretical Advances.* Academic Press, ISBN 0126372411

Shen, J.; Sun, H.; Zhao, H. & Jin, X. (2009). Bilateral filtering using fuzzy-median for image manipulations. *Proceedings 11th IEEE International Conference Computer-Aided Design and Computer Graphics.* pp. 158-161, ISBN 9781424436996, Huangshan, China, August 19-21, 2009

Shimada, T; Kato, K; Kamikouchi, A & Ito, K. (2005). Analysis of the distribution of the brain cells of the fruit fly by an automatic cell counting algorithm *Physica A: Statistical and Theoretical Physics. Vol.* 350, No. 1, (May 2005), pp. 144-149, ISSN 03784371

Starck, J. L.; Pantin, E. & Murtagh F. (2002). Deconvolution in astronomy: A Review. *The Publications of the Astronomical Society of the Pacific,* Vol. 114, No. 800, (October 2002), pp. 1051-1069, ISSN 00046280.

Sternberg, S. R. (1986). Grayscale morphology. *Computer Vision, Graphics, and Image Processing,* Vol. 35, No. 3, (September 1986), pp. 333-355, ISSN 0734189X

Svensson, S. (2007). A decomposition scheme for 3D fuzzy objects based on fuzzy distance information. *Pattern Recognition Letters.* Vol. 28, No. 2, (January 2007), pp. 224-232, ISSN 01678655

Thurfjell, L.; Bengtsson, E. & Nordin, B. (1992). A new three-dimensional connected components labeling algorithm with simultaneous object feature extraction capability. *CVGIP: Graphical Models and Image Processing,* Vol. 54, No. 4, (July 1992), pp. 357-364, ISSN 10499652

Tomasi, C. & Manduchi, R. (1998). Bilateral filtering for gray and color images. *Proceedings Sixth International Conference on Computer Vision,* Chandran, S. & Desai, U. (Eds.), pp. 839-846, ISBN 8173192219, Bombay, India, January 4-7, 1998

Vincent, L. & Soille, P. (1991). Watersheds in digital spaces: an efficient algorithm based on immersion simulations. *IEEE Transactions on Pattern Analysis and Machine Intelligence,* Vol. 13, No.6, (June 1991), pp. 583-598, ISSN 01628828

Vincent, L. (1992). Morphological grayscale reconstruction: definition, efficient algorithm and applications in image analysis. *IEEE Computer Society Conference on Computer Vision and Pattern Recognition,* pp. 633-635, ISSN 10636919, Champaign, IL, USA, June 15-18, 1992

Vincent, L. (1993). Morphological grayscale reconstruction in image analysis: applications and efficient algorithms. *IEEE Transactions on Image Processing*. Vol. 2, No. 2, (April 1993), pp. 176-201, ISSN 10577149

Wählby, C. (2003). PhD dissertation. Algorithms for applied digital image cytometry. *Upsala University*, (October 2003)

Wählby, C.; Sintorn, I.; Erlandsson, F.; Borgefors, G. & Bengtsson, E. et al. (2004). Combining intensity, edge and shape information for 2d and 3d segmentation of cell nuclei in tissue sections. *Journal of Microscopy*. Vol. 215, No. 1, (July 2004), pp. 67-76, ISSN 00222720

Wu, H.X. & Ji, L. (2005). Fully Automated Intensity Compensation for Confocal Microscopic Images. *Journal of Microscopy*. Vol.220, No.1, (October 2005), pp. 9-19, ISSN 00222720

Yu, W.; Lee, H. K.; Hariharan, S.; Bu, W. & Ahmed, S. (2009). Quantitative neurite outgrowth measurement based on image segmentation with topological dependence. *Cytometry A* Vol. 75A, No. 4 (April 2009), pp 289-297, ISSN 15524922

2

Multivariate Models and Algorithms for Learning Correlation Structures from Replicated Molecular Profiling Data

Lipi R. Acharya[1] and Dongxiao Zhu[1,2]
[1]*University of New Orleans, New Orleans*
[2]*Research Institute for Children, Children's Hospital, New Orleans*
U.S.A.

1. Introduction

Advances in high-throughput data acquisition technologies, e.g. microarray and next-generation sequencing, have resulted in the production of a myriad amount of molecular profiling data. Consequently, there has been an increasing interest in the development of computational methods to uncover gene association patterns underlying such data, e.g. gene clustering (Medvedovic & Sivaganesan, 2002; Medvedovic *et al.*, 2004), inference of gene association networks (Altay and Emmert-Streib, 2010; Butte & Kohane, 2000; Zhu *et al.*, 2005), sample classification (Yeung & Bumgarner, 2005) and detection of differentially expressed genes (Sartor *et al.*, 2006). However, outcome of any bioinformatics analysis is directly influenced by the quality of molecular profiling data, which are often contaminated with excessive noise. Replication is a frequently used strategy to account for the noise introduced at various stages of a biomedical experiment and to achieve a reliable discovery of the underlying biomolecular activities.

Particularly, estimation of the correlation structure of a gene set arises naturally in many pattern analyses of replicated molecular profiling data. In both supervised and unsupervised learning, performance of various data analysis methods, e.g. linear and quadratic discriminate analysis (Hastie *et al.*, 2009), correlation-based hierarchial clustering (Eisen *et al.*, 1998; de Hoon *et al.*, 2004; Yeung *et al.*, 2003) and co-expression networking (Basso *et al.*, 2005; Boscolo *et al.*, 2008) relies on an accurate estimate of the true correlation structure.

The existing MLE (maximum likelihood estimate) based approaches to the estimation of correlation structure do not automatically accommodate replicated measurements. Often, an *ad hoc* step of data preprocessing by averaging (either weighted, unweighted or something in between) is used to reduce the multivariate structure of replicated data into bivariate one (Hughes *et al.*, 2000; Yao *et al.*, 2008; Yeung *et al.*, 2003). Averaging is not completely satisfactory as it creates a strong bias while reducing the variance among replicates with diverse magnitudes. Moreover, averaging may lead to a significant amount of information loss, e.g. it may wipe out important patterns of small magnitudes or cancel out opposite patterns of similar magnitudes. Thus, it is necessary to design multivariate correlation estimators by treating each replicate exclusively as a random variable. In general, the experimental design that specifies replication mechanism of a gene set may be unknown (blind) or known (informed) to data analysts. The suite of multivariate models and algorithms offer flexible ways to capture the correlation structure of a gene set with diverse replication mechanisms and allow for further generalizations.

In this chapter, we present bivariate and multivariate approaches to estimate the correlation structure of a gene set with replicated measurements. We begin with two popular bivariate correlation estimators, Pearson's correlation (Eisen *et al.*, 1998; Kung *et al.*, 2005) and SD-weighted correlation (Hughes *et al.*, 2000; Yeung *et al.*, 2003) followed by a comprehensive discussion of three generalized multivariate models, blind-case model, informed-case model and finite mixture model introduced in (Acharya & Zhu, 2009; Zhu *et al.*, 2007; 2010) to estimate the correlation structure of a gene set with either blind or informed replication mechanism. We analyze the performance of various correlation estimators using synthetic and real-world replicated data sets.

2. Replicated molecular profiling data

Molecular profiling data in the present context refers to a numerical matrix of gene abundance levels, where rows correspond to genes and columns represent experiments (samples). High-throughput platforms, such as microarrays, enable the scientists to simultaneously interrogate the expression abundance of tens of thousands of genes in the living cell. A microarray experiment is typically performed by hybridizing target cRNA samples labeled with fluorescent dyes on a glass slide spotted with oligonucleotides. After hybridization, the glass slide is washed and scanned to detect the gene expression levels. Some of the popular microarray platforms include Affymetrix GeneChip, Agilent Microarray, Illumina BeadArray and housemade twocolor arrays. Based on the experimental design employed by a data acquisition platform, the replication mechanism underlying molecular profiling data can be either *blind* or *informed* to data analysts (Figure 1). For example, the measurements from Affymetrix GeneChip platform (Lokhart *et al.*, 1996) correspond to blind replication mechanism, where expression levels of a gene are measured by designing a set of 11 perfect match sibling probes against the 3-prime end of mRNA, although a mixture of gene isoforms can exist. On the other hand, some of the more recent Illumina hybridization-based BeadArray (Gunderson *et al.*, 2004) and deep sequencing based Genome Analyzer II (Shendure & Ji, 2008) platforms utilize an informed replication mechanism. Indeed, such platforms simultaneously profile $6-12$ samples of whole-genome gene expression in a chip, where both biological and technical replicates can be used in the experiment. Many studies also use a more general replication strategy of combining the two mechanisms, e.g. blind replication mechanism nested within the informed mechanism and *vice versa* (Kerr & Churchill, 2001). It is necessary to explicitly consider both blind and informed mechanisms for a robust pattern analyses of replicated data. For instance, Fig. 1 presents two gene sets with the same number of replicated measurements, however, their underlying correlation structures differ by incorporating the prior knowledge of replication mechanism. For a comprehensive correlation based analysis of replicated molecular profiling data with both blind and informed replication mechanism, we refer to (Zhu *et al.*, 2010).

3. Bivariate correlation estimators

In this section, we discuss two bivariate correlation estimators, Pearson's correlation (Eisen *et al.*, 1998; Kung *et al.*, 2005; Rengarajan *et al.*, 2005) and SD-weighted correlation (Hughes

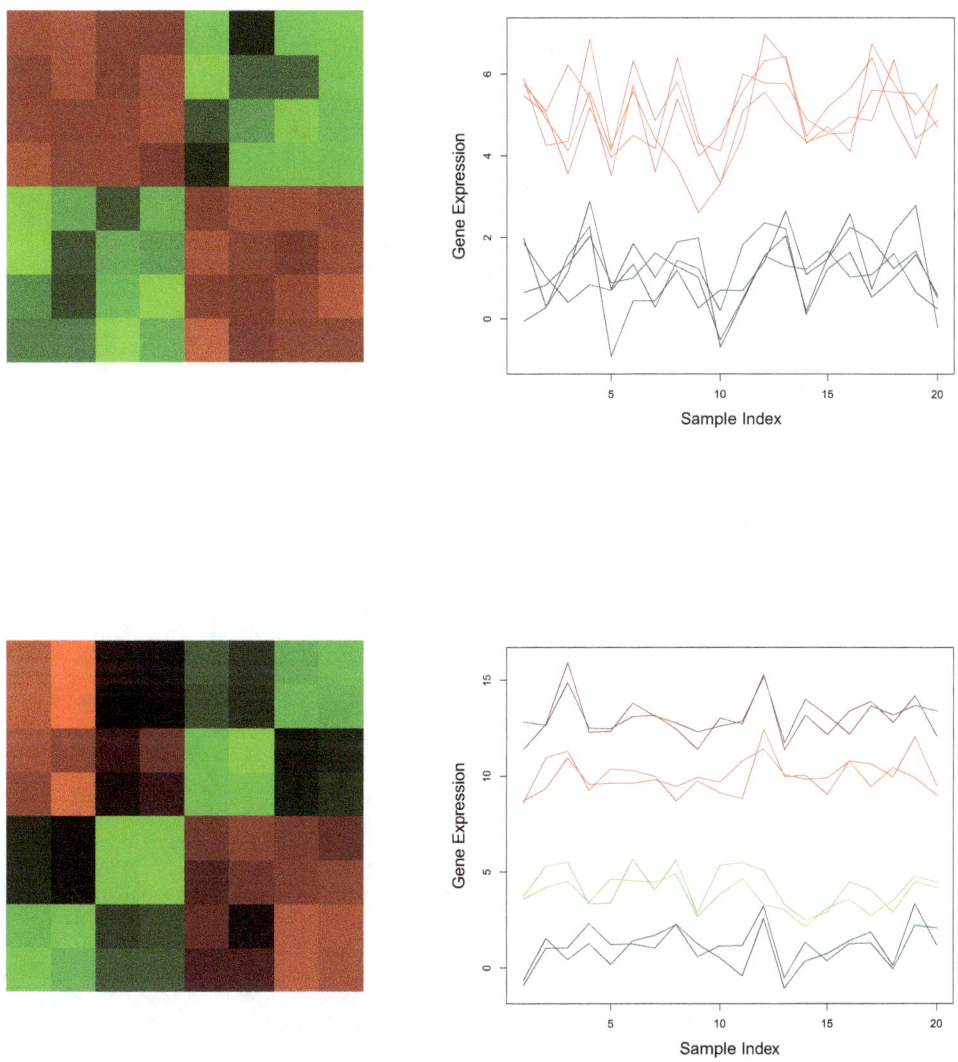

Fig. 1. Correlation structures (left) and molecular profiling data (right) corresponding to a pair of genes, each with 4 replicated measurements. The upper panels represent the correlation structure and molecular profiling data with blind replication mechanism, whereas the lower panels correspond to the ones with informed replication mechanism. In case of informed replication mechanism 2 biological replicate and 2 technical replicates nested within each biological replicates are used for a gene.

et al., 2000; van't Veer *et al.*, 2002; Yeung *et al.*, 2003), frequently used in the analysis of replicated molecular profiling data. We assume that the abundance levels of two genes X and Y with m_1 and m_2 replicated measurements respectively, are simultaneously measured over n independent experiments. If x_{ij} and y_{ij} denote the abundance levels of X and Y in the ith replicate and j^{th} sample respectively, we write

$$\bar{x}_j = \frac{1}{m_1} \sum_{i=1}^{m_1} x_{ij} \tag{1}$$

and

$$\bar{y}_j = \frac{1}{m_2} \sum_{i=1}^{m_2} y_{ij} \tag{2}$$

for the average measurements in the jth sample,

$$\bar{x} = \frac{1}{n} \sum_{j=1}^{n} \bar{x}_j \tag{3}$$

and

$$\bar{y} = \frac{1}{n} \sum_{j=1}^{n} \bar{y}_j \tag{4}$$

for the grand means of the measurements,

$$s_x^2(j) = \frac{1}{m_1 - 1} \sum_{i=1}^{m_1} (x_{ij} - \bar{x}_j)^2 \tag{5}$$

and

$$s_y^2(j) = \frac{1}{m_2 - 1} \sum_{i=1}^{m_2} (y_{ij} - \bar{y}_j)^2 \tag{6}$$

for the variances in the jth sample,

$$\bar{x}_w = \sum_{j=1}^{n} \frac{\bar{x}_j}{s_x^2(j)} \Big/ \sum_{j=1}^{n} \frac{1}{s_x^2(j)} \tag{7}$$

and

$$\bar{y}_w = \sum_{j=1}^{n} \frac{\bar{y}_j}{s_y^2(j)} \Big/ \sum_{j=1}^{n} \frac{1}{s_y^2(j)}, \tag{8}$$

for the SD-weighted average measurements corresponding to X and $Y, j = 1, \ldots, n$.

3.1 Pearson's correlation estimator

Pearson's correlation coefficient is a well-known similarity measure for clustering molecular profiling data (Eisen *et al.*, 1998). The estimate of correlation between X and Y is defined in terms of unweighted average of replicated measurements for a gene across different experiments (Kung *et al.*, 2005; Rengarajan *et al.*, 2005) and is given by

$$cor(X, Y) = \frac{\sum_{j=1}^{n} (\bar{x}_j - \bar{x})(\bar{y}_j - \bar{y})}{\sqrt{\sum_{j=1}^{n} (\bar{x}_j - \bar{x})^2 \sum_{j=1}^{n} (\bar{y}_j - \bar{y})^2}}. \tag{9}$$

In case of a gene set with k genes $X_1, \ldots, X_k$, where m_i replicated measurements are available for X_i, the correlation structure is defined by all pairwise correlations $cor(X_i, X_j)$, $i, j = 1, \ldots, k$. Due to its closed-form representation, Pearson's estimator enjoys computational simplicity. However, it is exclusively based on estimating bivariate correlation from a data with multivariate structure. Additionally, the estimator assigns equal weights to all replicates of a gene without considering the variation in their magnitudes, which is often large for data generated from high-throughput platforms. To overcome this problem, a number of more generalized correlation estimators have been proposed by considering weighted average of replicated measurements in place of simple average.

3.2 SD-weighted correlation estimator

The SD-weighted correlation estimator considers weighted average of replicated measurements, where weights are determined by standard deviations of the measurements across different experiments. The SD-weighted correlation between X and Y is defined as (Hughes *et al.*, 2000; Zhu *et al.*, 2010)

$$cor_w(X, Y) = \frac{\sum_{j=1}^{n} \left(\frac{\bar{x}_j - \bar{x}_w}{s_x(j)} \right) \left(\frac{\bar{y}_j - \bar{y}_w}{s_y(j)} \right)}{\sqrt{\sum_{j=1}^{n} \left(\frac{\bar{x}_j - \bar{x}_w}{s_x(j)} \right)^2 \sum_{j=1}^{n} \left(\frac{\bar{y}_j - \bar{y}_w}{s_y(j)} \right)^2}}. \tag{10}$$

Advantages of SD-weighted correlation have been demonstrated in terms of increased accuracy and stability in cluster analysis, compared with Pearson's estimator (Yeung *et al.*, 2003). Nevertheless, SD-weighted estimator also does not explicitly accommodate replicated measurements and requires a preprocessing of data by computing their weighted average. In averaging, many useful patterns of small magnitude may be wiped out or patterns of opposite magnitude may be canceled out. Moreover, standard deviation of replicated measurements may not be a faithful representation of their internal variation, specially when the number of replicates is small. This problem has been addressed by considering a shrinkage version of the correlation estimator (Yao *et al.*, 2008), however, none of the aforementioned estimators are ready to explicitly accommodate replicated data and exploit prior knowledge of experimental design that explains replication mechanism.

4. Multivariate correlation estimators

In this section, we review three multivariate models, blind-case model (Acharya & Zhu, 2009; Zhu *et al.*, 2007), informed-case model (Zhu *et al.*, 2010) and finite mixture model (Acharya & Zhu, 2009) for estimating the correlation structure from replicated measurements corresponding to a gene set with blind or informed replication mechanism. Throughout this section, we treat each replicated measurement individually as a random variable and assume that data are independently and identically distributed samples from a multivariate normal distribution. We discuss the parameter structures for each model and their estimation from replicated measurements corresponding to a pair of genes X and Y or a gene set with k genes $X_1, \ldots, X_k$. It is assumed that gene abundance levels are measured over n independent samples, where m_i replicated measurements of the ith gene X_i are available in each of them, $i = 1, \ldots, k$. We denote the n multivariate samples by Z_j, $j = 1, \ldots, n$.

4.1 Blind-case model

Blind-case model from (Acharya & Zhu, 2009; Zhu *et al.*, 2007) estimates the correlation structure of a gene set with replicated measurements by assuming a constrained set of parameters in the multivariate normal distribution. The model is designated as 'blind' since it imposes a fixed number of within-molecular and between-molecular correlation parameters in the underlying correlation structure. Throughout this section, we follow the notations from (Acharya & Zhu, 2009). The parameters, mean vector μ_B and the correlation matrix Σ_B, for the blind-case model are defined as

$$\mu_B = \begin{bmatrix} \mu_{x_1}^B e_{m_1} \\ \vdots \\ \mu_{x_k}^B e_{m_k} \end{bmatrix} \tag{11}$$

where $\mu_{x_i}^B$ is a scalar and $e_{m_i} = (1, \ldots, 1)^T$ is a vector of size $m_i \times 1$, for $i = 1, \ldots, k$. The correlation matrix Σ_B of size $\sum_{i=1}^k m_i \times \sum_{i=1}^k m_i$ has the following structure

$$\Sigma_B = \begin{bmatrix} 1 & \cdots \rho_{11} & \cdots \rho_{1k} & \cdots \rho_{1k} \\ \vdots & \ddots \vdots & \vdots & \ddots \vdots \\ \rho_{11} & \cdots 1 & \cdots \rho_{1k} & \cdots \rho_{1k} \\ \vdots & \ddots \vdots & \vdots & \ddots \vdots \\ \rho_{k1} & \cdots \rho_{k1} & \cdots 1 & \cdots \rho_{kk} \\ \vdots & \ddots \vdots & \vdots & \ddots \vdots \\ \rho_{k1} & \cdots \rho_{k1} & \cdots \rho_{kk} & \cdots 1 \end{bmatrix}$$

$$= \begin{bmatrix} \Sigma_{11}^B & \cdots & \Sigma_{1k}^B \\ \vdots & \vdots & \vdots \\ {\Sigma_{1k}^B}^T & \cdots & \Sigma_{kk}^B \end{bmatrix}, \tag{12}$$

where Σ_{ij}^B is a $m_i \times m_j$ submatrix defined in terms of a single parameter ρ_{ij}. The parameters ρ_{ij}'s correspond to either within-molecular correlation (case $i = j$) or between-molecular correlation (case $i \neq j$). As a correlation matrix is symmetric, it is assumed that $\rho_{ij} = \rho_{ji}$. For practical purposes, only between-molecular correlations are of interest, whereas within-molecular correlations indicate data quality. Indeed, higher values of within-molecular correlations correspond to cleaner data.

To estimate the model parameters, the path of maximum likelihood estimation is followed. Due to their asymptotic properties, the MLE's are frequently used in parameter estimation problems when the underlying distribution is multivariate normal (Casella & Berger, 1990). Suppose the n observations Z_j's are sampled from multivariate normal distribution $N(\mu, \Sigma)$ with parameters μ and Σ, where $n > \sum_{i=1}^k m_i$. Then the likelihood function is defined as

$$L(\mu, \Sigma) = \prod_{j=1}^n N(Z_j|\mu, \Sigma) = \frac{1}{(2\pi)^{\frac{1}{2}(\sum_{i=1}^k m_i)n} |\Sigma|^{\frac{1}{2}n}} \exp[-\frac{1}{2}\sum_{j=1}^n (Z_j - \mu)^T \Sigma^{-1} (Z_j - \mu)]. \tag{13}$$

The MLE's are estimated by maximizing L with respect to μ and Σ. In the present context, if the the abundance level of lth gene in its ith replicate and j^{th} sample is denoted by x_{ij}^{l}, the MLE's of μ_B and Σ_B are obtained by solving

$$d\mathcal{L}/d\mu_{x_l}^{B} = 0, \tag{14}$$

for $l = 1, \ldots, k$ and

$$d\mathcal{L}/d\Sigma = 0, \tag{15}$$

where $\mathcal{L} = \log L$. This results in

$$\hat{\mu}_{x_l}^{B} = \frac{1}{n}\frac{1}{m_l}\sum_{j=1}^{n}\sum_{i=1}^{m_l} x_{ij}^{l} \tag{16}$$

for $l = 1, \ldots, k$. Thus, the MLE of μ_B is

$$\hat{\mu}_B = \begin{bmatrix} \hat{\mu}_{x_1}^{B} e_{m_1} \\ \vdots \\ \hat{\mu}_{k}^{B} e_{m_k} \end{bmatrix}. \tag{17}$$

The MLE of Σ_B is given by

$$\hat{\Sigma}_B = \frac{1}{n}\sum_{j=1}^{n}(Z_j - \hat{\mu}_B)(Z_j - \hat{\mu}_B)^T. \tag{18}$$

As the parameters $\hat{\rho}_{ij}$'s may not be tractable in practice, they are estimated using

$$\hat{\rho}_{ij} = Avg(\hat{\Sigma}_{ij}^{B}),\ i, j = 1, \ldots, k. \tag{19}$$

Equations 17-19 are used to obtain the correlation structure from blind-case model. When $k = 2$, blind-case model is defined in terms of two within-molecular and one between molecular correlation parameters, as presented in (Zhu *et al.*, 2007). Further, if there are no replicates for X and Y or $m_1 = m_2 = 1$, blind-case model and Pearson's correlation coefficient (Eq. 9) are connected as follows (Zhu *et al.*, 2007)

$$\hat{\rho}_{12} = \frac{n-1}{n} cor(X, Y). \tag{20}$$

Overall, blind-case model presents a simple and parsimonious multivariate approach for estimating the correlation structure of a gene set with blind replication mechanism. As the MLE's of parameters have closed-form representation, the model is computationally very efficient, e.g. it is well known that the infinite Bayesian mixture model approach (Medvedovic & Sivaganesan, 2002; Medvedovic *et al.*, 2004) suffers from non-trivial computational complexity as the number of genes and replicated measurements increases. However, blind-case model always imposes a fixed number of parameters in the model. This may correspond to an oversimplified representation of the underlying correlation structure of a gene set or an overly constrained correlation structure in case of replicated data for which the underlying experimental design is known. Thus, it is desirable to consider more flexible multivariate models by explicitly incorporating prior knowledge of replication mechanisms in the correlation structure.

4.2 Informed-case model

Informed-case model introduced in (Zhu *et al.*, 2010) generalizes blind-case model by accommodating prior knowledge of replication mechanism. In many cases the number of biological and technical replicates used in the experimental design are known. Informed-case model utilizes this information and assigns different parameters for the biological replicates of a gene. For simplicity, we present the informed-case model for two genes X and Y, where 3 biological replicates and 2 technical replicates nested within each biological replicate are used for each of them. This representation can be naturally extended to the case of a gene set with a given number of biological and technical replicates. Throughout this section, we follow the notations from (Zhu *et al.*, 2010). The two parameters, mean vector μ_I and correlation matrix Σ_I, for the informed-case model are defined as

$$\mu^I = \left(\mu_x^1, \mu_x^1, \mu_x^2, \mu_x^2, \mu_x^3, \mu_x^3, \mu_y^1, \mu_y^1, \mu_y^2, \mu_y^2, \mu_y^3, \mu_y^3\right)^T \tag{21}$$

and

$$\Sigma^I = \begin{pmatrix}
1 & \rho^{tt} & \rho_x^{12} & \rho_x^{12} & \rho_x^{13} & \rho_x^{13} & \rho_{xy}^{11} & \rho_{xy}^{11} & \rho_{xy}^{12} & \rho_{xy}^{12} & \rho_{xy}^{13} & \rho_{xy}^{13} \\
\rho^{tt} & 1 & \rho_x^{12} & \rho_x^{12} & \rho_x^{13} & \rho_x^{13} & \rho_{xy}^{11} & \rho_{xy}^{11} & \rho_{xy}^{12} & \rho_{xy}^{12} & \rho_{xy}^{13} & \rho_{xy}^{13} \\
\rho_x^{21} & \rho_x^{21} & 1 & \rho^{tt} & \rho_x^{23} & \rho_x^{23} & \rho_{xy}^{21} & \rho_{xy}^{21} & \rho_{xy}^{22} & \rho_{xy}^{22} & \rho_{xy}^{23} & \rho_{xy}^{23} \\
\rho_x^{21} & \rho_x^{21} & \rho^{tt} & 1 & \rho_x^{23} & \rho_x^{23} & \rho_{xy}^{21} & \rho_{xy}^{21} & \rho_{xy}^{22} & \rho_{xy}^{22} & \rho_{xy}^{23} & \rho_{xy}^{23} \\
\rho_x^{31} & \rho_x^{31} & \rho_x^{32} & \rho_x^{32} & 1 & \rho^{tt} & \rho_{xy}^{31} & \rho_{xy}^{31} & \rho_{xy}^{32} & \rho_{xy}^{32} & \rho_{xy}^{33} & \rho_{xy}^{33} \\
\rho_x^{31} & \rho_x^{31} & \rho_x^{32} & \rho_x^{32} & \rho^{tt} & 1 & \rho_{xy}^{31} & \rho_{xy}^{31} & \rho_{xy}^{32} & \rho_{xy}^{32} & \rho_{xy}^{33} & \rho_{xy}^{33} \\
\rho_{xy}^{11} & \rho_{xy}^{11} & \rho_{xy}^{21} & \rho_{xy}^{21} & \rho_{xy}^{31} & \rho_{xy}^{31} & 1 & \rho^{tt} & \rho_y^{12} & \rho_y^{12} & \rho_y^{13} & \rho_y^{12} \\
\rho_{xy}^{11} & \rho_{xy}^{11} & \rho_{xy}^{21} & \rho_{xy}^{21} & \rho_{xy}^{31} & \rho_{xy}^{31} & \rho^{tt} & 1 & \rho_y^{12} & \rho_y^{12} & \rho_y^{13} & \rho_y^{12} \\
\rho_{xy}^{12} & \rho_{xy}^{12} & \rho_{xy}^{22} & \rho_{xy}^{22} & \rho_{xy}^{32} & \rho_{xy}^{32} & \rho_y^{21} & \rho_y^{21} & 1 & \rho^{tt} & \rho_y^{23} & \rho_y^{23} \\
\rho_{xy}^{12} & \rho_{xy}^{12} & \rho_{xy}^{22} & \rho_{xy}^{22} & \rho_{xy}^{32} & \rho_{xy}^{32} & \rho_y^{21} & \rho_y^{21} & \rho^{tt} & 1 & \rho_y^{23} & \rho_y^{23} \\
\rho_{xy}^{13} & \rho_{xy}^{13} & \rho_{xy}^{23} & \rho_{xy}^{23} & \rho_{xy}^{33} & \rho_{xy}^{33} & \rho_y^{31} & \rho_y^{31} & \rho_y^{32} & \rho_y^{32} & 1 & \rho^{tt} \\
\rho_{xy}^{13} & \rho_{xy}^{13} & \rho_{xy}^{23} & \rho_{xy}^{23} & \rho_{xy}^{33} & \rho_{xy}^{33} & \rho_y^{31} & \rho_y^{31} & \rho_y^{32} & \rho_y^{32} & \rho^{tt} & 1
\end{pmatrix}, \tag{22}$$

where ρ_x^{ij}, ρ_y^{ij} and ρ_{xy}^{ij} denote within-molecular and between-molecular correlations between i^{th} and j^{th} biological replicates. As the technical replicates of a biological replicate are often highly correlated, we use a single parameter ρ^{tt} to represent their correlation.
Analogous to the case of blind-case model (Eq. 14 and Eq. 15), the MLE's $\hat{\mu}^I$ and $\hat{\Sigma}^I$ are given by the following sets of equations

$$\hat{\mu}_x^{j_{m_1}} = \frac{1}{I_{m_1}^j n} \sum_{k=1}^{n} \sum_{i=\sum_{l=1}^{j} I_{m_1}^{l-1}+1}^{\sum_{l=1}^{j} I_{m_1}^{l}} x_{ik}, \; 1 \leq j_{m_1} \leq J_{m_1} \tag{23}$$

$$\hat{\mu}_y^{j_{m_2}} = \frac{1}{I_{m_2}^j n} \sum_{k=1}^{n} \sum_{i=\sum_{l=1}^{j} I_{m_2}^{l-1}+1}^{\sum_{l=1}^{j} I_{m_2}^{l}} y_{ik}, \; 1 \leq j_{m_2} \leq J_{m_2} \tag{24}$$

$$\hat{\mu}^I = \left(\hat{\mu}_x^1, \ldots, \hat{\mu}_x^1, \ldots, \hat{\mu}_x^{J_{m_1}}, \ldots, \hat{\mu}_x^{J_{m_1}}, \hat{\mu}_y^1, \ldots, \hat{\mu}_y^1, \ldots, \hat{\mu}_y^{J_{m_2}}, \ldots, \hat{\mu}_y^{J_{m_2}}\right)^T \tag{25}$$

and

$$\hat{\Sigma}^I = \frac{1}{n}\sum_{j=1}^{n}(Z_j - \hat{\mu}_I)(Z_j - \hat{\mu}_I)^T. \tag{26}$$

Here, J_{m_1}, J_{m_2} denote the number of biological replicates for X and Y, whereas $I_{m_1}^j$, $I_{m_2}^j$, $1 \leq j_{m_1} \leq J_{m_1}$, $1 \leq j_{m_2} \leq J_{m_2}$, represent the number of technical replicates nested within $j_{m_1}^{th}$ and $j_{m_2}^{th}$ biological replicate respectively, where $\sum_{j=1}^{J_{m_1}} I_{m_1}^j = m_1$ and $\sum_{j=1}^{J_{m_2}} I_{m_2}^j = m_2$. However, on averaging the off-diagonal block of $\hat{\Sigma}^I$ to estimate a single correlation value, as in the case of blind-case model (Eq. 19), between-molecular correlations from informed-case model and blind-case model become identical (see (Zhu *et al.*, 2010) for proof). To exploit the informed replication mechanism and compare model performances, likelihood ratio test based methods (Anderson, 1958) are used. Indeed, the hypothesis

$$H_0 : Z \in N(\mu, \Sigma_0) \;\text{ versus }\; H_\alpha : Z \in N(\mu, \Sigma)$$

is tested by considering $(\mu, \Sigma) = (\mu_B, \Sigma_B)$ and $(\mu, \Sigma) = (\mu_I, \Sigma_I)$. Matrix Σ_0 is obtained by setting the off-diagonal entries in Σ to 0. Likelihood ratio test statistics for blind-case and informed-case models are calculated using

$$\Psi = -2\,\log(\wedge) \tag{27}$$

where

$$\wedge = \frac{|\hat{\Sigma}_0|^{-n/2}\exp(\frac{-1}{2}\sum_{j=1}^{n}(Z_j - \hat{\mu})^T\hat{\Sigma}_0^{-1}(Z_j - \hat{\mu}))}{|\hat{\Sigma}|^{-n/2}\exp(\frac{-1}{2}\sum_{j=1}^{n}(Z_j - \hat{\mu})^T\hat{\Sigma}^{-1}(Z_j - \hat{\mu}))}. \tag{28}$$

Under null hypothesis, the two statistics $\Psi^B = -2\log\wedge^B$ and $\Psi^I = -2\log\wedge^I$ corresponding to blind-case and informed-case model follow an asymptomatic chi-square distribution with 1 and $J_{m_1}J_{m_2}$ degrees of freedom, respectively. Thus, the model performances can be evaluated by comparing the P-values (P) from blind-case and informed-case models or directly comparing the difference $\Psi^I - \Psi^B$ to the chi-square distribution with $J_{m_1}J_{m_2} - 1$ degrees of freedom. For a more detailed study on informed-case model, we refer to (Zhu *et al.*, 2010).

It is clear that informed-case correlation estimator generalizes blind-case model by explicitly considering prior knowledge of experimental design. When there is only one biological replicate for each gene in replicated data, the two models become identical. Although informed-case model is useful, it is not practical to design a correlation structure that will fit for any replicated molecular profiling data. A key is to adaptively determine the underlying correlation structure by balancing between a model with a constrained set of parameters and the one without any constraints. This situation can be translated into the Expectation-Maximization (EM) framework (Dempster *et al.*, 1977), where we seek for the missing membership of a multivariate observation in either a component with a constrained set of parameters or the one with an unconstrained set of parameters. EM algorithm plays a crucial role in the following generalization of blind-case or informed-case model.

4.3 Finite mixture model

In the finite mixture model approach (Fraley & Raftery, 2002; McLachlan & Peer, 2000), density of an observation is modeled as mixture of a finite number of component densities. Such an approach can be used to shrink the correlation structure of a gene set between a constrained correlation structure and an unconstrained one. Advantages of shrinkage approach have been demonstrated in many related studies (Schäfer & Strimmer, 2005; Zhu & Hero, 2007). In the following discussion, we consider the two-component mixture model approach from (Acharya & Zhu, 2009), where the density of each multivariate observation Z_j is modeled as a mixture of two component densities denote by $f_1(Z_j)$ and $f_2(Z_j)$. This is expressed as

$$f(Z_j, \Psi) = \pi_1 f_1(Z_j) + \pi_2 f_2(Z_j), \tag{29}$$

where π_1 and π_2 stand for mixture proportions with $\pi_1 + \pi_2 = 1$ and Ψ denotes the set of all parameters in the mixture model, $j = 1, \ldots, n$. The first component in the mixture represents either blind-case or informed-case estimator, whereas the second component corresponds to the unconstrained $\sum_{i=1}^{k} m_i$-variate multivariate normal distribution. Let $\theta_i = \{\mu_i, \Sigma_i\}$ denote the set of parameters for the ith component, $i = 1, 2$, where $\theta_1 = \{\mu_B, \Sigma_B\}$ or $\theta_1 = \{\mu_I, \Sigma_I\}$. Finite mixture model employs EM algorithm (McLachlan & Peer, 2000) to estimate the posterior probability that the jth observation belongs to the ith component of the mixture. Thus, incompleteness in the EM framework is incorporated by considering the component-indicator vectors z_j's, $j = 1, 2, \ldots, n$, where $(z_j)_i = z_{ij} = 1$ if Z_j is sampled from the ith component, as unobserved. Complete data is comprised of the observations Z_j's together with the component-indicator vectors z_j's. The E step and M step at the $(k+1)^{th}$ iteration are defined as

E-step: For $i = 1, 2,$

$$\tau_i(Z_j; \Psi^{(k)}) = \frac{\pi_i^{(k)} f_i(Z_j; \theta_i^{(k)})}{\sum_{h=1}^{2} \pi_h^{(k)} f_h(Z_j; \theta_h^{(k)})} \tag{30}$$

where $\tau_i(Z_j; \Psi^{(k)})$ is the posterior probability that Z_j belongs to the ith component.

M-step: For $i = 1, 2,$

$$\pi_i^{k+1} = \frac{1}{n} \sum_{j=1}^{n} \tau_i(Zj; \Psi^{(k)}) \tag{31}$$

$$\mu_i^{k+1} = \frac{\sum_{j=1}^{n} \tau_{ij}^{(k)} Z_j}{\sum_{j=1}^{n} \tau_{ij}^{(k)}} \tag{32}$$

$$\Sigma_i^{k+1} = \frac{\sum_{j=1}^{n} \tau_{ij}^{(k)} (Z_j - \mu_i^{(k+1)})(Z_j - \mu_i^{(k+1)})^T}{\sum_{j=1}^{n} \tau_{ij}^{(k)}} \tag{33}$$

where $\tau_{ij}^{(k)} = \tau_i(Z_j; \Psi^{(k)})$. EM algorithm iterates between the E step and the M step until convergence. Finally, an observation Z_j corresponds to a component model for which it has higher posterior probability of belonging, $j = 1, 2, \ldots, n$. However, in many cases the sequence $\{\log L(\Psi^k)\}$ of log-likelihood values generated in the iterative procedure may not be bounded or it may be trapped in a local solution (McLachlan & Peer, 2000). Consequently,

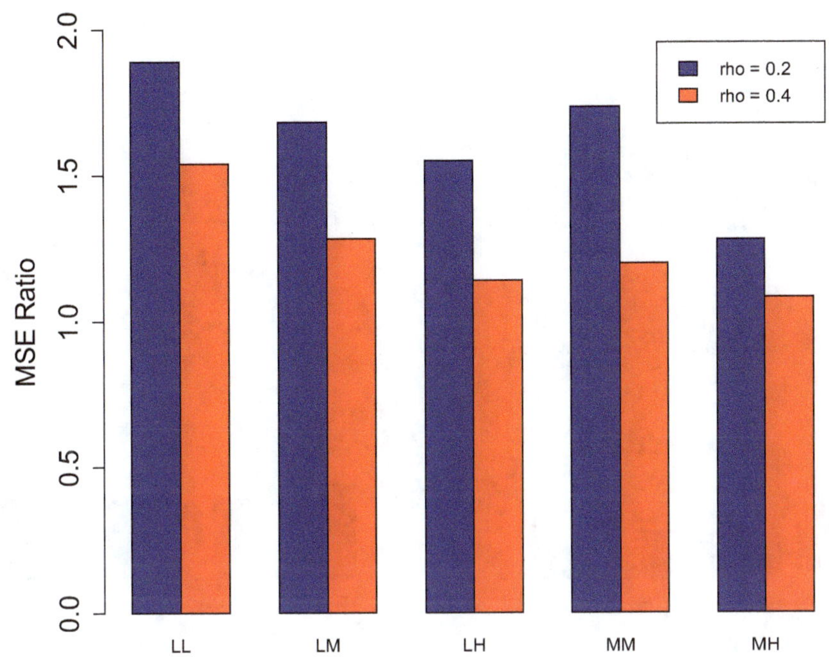

Fig. 2. Comparison of the multivariate blind-case model and bivariate Pearson's correlation estimator. In the figure, the x-axis corresponds to data quality and y-axis represents MSE ratio, which is the ratio MSE from Pearson's estimator/MSE from blind-case model. Pair of genes, each with 4 replicated measurements across 20 samples, were considered in the comparison. The between molecular correlation parameter (rho) was set at 0.2 (low) and 0.4 (medium), respectively.

the unconstrained EM algorithm presented above may not necessarily converge to the MLE $\hat{\Psi}$. To reduce various problems associated with the convergence of EM algorithm, remedies have been proposed by constraining the eigenvalues of the component correlation matrices (Ingrassia, 2004; Ingrassia & Rocci, 2007). For example, the constrained EM algorithm presented in (Ingrassia, 2004) considers two strictly positive constants a and b such that $a/b \geq c$, where $c \in (0\ 1]$. In each iteration of the EM algorithm, if the eigenvalues of the component correlation matrices are smaller than a, they are replaced with a and if they greater than b, they are replaced with b. Indeed, if the eigenvalues of the component correlation matrices satisfy $a \leq \lambda_j(\Sigma_i) \leq b$, for $i = 1,2, j = 1,2,\ldots,\sum_{i=1}^{k} m_i$, then the condition $\lambda_{\min}(\Sigma_1 \Sigma_2^{-1}) \geq c$ (Hathaway, 1985) is also satisfied, and results in constrained (global) maximization of the likelihood.

5. Results

5.1 Simulations

In this section, we evaluate the performance of multivariate and bivariate correlation estimators using synthetic replicated data. In Figure 2, we compare multivariate blind-case model and bivariate Pearson's correlation estimator by simulating 1000 synthetic data sets corresponding to a pair of genes, each with 4 replicated measurements and 20 observations.

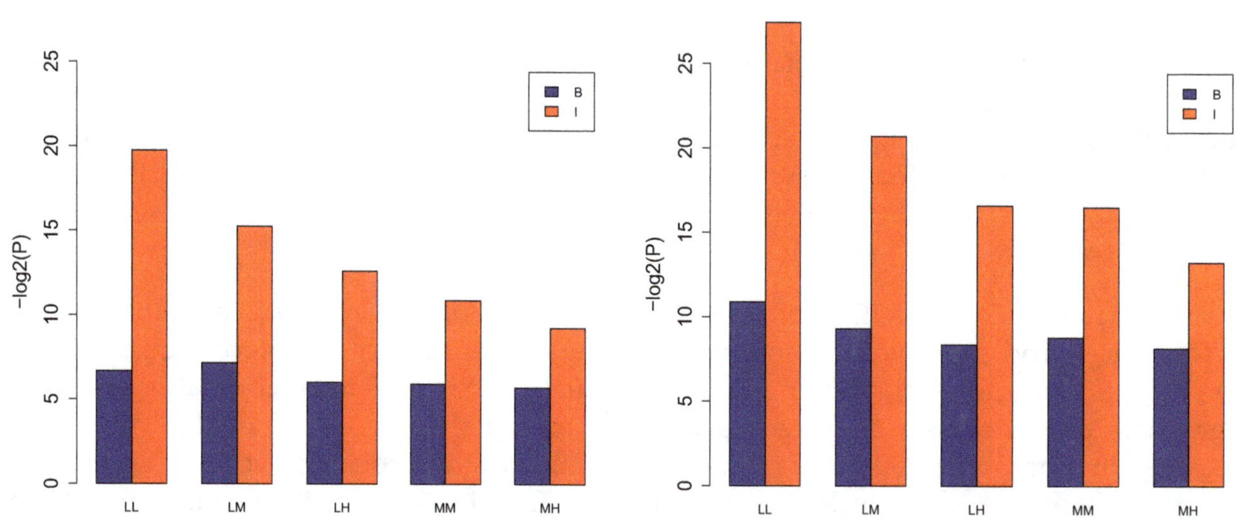

Fig. 3. Comparison of the multivariate blind-case model and informed-case model with increasing data quality and sample size, as presented in (Zhu *et al.*, 2010). Pair of genes, each with 3 biological replicates and 2 technical replicates nested within a biological replicate, were considered in the comparison. The range of between-molecular correlation parameters was set at M (0.3-0.5). Two upper panels correspond to replicated data with sample size $n = 20$ (left) and $n = 30$ (right), and the lower panels correspond to the ones with $n = 40$ (left) and $n = 50$ (right).

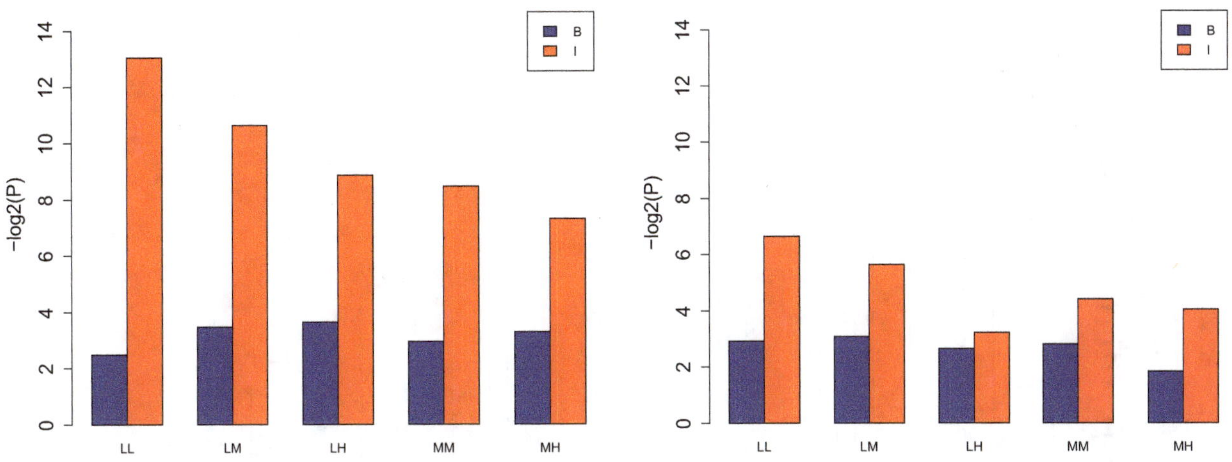

Fig. 4. Comparison of the multivariate blind-case model and informed-case model with increasing number of technical replicates, as presented in (Zhu *et al.*, 2010). Pair of genes, each with 3 biological replicates and 20 observations were considered in the comparison. The range of between-molecular correlation parameters was set at M (0.3-0.5). The left and right panels correspond to 1 and 2 technical replicates nested within a biological replicate, respectively.

Along the x-axis, L (low: $0.1-0.3$), M (medium: $0.3-0.5$) and H (high: $0.5-0.7$) represent the range of within-molecular correlations for each of the two genes. The y-axis corresponds to MSE (mean squared error) ratio, which is the ratio of MSE from Pearson's estimator over MSE from blind-case model. Thus, MSE ratio greater than 1 indicates the superior performance of blind-case model. We fixed the between molecular correlation parameter at 0.2 (low) and 0.4 (medium), respectively. As shown in Fig. 2, all examined MSE ratios were found greater than 1. Figure 2 also demonstrates that the performance of blind-case model is a decreasing function of data quality. This observation makes blind-case model particularly suitable for analyzing real-world replicated data sets, which are often contaminated with excessive noise. Figure 3 and Figure 4 represent parts of more detailed studies conducted in (Zhu *et al.*, 2010) to evaluate the performances of multivariate correlation estimators. For instance, Figure 3 compares the multivariate blind-case model and informed-case model with increasing data quality and sample size. Synthetic data sets corresponding to a pair of genes, each with 3 biological replicates and 2 technical replicates nested within a biological replicate in 20 experiments were used in the comparison. The model performances were estimated in terms of $-\log_2(P)$ values. Higher $-\log_2(P)$ values indicate better performance by a model. As demonstrated in Fig. 3, informed-case model significantly outperformed the blind-case model in estimating pairwise correlation from replicated data with informed replication mechanisms. It is also observed in Figure 3 that blind-case and informed-case models are increasing functions of sample size and decreasing functions of data quality. The two models were also compared in terms of increasing number of technical replicates of a biological replicate, as demonstrated in Figure 4. We conclude from Figure 4 that blind-case and informed-case models are decreasing functions of the number of technical replicates nested with a biological replicate.

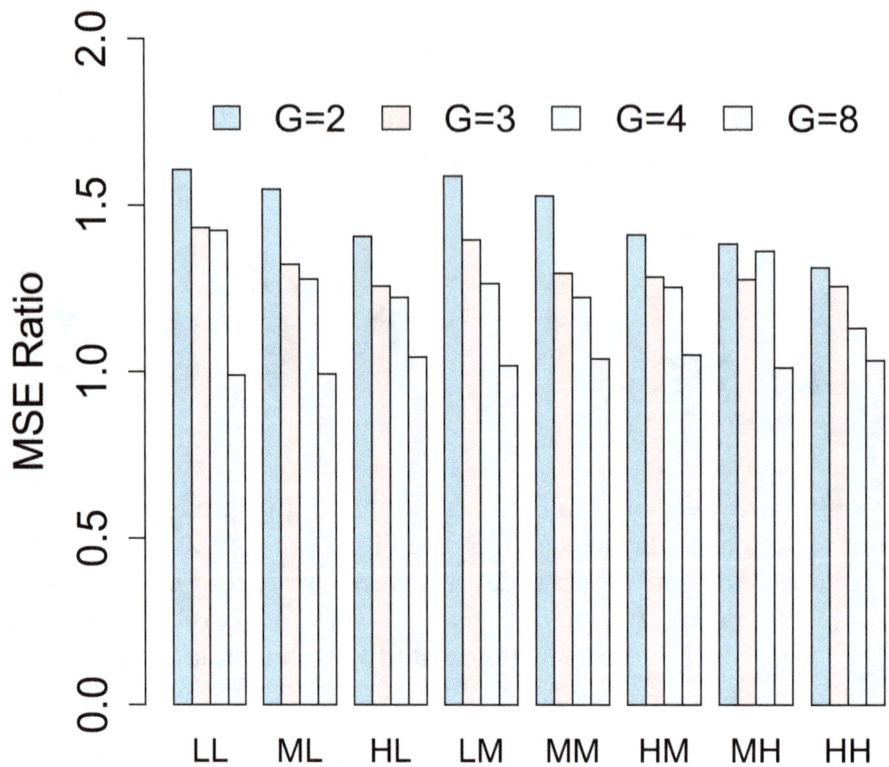

Fig. 5. Comparison of the multivariate blind-case model and two-component finite mixture model in terms of MSE ratio, as presented in (Acharya & Zhu, 2009). MSE ratio is calculated as MSE from blind-case model/MSE from mixture model. Gene sets with 2, 3, 4 and 8 genes, each with 4 replicated measurements across 20 samples were considered in the comparison.

Fig. 5, originally from (Acharya & Zhu, 2009), compares the performance of blind-case model and two component finite mixture model in estimating the correlation structure of a gene set. The constrained component in the mixture model corresponds to blind-case correlation estimator. Fig. 5 plots the model performances in terms of MSE ratio defined as MSE from blind-case model/MSE from mixture model. The number of genes in a gene set are fixed at $G = 2$, 3, 4 and 8. In Fig. 5, almost all examined MSE ratios greater than 1 indicate an overall better performance of the mixture model approach compared with blind-case model. Fig. 5 also indicates that the performance of finite mixture model is a decreasing functions of data quality and number of genes in the input.

5.2 Real-world data analysis

In Figure 6-8, we present real-world studies conducted in (Acharya & Zhu, 2009), where blind-case model and finite mixture model were used to analyze two publically available replicated data sets, spike-in data from Affymetrix (`http://www.affymetrix.com`) and yeast galactose data (`http://expression.washington.edu/publications/kayee`) from (Yeung *et al.*, 2003). Spike-in data comprises of the gene expression levels of 16 genes

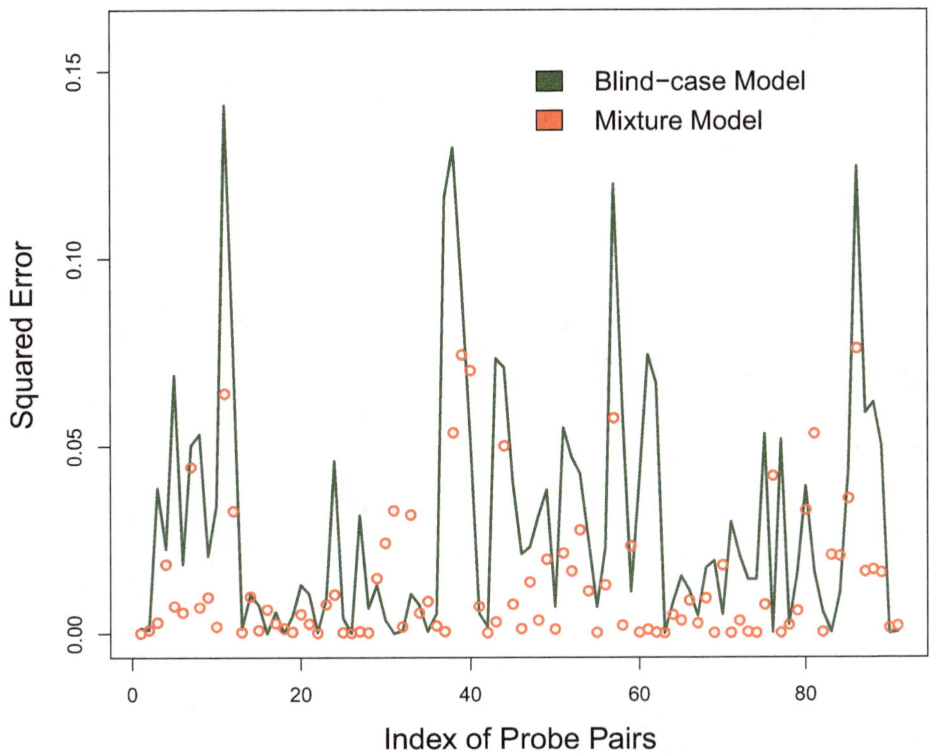

Fig. 6. Comparison of two multivariate models, blind-case model and finite mixture model, in estimating pairwise correlations among genes in spike-in data, as presented in (Acharya & Zhu, 2009).

in 20 experiments, where 16 replicated measurements are available for a gene. Correlation structures estimated using spike-in data were compared with the nominal correlation structure obtained from a prior known probe-level intensities. On the other hand, yeast data contains the gene expression levels of 205 genes, each with 4 replicated measurements. Yeast data was used to assess model performances in hierarchial clustering by utilizing a prior knowledge of the class labels of 205 genes.

Figure 6 compares the performance of blind-case model and mixture model in estimating pairwise correlation between genes present in spike-in data. We observed that for almost 82% of the probe pairs, mixture model provided a better approximation to the nominal pairwise correlation compared with blind-case model. The two models were further employed to estimate the correlation structure of a gene set. Figure 7 corresponds to the correlation structure of a collection of 10 randomly selected probe sets from spike-in data. As demonstrated in Figure 7, an overall better performance of mixture model approach was given by lower squared error in comparison to blind-case model.

Finally, blind-case model and mixture model were utilized to estimate the correlation structures from 150 subsets of yeast data, each with 60 randomly selected probe sets. The estimated correlation structures were used to perform correlation based hierarchial clustering. Figure 8 compares the clustering performance of blind-case model and mixture model in terms of Minkowski score. Minkowski score is defined as $\|C - T\| / \|T\|$, where C and T are binary matrices constructed from the predicted and true labels of genes, respectively. C_{ij}

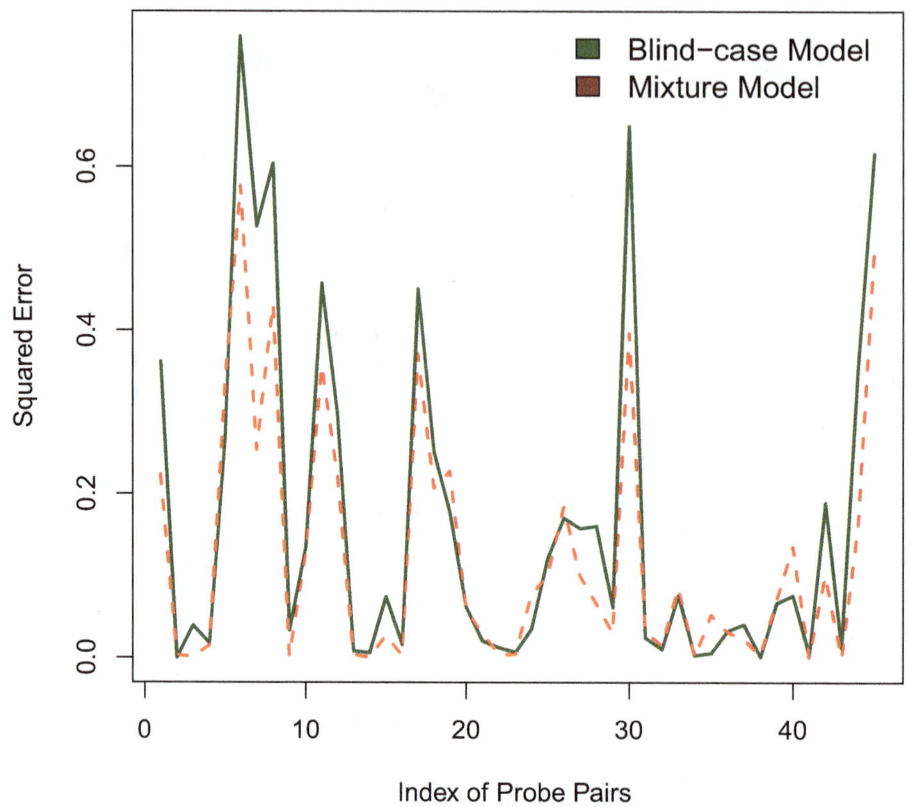

Fig. 7. Comparison of the multivariate blind-case model and finite mixture model in estimating the correlation structure of a gene set, as presented in (Acharya & Zhu, 2009). The figure corresponds to a gene set comprising of 10 randomly selected probe sets in spike-in data. Each index along the x-axis represents a probe set pair and y-axis plots squared error values in estimating nominal correlations.

=1, if i^{th} and j^{th} gene belong to the same cluster in the solution and 0 otherwise. Matrix T is obtained analogously using the true labels. A lower Minkowski score indicates higher clustering accuracy. In Figure 8, an overall better performance of two-component mixture model approach was observed in almost 73% cases.

6. Conclusions

Rapid developments in high-throughput data acquisition technologies have generated vast amounts of molecular profiling data which continue to accumulate in public databases. Since such data are often contaminated with excessive noise, they are replicated for a reliable pattern discovery. An accurate estimate of the correlation structure underlying replicated data can provide deep insights into the complex biomolecular activities. However, traditional bivariate approaches to correlation estimation do not automatically accommodate replicated measurements. Typically, an *ad hoc* step of data preprocessing by averaging (weighted, unweighted or something in between) is needed. Averaging creates a strong bias while reducing variance among the replicates with diverse magnitudes. It may also wipe out

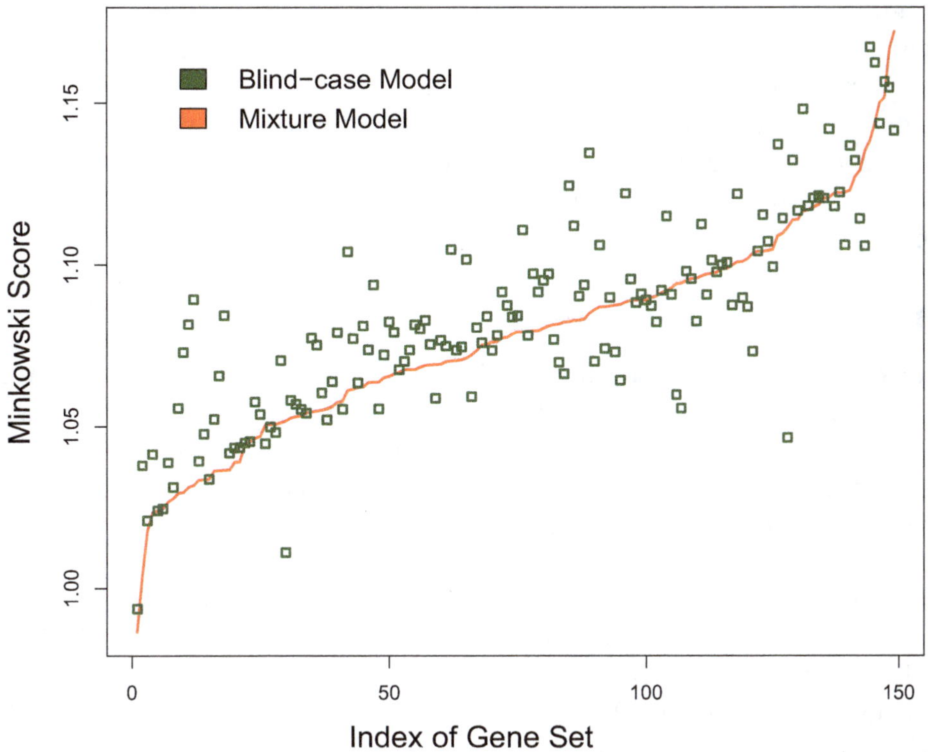

Fig. 8. Performance of the multivariate blind-case model and finite mixture model in clustering yeast data, as presented in (Acharya & Zhu, 2009). Each index along the x-axis corresponds to a subset of yeast data comprising of 60 randomly selected probe sets. The y-axis plots model performances in terms of Minkowski score. An overall better performance of the mixture model approach is given by lower Minkowski scores in almost 73% cases.

important patterns of small magnitudes or cancel out patterns of similar magnitudes. In many cases prior knowledge of the underlying replication mechanism might be known. However, this information can not be exploited by averaging replicated measurements. Thus, it is necessary to design multivariate approaches by treating each replicate as a variable. In this chapter, we reviewed two bivariate correlation estimators, Pearson's correlation and SD-weighted correlation, and three multivariate models, blind-case model, informed-case model and finite mixture model to estimate the correlation structure from replicated molecular profiling data corresponding to a gene set with blind or informed replication mechanism. Each of the three multivariate models treat a replicated measurement individually as a random variable by assuming that data as independently and identically distributed samples from a multivariate normal distribution. Blind-case model utilizes a constrained set of parameters to define the correlation structure of a gene set with blind replication mechanism, whereas informed-case model generalizes blind-case model by incorporating prior knowledge of experimental design. Finite mixture model presents a more general approach of shrinking between a constrained model, either blind-case model or informed-case model, and the unconstrained model. The aforementioned multivariate models were used to analyze synthetic and real-world replicated data sets. In practice, the choice of a multivariate correlation estimator may depend on various factors, e.g. number of genes, number of replicated measurements available for a gene, prior knowledge of experimental design etc. For instance, blind-case and informed-case models are more stable and computationally more efficient than iterative EM based finite mixture model approach. However, considering the real-world scenarios, finite mixture model assumes a more faithful representation of the underlying correlation structure. Nonetheless, the multivariate models presented here are sufficiently generalized to incorporate both blind and informed replication mechanisms, and open new avenues for future supervised and unsupervised bioinformatics researches that require accurate estimation of correlation, e.g. gene clustering, gene networking and classification problems.

7. References

Acharya LR and Zhu D (2009). Estimating an Optimal Correlation Structure from Replicated Molecular Profiling Data Using Finite Mixture Models. In the Proceedings of *IEEE International Conference on Machine Learning and Applications*, 119-124.

Altay G and Emmert-Streib F (2010). Revealing differences in gene network inference algorithms on the network-level by ensemble methods. *Bioinformatics*, 26(14), 1738-1744.

Anderson TW (1958). *An introduction to mutilvariate statistical analysis*, Wiley Publisher, New York.

Basso K, Margolin AA, Stolovitzky G, Klein U, Dalla-Favera R and Califano, A (2005). Reverse engineering of regulatory networks in human B cells. *Nature Genetics*, 37:382-390.

Boscolo R, Liao J, Roychowdhury VP (2008). An Information Theoretic Exploratory Method for Learning Patterns of Conditional Gene Coexpression from Microarray Data. *IEEE/ACM Transactions on Computational Biology and Bioinformatics*, 15-24.

Butte AJ and Kohane IS (2000). Mutual information relevance networks: functional genomic clustering using pairwise entropy measurements. *Pacific Symposium on Biocomputing*, 5, 415-426.

Casella G and Berger RL (1990). *Statistical inference*, Duxbury Advanced Series.

Dempster AP, Laird NM and Rubin DB (1977). Maximum Likelihood from incomplete data via the EM algorithm. *Journal of the Royal Statistical Society B*, 39(1):1-38.

Eisen M, Spellman P, Brown PO, Botstein D (1998). Cluster analysis and display of genome-wide expression patterns. *Proceedings of the National Academy of Sciences*, 95:14863-14868.

Fraley C and Raftery AE (2002). Model-based clustering, discriminant analysis, and density estimation. *Journal of the American Statistical Association*, 97, 611-631.

Gunderson KL, Kruglyak S, Graige MS, Garcia F, Kermani BG, Zhao C, Che D, Dickinson T, Wickham E, Bierle J, Doucet D, Milewski M, Yang R, Siegmund C, Haas J, Zhou L, Oliphant A, Fan JB, Barnard S and Chee MS (2004). Decoding randomly ordered DNA arrays. *Genome Research*, 14:870-877.

Hastie T, Tibshirani R and Friedman J (2009). *The Elements of Statistical Learning: Prediction, Inference and Data Mining*, Springer-Verlag, New York.

Hathaway RJ (1985). A constrained formulation of maximum-likelihood estimation for normal mixture distributions. *Annals of Statistics*, **13**, 795-800.

de Hoon MJL, Imoto S, Nolan J and Miyano S (2004). Open source clustering software. *Bioinformatics*, 20(9):1453-1454.

Hughes TR, Marton MJ, Jones AR, Roberts CJ, Stoughton R, Armour CD, Bennett HA, Coffey E, Dai H and He YD (2000). Functional discovery via a compendium of expression profiles. *Cell*, 102:109-126.

Ingrassia S (2004). A likelihood-based constrained algorithm for multivariate normal mixture models. *Statistical Methods and Applications*, 13, 151-166.

Ingrassia S and Rocci R (2007). Constrained monotone EM algorithms for the finite mixtures of multivariate Gaussians. *Computational Statistics and Data Analysis*, 51, 5399-5351.

Kerr MK and Churchill GA (2001). Experimental design for gene expression microarrays. *Biostatistics*, 2:183-201.

Kung C, Kenski DM, Dickerson SH, Howson RW, Kuyper LF, Madhani HD, Shokat KM (2005). Chemical genomic profiling to identify intracellular targets of a multiplex kinase inhibitor. *Proceedings of the National Academy of Sciences*, 102:3587-3592.

Lockhart DJ, Dong H, Byrne MC, Follettie MT, Gallo MV, Chee MS, Mittmann M, Wang C, Kobayashi M, Horton H and Brown EL (1996). Expression monitoring by hybridization to high-density oligonucleotide arrays. *Nature Biotechnology*, 14:1675-1680.

McLachlan GJ and Peel D (2000). *Finite Mixture Models*. Wiley series in Probability and Mathematical Statistics, John Wiley & Sons.

McLachlan GJ and Peel D (2000). On computational aspects of clustering via mixtures of normal and t-components. *Proceedings of the American Statistical Association*, Bayesian Statistical Science Section, Indianapolis, Virginia.

Medvedovic M and Sivaganesan S (2002). Bayesian infinite mixture model based clustering of gene expression profiles. *Bioinformatics*, 18:1194-1206.

Medvedovic M, Yeung KY and Bumgarner RE (2004). Bayesian mixtures for clustering replicated microarray data. *Bioinformatics*, 20:1222-1232.

Rengarajan J, Bloom BR and Rubin EJ (2005). From The Cover: Genomewide requirements for Mycobacterium tuberculosis adaptation and survival in macrophages. *Proceedings of the National Academy of Sciences*, 102(23):8327-8332.

Sartor MA, Tomlinson CR, Wesselkamper SC, Sivaganesan S, Leikauf GD and Medvedovic, M (2006) Intensity-based hierarchical Bayes method improves testing for differentially expressed genes in microarray experiments. *BMC Bioinformatics*, 7:538.

Schäfer J and Strimmer K (2005). A shrinkage approach to large-scale covariance matrix estimation and implications for functional genomics. *Statistical Applications in Genetics and Molecular Biology*, 4, Article 32.

Shendure J and Ji H (2008). Next-generation DNA sequencing. *Nature Biotechnology*, 26, 1135-1145.

van't Veer LJ, Dai HY, van de Vijver MJ, He YDD, Hart AAM, Mao M, Peterse HL, van der Kooy K, Marton MJ, Witteveen AT, Schreiber GJ, Kerkhoven RM, Roberts C, Linsley PS, Bernards R, Friend SH (2002). Gene expression profiling predicts clinical outcome of breast cancer. *Nature*, 415:530-536.

Yao J, Chang C, Salmi ML, Hung YS, Loraine A and Roux SJ (2008). Genome-scale cluster analysis of replicated microarrays using shrinkage correlation coefficient. *BMC Bioinformatics*, 9:288.

Yeung KY, Medvedovic M and Bumgarner R. (2003). Clustering gene expression data with repeated measurements. *Genome Biology*, 4:R34.

Yeung KY and Bumgarner R (2005). Multi-class classification of microarray data with repeated measurements: application to cancer. *Genome Biology*, 6(405).

Zhu D, Hero AO, Qin ZS and Swaroop A (2005). High throughput screening co-expressed gene pairs with controlled biological significance and statistical significance. *Journal of Computational Biology*, 12(7):1029-1045.

Zhu D, Li Y and Li H (2007). Multivariate correlation estimator for inferring functional relationships from replicated genome-wide data. *Bioinformatics*, 23(17):2298-2305.

Zhu D and Hero AO (2007). Bayesian hierarchical model for large-scale covariance matrix estimation. *Journal of Computational Biology*, 14(10):1311-1326.

Zhu D, Acharya LR and Zhang H (2010). A Generalized Multivariate Approach to Pattern Discovery from Replicated and Incomplete Genome-wide Measurements, *IEEE/ACM transaction on Computational Biology and Bioinformatics*, (in press).

3

Diffusion of Methylene Blue in Phantoms of Agar Using Optical Absorption Techniques

Lidia Vilca-Quispe, Alejandro Castilla-Loeza,
Juan José Alvarado-Gil and Patricia Quintana-Owen
Centro de Investigación y de Estudios Avanzados del IPN, Unidad Mérida
Mérida, Yucatán
México

1. Introduction

Diffusion of substances in tissue is an extremely complex process. Various phantoms have been proposed as a model to simulate biological organs and to study physicochemical effects on the human body. Low concentration aqueous agar phantoms systems are specially suited for this purpose (Madsen et al., 2005), because they resemble the desired tissue, and are inexpensive to prepare (Bauman et al., 2004). Recently, they have been suggested for the study of the treatment of neurodegenerative diseases of the central nervous system (CNS) by implantation of nanoreservoirs, for controlled drug release into the brain (Staples et al., 2006). A variety of experimental methods have been developed for the study of drug diffusion phenomena in such a complex system. Methylene blue can be used to monitor the diffusion processes inside a gel-like material to simulate the actual process that takes place in the living tissue, since the size of this molecule is similar to that of some chemotherapeutic drugs (Buchholz et al., 2008). Methylene blue is a heterocyclic aromatic chemical compound with the molecular formula $C_{16}H_{18}N_3SCl$, a scheme of the molecule is shown in Figure 1. Additionally, methylene blue is a molecule that has played important roles in microbiology and pharmacology. It has been widely used to stain living organisms, to treat methemoglobinemia, and recently it has been considered as a drug for photodynamic therapy (Tardivo et al., 2005). This compound shows in-vivo activity against several types of tumors, when locally injected and illuminated with read laser light (Tardivo et al., 2005). Orth and coauthors have demonstrated that intratumoral injection of 1% methylene blue followed by illumination by an argon-pumped dye laser, was able to kill xenotransplanted tumors in animals and recurrent esophageal tumors in patients (Orth et al., 1998).

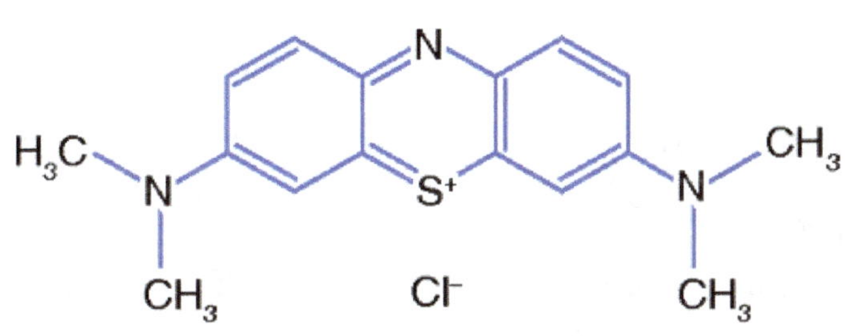

Fig. 1. Molecular structure scheme of the methylene blue.

Various techniques have been developed to study this kind of process using microscopy, optical techniques, electrical analysis, etc. (Bauman et al., 2004). For the experimenter it is always important to have access to new, simple, and reliable methodologies. Optical techniques have been also used successfully to study diffusion processes (Almond & Patel, 1996). These techniques are in general based in the study of light transmission at a fixed height of a sample column or illuminating the whole column to detect the change of the system. In this case, the results have been interpreted as a consequence of variations in the optical properties of the system. Photoacoustic effect has been demonstrated to be a useful tool for materials characterization, and in the study of diverse phenomena (Almond & Patel, 1996; Mandelis, 1993; Vargas & Miranda, 1988). Photoacoustics have been also used recently in the study of the evolution of dynamic systems, such as oxygen release in plants, blood sedimentation, evaporation of liquids, etc. (Acosta et al., 1996; Frandas et al., 2000; Landa et al., 2003; Martinez-Torres & Alvarado-Gil, 2007). The photoacoustic (PA) signal is not only directly related to the time evolution of the optical and thermal properties, but also with various physical processes leading to modulated heat and additional changes in the geometry of the sample (Bialkowski, 1996). The PA technique is based on the periodic heating of a sample illuminated with modulated optical radiation. In a gas-microphone configuration, the sample is in contact with the gas-tight cell. In addition to a steady-state temperature gradient, a thermal wave in the material couples back to the gas around the sample and this will result in a periodic fluctuation of the temperature of a thin layer of gas, close to the sample surface. This thin layer of gas will act as an acoustic piston, which will result in the production of a periodic pressure change in the cavity. A sensitive microphone coupled to the sample chamber can be used to detect this pressure fluctuation.

In this work the diffusion of an aqueous solution of methylene blue into an agar gel using a novel optical technique and photoacoustic spectroscopy are presented. The optic study was performed illuminating with a laser a transparent tube containing the sample of agar, simultaneously the data acquisition of the transmission is done using eight photodiodes. This technique allows measuring the diffusion of methylene blue into the agar as a function of the position and time. Additionally, the diffusion process is monitored applying the photoacoustic technique using a modified Rosencwaig photoacoustic cell (Fernelius, 1980; Quimby & Yen, 1980), in which the sample is illuminated with a modulated red laser beam at a fixed frequency (Teng & Royce, 1980; Wetsel & McDonald, 1977). For both techniques, simple theoretical analyses allow the determination of the evolution of the effective optical properties. The stabilization time of the process, is presented, and it is shown that the characteristic time, in which the dye diffusion process stabilizes, increases with the agar concentration.

2. Materials and methods

2.1 Materials preparation

Samples were prepared using agar powder (BD Bioxon hygroscopic bacteriologic agar) and 17.4 MΩ.cm of de-ionized water. The following agar powder concentration in water is used for the optical analysis [100 × mass of agar powder / (mass of agar powder + mass of water)] and fixed at 0.1 %, 0.2 %, 0.3 %, 0.4 % and 0.5 % mass/volume (w/v) and for photoacoustic technique measurement 0.01 % and 0.05 % mass/volume (w/v), were analyzed. This difference is due to the size of the agar column analyzed in each case. Optical measurements were made in containers much larger than the ones used in photoacoustics.

The mixture of agar in water was heated up to 80 °C and stirred during 4 min in such a way that all the agar powder is completely dissolved. The resulting solutions were deposited in containers, cooled to room temperature and the containers were sealed.

2.2 Optical detection technique

In order to evaluate the diffusion processes, a simple optical system was developed. The experimental arrangement is shown in Fig. 2. In this case, the samples were contained inside glass tubes (10 cm long × 3 mm diameter). As the light source, a 635 nm and 4 mW laser diode with a uniformly opened elliptical spot, with an approximate area of 1.8 cm long and 3 mm wide, was used to illuminate the glass tube. The light transmitted through the sample is collected on the opposite side of the tube using a Judson PA-7: 16C detector (with a working range of wavelengths from 500 nm to 5.0 μm). This detector consists of a linear array of sixteen photodiodes (Fig. 3), with a cross section of 1 mm^2 with a separation of 2 mm between two consecutive photodiodes. The detector output is connected to homemade electronics and from that to a National Instruments BNC-2090 device allowing the detection of eight simultaneous signals along the tube. The analog signals are captured using a data acquisition Analog-Digital card PCI-6035. This information is sent to a PC for storage and subsequent analysis.

The diffusion process was induced by adding 4 mL of methylene blue solution (0.0125 $g.mL^{-1}$) on the upper side of the tube. As a consequence, the methylene solution starts to migrate downwards through the sample and the agar slowly changes color and becomes dyed by the methylene blue. The light transmitted through the sample changes when the dye absorbs the light and this is registered by the photodiodes array detector. In this way, the transmitted light is a direct measurement of the changes in concentration and provides the parameters associated with the kinetic diffusion process. The first photodiode was at 2 mm below the surface of the agar sample.

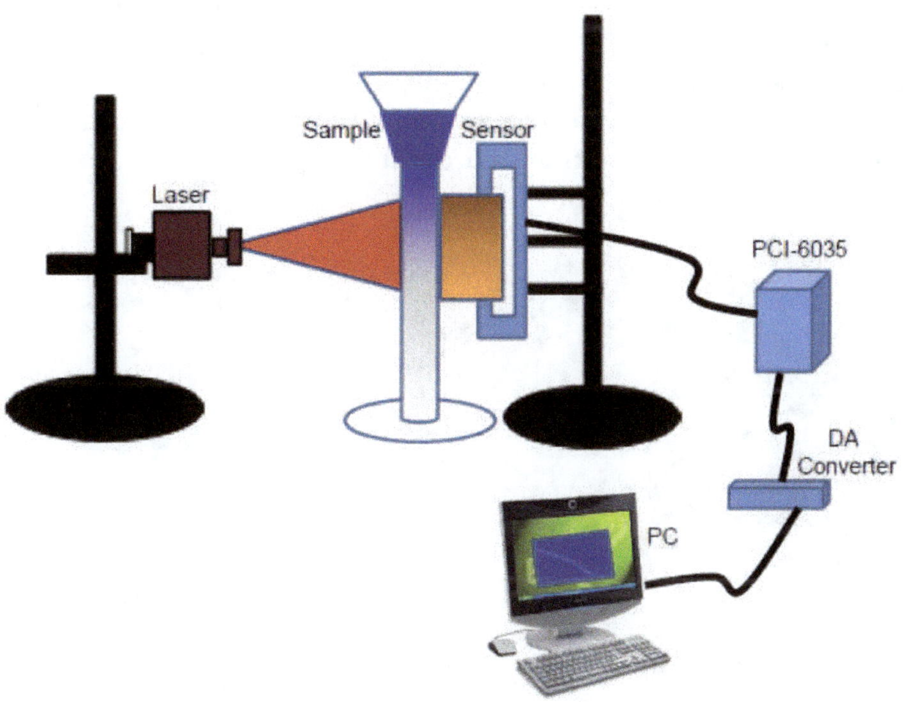

Fig. 2. Experimental arrangement for the light transmission measurement system.

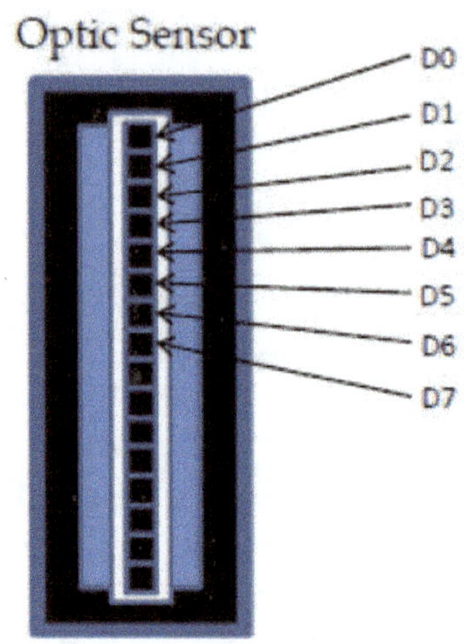

Fig. 3. Cross section of the optic detector, only the indicated upper eight photodiodes, was used.

2.3 Photoacoustic technique

The diffusion process of methylene blue aqueous solutions in agar samples was also using the photoacoustic technique (PA). It consists of a conventional PA cell (Figs. 4 and 5), closed on one side by a transparent quartz window and on the opposite side by a transparent polyvinyl acetate foil, used as a backing material, with a thickness of 98 µm (Vargas-Luna et al., 2002). On top of this foil, the agar gel sample was deposited. The polyvinyl acetate and the sample was illuminated through the quartz transparent window. An electret microphone is used, coupled to the cavity wall, to detect the pressure fluctuations in the PA chamber, generated by the periodic light beam of a 160 mW diode laser at 658 nm (ML120G21) modulated at a constant frequency. The microphone signal is fed into a lock-in amplifier (SR830), from where the output signal amplitude is recorded, as a function of time, in a personal computer. At the beginning of the experiment, 100 µL of agar solution are deposited; when the signal stabilizes, 10 µL of methylene blue solution (0.0125 $g.mL^{-1}$) are added to the surface of the agar with a micropipette. Due to the methylene blue diffusion inside the agar, the PA signal changes in the subsequent stages. In order to get data independent of the microphone characteristics, the PA signal amplitude at any time was normalized dividing it by the maximum value of the PA signal amplitude for a given experiment.

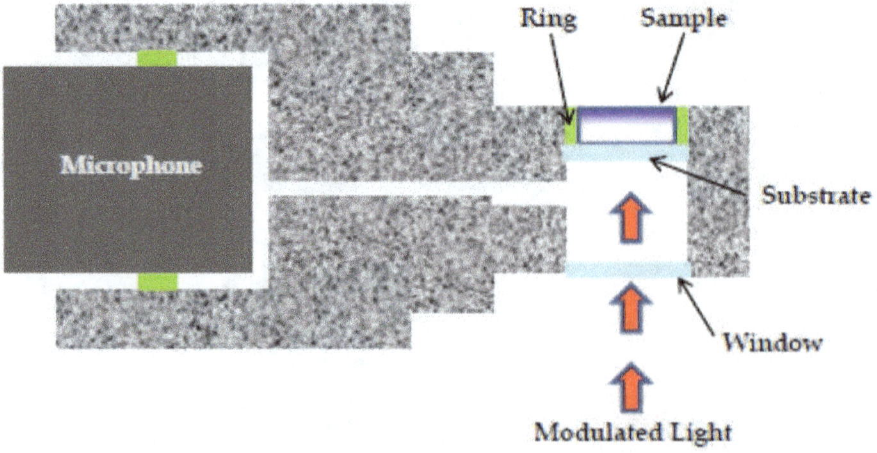

Fig. 4. Schematic cross-section of the used conventional PA cell.

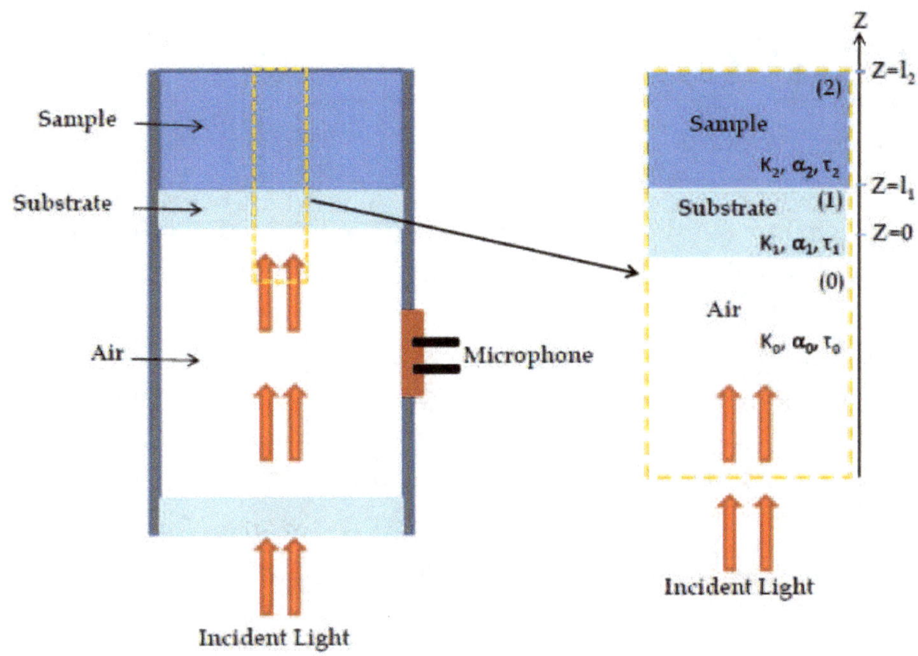

Fig. 5. Cross-section of the cylindrical photoacoustic cell, showing the positions of the sample, backing material, and gas column.

In order to understand the evolution of the PA signal, a theoretical methodology is used, in which it is considered that the system has homogeneous optical and thermal properties at any given time (Vilca et al., 2010). The formalism consists in finding the temperature of the layered system shown in Fig. 5. Using the heat conduction equation with a modulated heat source at modulation frequency f (Carslaw, 2005; Almond & Patel, 1996):

$$\frac{\partial^2 T(z,t)}{\partial z^2} - \frac{1}{\alpha}\frac{\partial T(z,t)}{\partial t} = -\frac{1}{k}F(z)\left(\frac{1+\cos(\omega t)}{2}\right), \tag{1}$$

where z is the spatial coordinate, t is the time, T is the absolute temperature, α_j (k_j) is the thermal diffusivity (thermal conductivity) of layer j, $\omega = 2\pi f$ and $F(z)$ is the spatial distribution of the deposited energy over the sample, per unit volume and unit time. Under these conditions, the temperature at any point inside the sample ($z \geq 0$) is given by

$$T(z,t) = T_{\mathrm{amb}} + T_{\mathrm{dc}}(z) + T_{\mathrm{ac}}(z,t), \tag{2}$$

with T_{amb} being the ambient temperature. $T_{\mathrm{dc}}(z)$ and $T_{\mathrm{ac}}(z,t) = \mathrm{Re}\left[\theta(z)e^{i\omega t}\right]$ are the stationary raising and periodic components of the temperature, due to the first and second terms of the heat source, respectively. From now on, the operator will be omitted, taking into account the convention that the real part of the expression must be taken to obtain physical quantities. We will focus our attention on the oscillatory part of the temperature, since it is the quantity of interest in lock-in and similar detection techniques.
It can be shown that when the layers T_{amb} have an ideal perfect thermal contact (Pichardo & Alvarado-Gil, 2001), and considering that layer 2 is sufficiently thick, to avoid the presence of thermal waves traveling in the $-z$ direction inside it, the following result is obtained for $z \leq 0$:

$$\theta(z)=\Theta\frac{\eta_1 r_1\left(\frac{\varepsilon_{21}+1}{r_1+1}\mathrm{e}^{\sigma_1 l_1}-\frac{\varepsilon_{21}-1}{r_1-1}\mathrm{e}^{-\sigma_1 l_1}+2\frac{\varepsilon_{21}-r_1}{r_1^2-1}\mathrm{e}^{-\beta_1 l_1}\right)+2(1-R_2)\frac{\eta_2 r_2}{r_2+1}\mathrm{e}^{-(\beta_1+\beta_2)l_1}}{(\varepsilon_{01}+1)(\varepsilon_{21}+1)\mathrm{e}^{\sigma_1 l_1}-(\varepsilon_{01}-1)(\varepsilon_{21}-1)\mathrm{e}^{-\sigma_1 l_1}}\mathrm{e}^{\sigma_0 z} \quad (3)$$

Where $\Theta=(1-R_1)I/(2\varepsilon_1(1+i)(\pi f)^{1/2})$, $\sigma_j=(1+i)(\pi f/\alpha_j)^{1/2}$, $\varepsilon_{mn}=\varepsilon_m/\varepsilon_n$, $\varepsilon_j=k_j/(\alpha_j)^{1/2}$, and $r_m=\beta_m/\sigma_m$, with β_j the absorption coefficient, η_j the efficiency at which the absorbed light is converted into heat, R_j is the reflection coefficient, of the corresponding layer *j*, with $j=1,\ 2$ (Almond & Patel, 1996).

Taking into account that under our experimental conditions, layer 1 can be considered as thermally thick and optically transparent ($\mu_1 << l_1 << 1/\beta_1$), $R_2 \approx 0$, which is a reasonable assumption for layer 2 (agar combined with methylene blue), $\eta_1 \approx \eta_2$ as usual (Almond & Patel, 1996), and $\beta_2 l_1 << 1$; therefore Eq. 3 takes the form of,

$$\theta(z)\approx\frac{\eta_1(1-R_1)I\beta_1\sqrt{\alpha_1}}{4\pi\mathrm{i}\varepsilon_1 f}\left(1+T_{21}\sqrt{\alpha_{21}}\beta_{21}\mathrm{e}^{-\sigma_1 l_1}\right)\mathrm{e}^{\sigma_0 z}, \quad (4)$$

where $T_{21}=2/(1+\varepsilon_{21})$, $\beta_{21}=\beta_2/\beta_1$, and $\alpha_{21}=\alpha_2/\alpha_1$. It will be assumed that the thermal properties of layer 1 are constant along the entire experiment and assuming that only the optical absorption coefficient β_2 of layer 2 is changing appreciably, during the process of diffusion of the methylene blue into the agar. This last assumption is valid for low concentrations of methylene blue only; it is convenient to define the normalized signal Ω as follows:

$$\Omega=\frac{\theta(z,\beta)}{\theta(z,\beta_0)}=\frac{\left(1+T_{21}\sqrt{\alpha_{21}}\beta\mathrm{e}^{-\sigma_1 l_1}\right)}{\left(1+T_{21}\sqrt{\alpha_{21}}\beta_0\mathrm{e}^{-\sigma_1 l_1}\right)}, \quad (5)$$

where $\beta_0=\beta_{21}(t=0)$ is the normalized optical absorption coefficient at the beginning of the diffusion process and $\beta=\beta_{21}(t)$ is the normalized optical absorption coefficient at some subsequent time $t>0$. Expressing Eq. 5 as a complex function in its polar form, it can be shown that its amplitude $A(f)$ is given by

$$A(f)=\sqrt{\frac{1+\left(T_{21}\sqrt{\alpha_{21}}\beta\right)^2\mathrm{e}^{-2\sqrt{f/f_c}}+2T_{21}\sqrt{\alpha_{21}}\beta\mathrm{e}^{-\sqrt{f/f_c}}\cos(\sqrt{f/f_c})}{1+\left(T_{21}\sqrt{\alpha_{21}}\beta_0\right)^2\mathrm{e}^{-2\sqrt{f/f_c}}+2T_{21}\sqrt{\alpha_{21}}\beta_0\mathrm{e}^{-\sqrt{f/f_c}}\cos(\sqrt{f/f_c})}}, \quad (6)$$

where $f_c=\alpha_1/\pi l_1^2$ is the cut-off frequency of layer 1. In this way, after determining experimentally the normalized amplitude given in Eq. 6, by means of a fitting procedure, the relative optical absorption coefficients β can be determined for a fixed time during the diffusion process, if the thermal diffusivity and effusivity of layers 1 and 2 are known.

3. Results and discussion

3.1 Optic technique

The signals for the eight photodiodes are presented in Fig. 6, for the five studied agar concentrations. As can be observed from this Figure, all the measurements show similar behavior as a function of time. The transmitted light signal shows small changes in the first seconds, after some time it exhibits a strong decrease and in the last stage the rate of change of the signal slows down. For a fixed concentration, the shift of the curve is higher when the measurement is made further away from the top of the glass tube. An additional displacement is observed for a fixed photodiode when the agar concentration increases. In particular, for the lowest concentration (0.1%), the first photodiode (D0) signal reaches the stabilization after 20 h, and for the lower sensor (D7) the signal reaches a constant value after 55 h. In contrast for a higher concentration (0.5%) the first photodiode shows a constant value after 80 h and the last sensor shows a stable signal after 140 h.

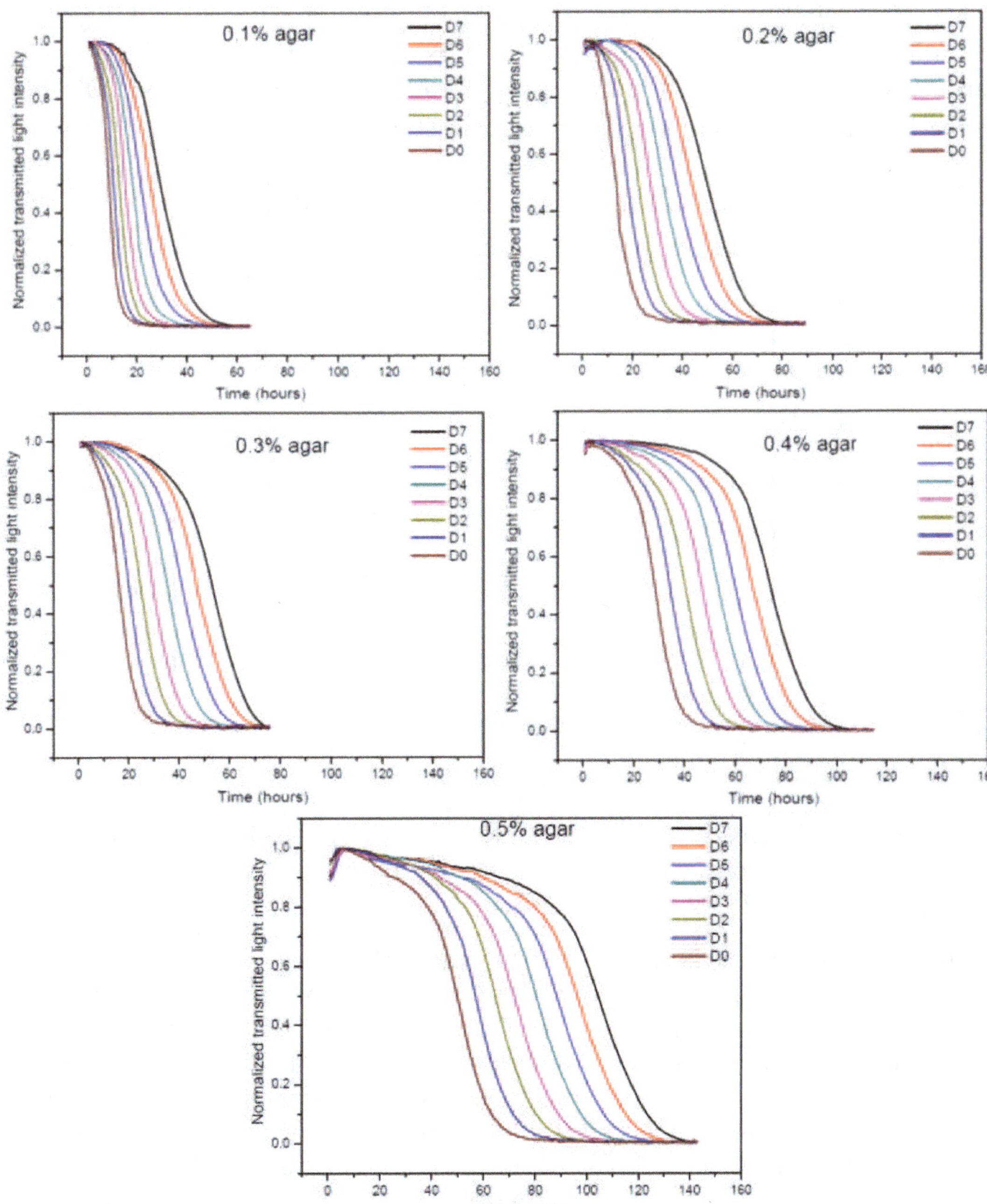

Fig. 6. Light transmission measured with eight optical photodiodes in the linear array for different concentrations during methylene blue diffusion on 0.1, 0.2, 0.3, 0.4 and 0.5 % w/v of agar concentration.

In order to get usable numerical parameters, the experimental data were analyzed using a sigmoidal fitting function applying the following equation,

$$I = I_0 + \frac{\Delta I}{\left(1 + e^{(t-t_0)/\tau}\right)}, \tag{7}$$

Where t is the time, I_0 is the initial value for the normalized transmitted light intensity, ΔI is the maximum change of the signal, and t_0 is the time at which the sigmoidal process reaches its minimum derivative. τ is the mean time in which the sigmoidal process occurs. In the particular case of 0.3% agar concentration and using the photodiode D2 (Fig. 7) the results were $t_0 = 41.4$ hours and $\tau = 6.02$ hours ($r^2 = 0.99$)

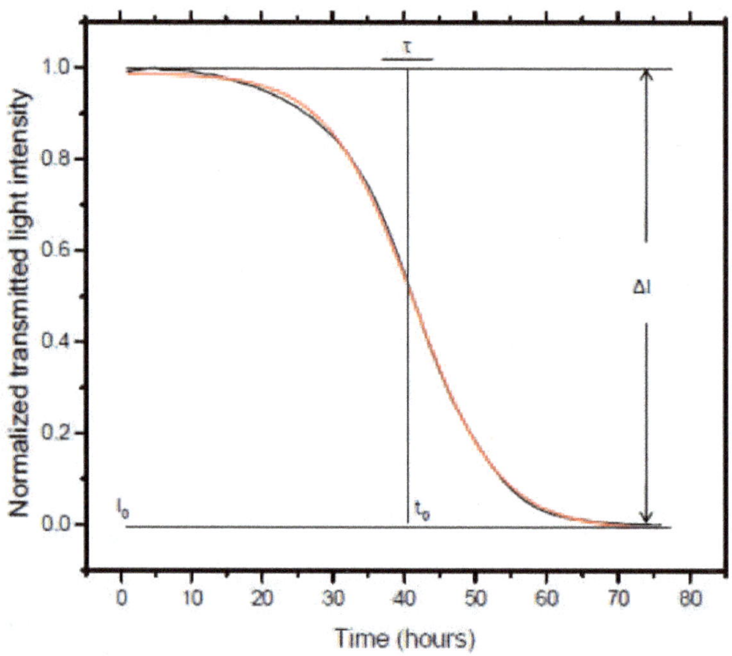

Fig. 7. Effect of the methylene blue diffusion into agar on the setting down time as a function of the distance, measured on the top surface of the phantom of agar column for five different agar concentrations (0.1, 0.2, 0.3, 0.4 and 0.5 %w/v) of agar.

Studies of general diffusion processes, has been shown that a good approximation consists in considering the diffusion coefficient as, the relation between the cross section of the window through which the phenomenon is observed divided by the settle-down time (Crank, 1975). In this case the size of the window is 1 mm^2. Following this procedure the diffusion coefficient can be estimated. In order to get comparative values a normalization process was performed. For each sensor the diffusion coefficient was normalized with respect to the coefficient of the lower concentration. In Figure 8 the normalized diffusion coefficient was calculated for all agar concentrations for D7 photodiode. The result show that the diffusion coefficient diminishes three times from the initial value when the agar concentration increases. The D7 photodiode was chosen because it is located far away from the methylene blue source and can be expected that provide a more realistic value of the diffusion coefficient.

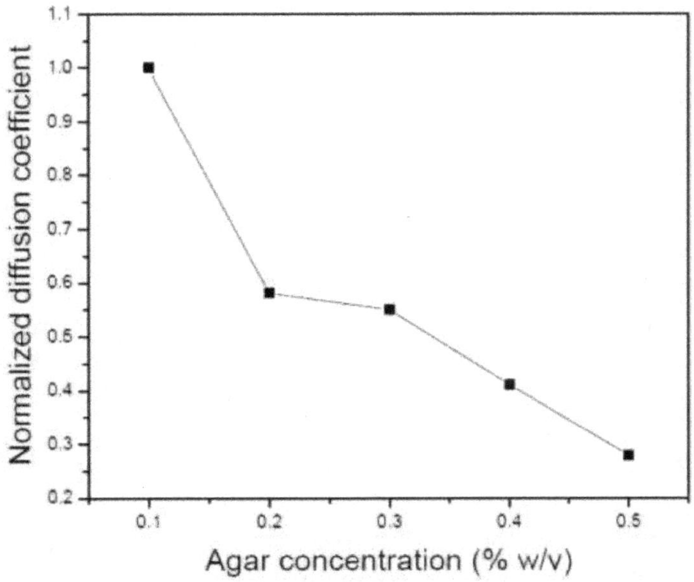

Fig. 8. Normalized diffusion coefficient behavior with the agar concentrations (0.1, 0.2, 0.3, 0.4 and 0.5 %w/v), determined for D7 photodiode.

3.2 Photoacoustic technique

The results for the PA measurements for 0.01 % and 0.05 % w/v concentrations of agar phantoms are presented in Figs. 9a and 9b. It can be observed that in the first seconds, the PA signal diminishes gradually, due to the progressive diffusion of the dye that induces a decrease of the light absorption; and the signal for the sample with higher agar concentration shows a slower decay. Also, the low frequency option provides a better measurement due to a higher thermal diffusion length of the PA system. These effects have been studied for different frequencies indicating that thermal wave phenomena, is more sensitive when the thermal wave monitors the changes occurring through the column detector that contains the sample (Vilca et al., 2010).

In Figs. 10a and b, the time dependence of the normalized signal amplitude is shown. These data were obtained dividing the PA signal by its maximum for the specific experiment. It can be observed that higher modulation frequencies are more sensitive to the changes induced by the diffusion process. It is important to mention that the normalization procedure is useful to obtain independent results of the specific characteristics of the microphone and substrate; this is desirable if we want to focus our attention on the changes of the optical properties of the sample. This method also cancels the *1/f* frequency dependence of the PA signal, leaving unaffected the frequency in the exponential terms. The effect of the normalization procedure magnifies the observation of the dye diffusion process, without affecting the settle-down time and the net change of the signal. From the point of view of thermal wave theory, the thermal diffusion length is mainly related to the exponential decay. In this way the normalization procedure is not eliminating the most important dependence on the frequency that represents the basic advantage of photoacoustic spectroscopy. In order to discard the effect of the evolution of the thermal properties in the photoacoustic measurements, the thermal diffusivities of the samples were measured using the thermal wave resonator cavity technique. The values for 0.01 % and 0.05 % w/v concentrations were 1.460 x 10^{-4} $cm^2.s^{-1}$ and 1.466 x 10^{-4} $cm^2.s^{-1}$, respectively. These values are very close to the thermal diffusivity for pure water (Almond & Patel, 1996).

Additionally, the measurements of agar samples in which the dye solution was completely diluted did not show considerable differences with the samples without the dye, being 1.453×10^{-4} $cm^2.s^{-1}$ and 1.455×10^{-4} $cm^2.s^{-1}$ for 0.01 % and 0.05 % w/v agar concentrations, respectively. Using these values and considering the changes in the thermal diffusivity of agar due to the addition of the dye, an estimation of the effects using Eq. 4 was performed. It was found that the magnitude of the PA signal is not affected appreciably. Therefore, the influence of the dye solution and its diffusion inside the agar gel on the thermal diffusivity values can be considered negligible. Based on these results, the variation in the PA signal can be exclusively related to the optical properties changes of the sample and can be appropriately parameterized as an effective optical absorption coefficient $\beta_{eff,}$, that would measure the light that is being converted into heat during the diffusion process. Experimental data shown in Fig. 10 were fitted with Eq. 6, considering the thermal diffusivity values measured using the thermal wave resonator for the agar and gel mentioned above, thermal effusivity is ε_2 = 1.588 $W.s^{1/2}.cm^{-2}.K^{-1}$, and for the polyvinyl acetate is, $\alpha_1 = 1.95 \times 10^{-4}$ $cm^2.s^{-1}$ and ε_1 = 0.0490 $W.s^{1/2}.cm^{-2}.K^{-1}$. With this procedure, the values of the effective optical absorption coefficients are obtained, as shown in Fig. 11.

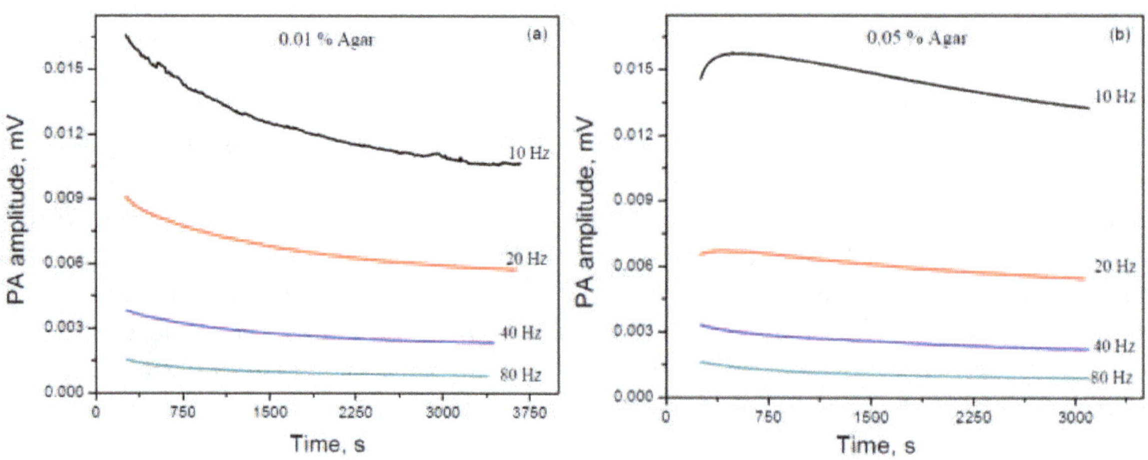

Fig. 9. PA signal behavior as a function of time during the diffusion processes through the solution, in (a) 0.01 % and (b) 0.05 % w/v, of agar phantoms after the application of the methylene blue solution.

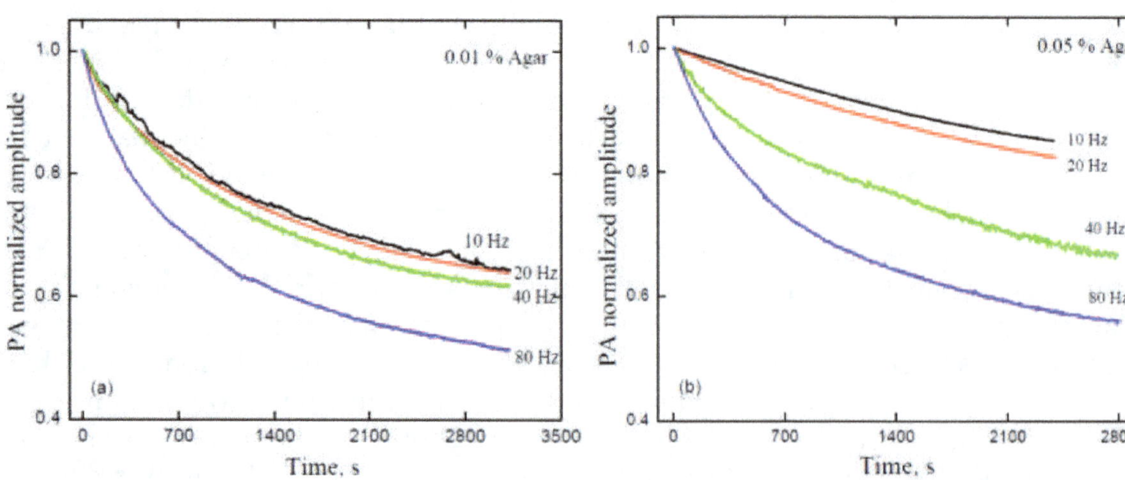

Fig. 10. Normalized photoacoustic signal for (a) 0.01 % and (b) 0.05 % w/v of agar.

The effective absorption coefficient shows a systematic decay on a time scale of 1000 s for both samples. In order to get usable numerical data, a fitting procedure can be performed using an exponential decay, parameterized in the form,

$$y = y_0 + A_1 e^{-(t-t_0)/\tau} \tag{8}$$

where t is the time, y_0 is the value of the absorption coefficient when the time is very large, A_1 measures the size of the decay of the absorption, t_0 is the initial time and τ is the characteristic time decay of the process that measures the time interval needed in the process of dilution for the methylene blue solution in the agar sample to be stabilized. The characteristic decay times for 0.01 % and 0.05 % w/v agar samples are 1111 s and 1232 s, respectively. This can be understood taking into account that, when the concentration of agar grows the agar gel becomes harder; therefore, it is more difficult for methylene blue to penetrate the solution. These results show that the PA technique is sensitive and useful in the measurement of the decay time, and secondly, it provides the difference in time in which the methylene blue solution diffuses for two different agar concentrations. These differences supply important results for biomedical sciences in which agar gels are used as phantoms resembling some of the properties of living organs and tissues.

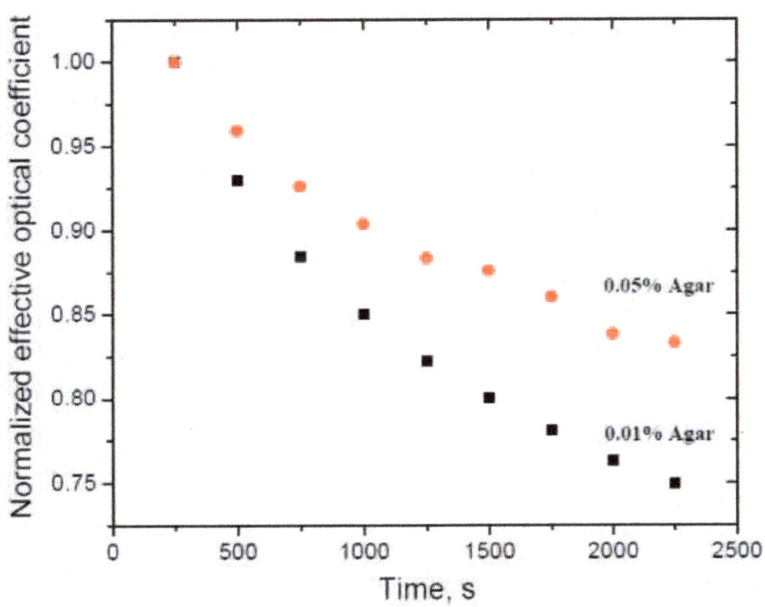

Fig. 11. Normalized effective optical absorption coefficient as a function of time, for two gel phantoms with concentrations of 0.01 and 0.05 % w/v of agar during the dye diffusion.

This work shows that increasing five times the concentration of agar in water, stabilization time only grows around 10 %; this behavior, is expected to occur only at low agar concentrations. At higher agar concentrations, stabilization of the processes would take longer time intervals. At these concentrations the link among the agar molecules generates a strong structure that is harder to penetrate by the dye.

From the optical and photoacoustic methodologies, it can be inferred that each option presented in this work, has its limitations and advantages. The optical experiment design provide a direct and position resolved measurement, having the possibility of studying in the laboratory the process of any substance applied on a given phantom, being highly useful in the diagnosis and time that a given medication can reach the desired zone. The optical technique can also provide useful information on which wavelength of the illuminating laser must be used. In the simple case of methylene blue, one of the reasons that explain the good quality of the experimental data obtained is the fact that a red laser for monitoring, has been used. For any other substance the wavelength at which it absorbs must be known to choose the right illuminating source. After that, using this optic technique previous conjecture can be corroborated and applied to optimize the measurements. In contrast, the photoacoustic technique would be more useful in the analysis of fast process with low agar concentrations (tissues of low density) providing an average optical absorption coefficient. This would be highly useful when studying samples as living tissue in which the lateral profile of the optical measurements is not possible. In this case, these measurements could be helpful in designing instruments with applications for clinical diagnosis.

The use of both measurements allow to obtain an integrated analysis of the diffusion process in which the optical measurements provide crucial data, as the evolution of optical absorption coefficient that can be useful in the comprehension of the data obtained with the photoacoustic technique.

4. Conclusions

The process of diffusion in methylene blue in phantoms of agar gels has been studied using two techniques, namely a novel optical methodology and photoacosutic spectroscopy using a conventional cell. Both techniques provide a useful analysis of the diffusion process. In both techniques it was found that an increase of the agar concentration slows down the methylene blue diffusion process. The optical measurement allows obtaining direct results and the monitoring of optical absorption coefficient as a function of the position. Given the close relationship of the optical absorption coefficient with concentration, we can infer that a direct measurement of the concentration of the dye as a function of time and position is possible. In contrast, the photoacoustic measurement would be more useful in the analysis of fast processes with low agar concentrations (tissues of low density) giving an average optical absorption coefficient. This would be highly useful when studying samples as living tissue in which the lateral profile of the optical measurements is not possible. In this case these measurements could be helpful in designing instruments with applications with *in situ* applications as in the case of clinical diagnosis.

5. Acknowledgments

This work was partially supported by CONACYT 49275-F (24214), 105816, 123913 Multidisciplinary-Cinvestav 2009, FONCICYT 96095, FOMIX No.108160 projects. The authors want to express their acknowledgments to M.S. J. Bante for his valuable help in the cells and electronic construction.

6. References

Acosta-Avalos, D.; Alvarado-Gil, J.J.; Vargas, H.; Frías-Hernández, J.; Olalde-Portugal, V.; Miranda, L.C.M., (1996). Photoacoustic monitoring of the influence of arbuscular mycorrhizal infection on the photosynthesis of corn (Zea mays L.). *Plant. Sci.*, 119 (1), 183-190

Almond, D. & Patel, P. (1996) *Photothermal Science and Techniques*, 0412578808, (Chapman and Hall, London)

Bauman, M.; Gillies, G.; Raghavan, R.; Brady, M.; Pedain, C., (2004). Physical characterization of neurocatheter performance in a brain phantom gelatin with nanoscale porosity: steady-state and oscillatory flows. *Nanotechnol.*, 15, 92-97

Bialkowski, S.E., (1996). *Photothermal Spectroscopy Methods for Chemical Analysis*. (John Wiley & Sons, New York)

Buchholz, K.; Marcelo, A.; Wissenbach, D.; Schirmer, H.; Krauth-Sieguel, L.; Gromer, S. Molec., (2008). Cytotoxic interactions of methylene blue with trypanosomatid-specific disulfide reductases and their dithiol products. *Biotechem. Parasitol.*, 160 (1), 65-69

Carslaw, H.S., (2005). *Introduction to the Theory of Fourier's Series and Integrals*. (University of Michigan, Michigan)

Crank, J., (1975). *The Mathematics of Diffusion*. (Clarendon Press, Oxford)

Fernelius, N.C., (1980). Photoacoustic signal variations with chopping frequency for ZnSe laser windows. *J. Appl. Phys.*, 51(3), 1756-1768

Frandas, A.; Paris, D.; Bissieux, C. ; Chirtoc, M.; Antoniow, J.S.; M. Egée, (2000). Classical and photopyroelectric study and optical thermophysics properties of starch sheets function of water content and temperature. *Appl. Phys. B.*, 71, 69-76

Koning, K.; Bockhorn, V.; Dietel, W.; Schubert, H., (1987). Photochemotherapy of animal tumors with photosensitizer methylene blue using a krypton laser. *Cancer Res Clin. Oncol.*, 3, 113:301

Landa, A.; Alvarado-Gil, J.J.; Gutiérrez-Juárez, J.; Vargas-Luna, M., (2003). Photoacoustic monitoring of real time blood and hemolymph sedimentation. *Rev. Sci. Instrum.*, 74, 377-380

Madsen, E.; Hobson, M; Shi, H.; Varghese, T. & Frank, G., (2005) Tissue-mimicking agar/gelatin materials for use in heterogeneous elastography phantoms. *Phys. Med. Biol.*, 50(23),5597-5618

Mandelis, A., (1993). *Non-Destructive Evaluation: Progress in Photothermal and Photoacoustic Science and Technology*, vol. 2. (PTR Prentice Hall, Englewood Cliffs, NJ,)

Martínez-Torres, P.; Alvarado-Gil, J.J., (2007). Monitoring the Formation of Thin Films by Photothermal Technique. *Int. J. Thermophys.*, 28, 996-1003

Orth, K.; Russ, D.; Beck, G.; Ruck, A.; Berger, HG., (1998). Photochemotherapy of experimental colonic tumours with intra-tumorally applied methylene blue. *Langenbecks Arch. Surg.*, 383, 276-281.

Pichardo, J.; Alvarado-Gil, J.J.; J., (2001). Open photoacoustic cell determination of the thermal interface resistance in two layer systems. *Appl. Phys.*, 89, 4070-4076

Quimby, R.; Yen, W.J., (1980). Photoacoustic measurement of the ruby quantum efficiency. *J. Appl. Phys.*, 51, 1780-1782

Singh, S., (2010). Nanomedicine-nanoscale drugs and delivery systems. *J. Nanosci. Nanotechnol.*, 10(12), 7906-7918

Staples, M.; Daniel, K.; Michael, J.C. & Langer, R., (2006), Application of Micro- and Nano-Electromechanical Devices to Drug Delivery. *Pharm. Res.*, 23(5), 847-863

Tardivo, J.; Del Giglio, A.; Santos de Oliveira, C.; Santesso, D.; Couto, H.; Batista, D.; Severino, D.; Turchiello, R.; Baptista, M., (2005). Photodiagnosis and Photodynamic

Therapy: From basic mechanisms to clinical applications. *Photodiagn. Photodyn. Ther.*, 2(3), 175-191

Teng, Y.C.; Royce, B.S.H., (1980). Absolute optical absorption coefficient measurements using photoacoustic spectroscopy amplitude and phase information. *J. Opt. Soc. Amer.*, 70, 557-560

Vargas, H.; Miranda, L.C.M., (1988). Photoacoustic and related photothermal techniques. *Phys. Rep.*, 161(2), 43-101

Vargas-Luna, M.; Gutiérrez-Juárez, G.; Rodríguez-Vizcaíno, J.M.; Varela-Nájera, J.B.; Rodríguez-Palencia, J.M.; Bernal-Alvarado, J.; Sosa, M.; Alvarado-Gil, J.J., (2002). Photoacoustic monitoring of inhomogeneous curing processes in polystyrene emulsions. *J. Phys. D: Appl. Phys.*, 35(13), 1532-1537

Vilca-Quispe, L.; Alvarado-Gil, J.J.; Quintana, P.; Ordonez-Miranda, J., (2010). Diffusion of Methylene Blue in Phantoms of Agar Using a Photoacoustic Technique. *Int. J. Thermophys*, 31, 987-997

Wetsel, G.C.; McDonald, Jr., F.A., (1977). Photoacoustic determination of absolute optical absorption coefficient. *Appl. Phys. Lett.*, 30(5), 252-254

4

Recent Developments in Cell-Based Microscale Technologies and their Potential Application in Personalised Medicine

Gregor Kijanka, Robert Burger, Ivan K. Dimov, Rima Padovani,
Karen Lawler, Richard O'Kennedy and Jens Ducrée
Biomedical Diagnostics Institute – Dublin City University
Ireland

1. Introduction

It is becoming increasingly apparent that some individuals are more susceptible to disease than others and more importantly some patients respond to prescribed therapies better than others. One of the main reasons for differences in disease susceptibility and the effectiveness of drug treatment lies in the genetic makeup of the patient. In addition to many environmental factors, genetic variations such as mutations, DNA polymorphisms and epigenetic gene regulation are the key players involved in the fate of a person's health. Recent advances in genomics and proteomics are providing novel insights into the complex biological process of disease. These insights will ultimately help to tailor personalised approaches to the treatment of disease based upon individual molecular "blueprints" of their genome and proteome.

Personalised medicine extends beyond the traditional medical approach in the treatment of patients as it aims to identify and target molecular factors contributing to the illness of individual patients. The personalised medicine approach is already playing a significant role in the way we treat and monitor disease. As many as 10 out of 36 anti-cancer drugs approved by the European Union in the last 10 years are considered to be personalised medicines (Eicheler, 2010). Breast cancer is one of the best examples whereby a personalised medical approach is adopted to detect the expression status of an oestrogen receptor called ESR1 in the nucleus of breast cancer cells. Approximately 70% of breast cancer patients overexpress this protein which is an important prognostic and predictive marker. Outcomes for these patients have been significantly improved by targeting the ESR1 using a hormonal treatment known as Tamoxifen. Interestingly this is the most commonly prescribed anti-cancer treatment in the world, highlighting the importance of a personalised approach in the management of disease.

Microscale technologies are emerging as an enabling platform for the development of novel personalised medicines and their broad accessibility. Miniaturised devices have the potential to process minute clinical samples and perform extensive genetic, molecular and cellular analyses directly on a microfluidic chip. The integration of pre-analytical sample handling with a subsequent sample analysis on a single microfluidic device will help to achieve highest reproducibility of results and minimise inter-laboratory bias and operators errors. This will enable rapid investigation of drug effects on normal and diseased cells and help to assess the optimal dosage and the combinations of drugs to be prescribed for each individual patient. Furthermore, modern microfabrication processes enable mass-production of low-cost and disposable microfluidic devices making the new therapies more affordable.

In this chapter we discuss the emerging microscale technologies and their potential impact on the future of healthcare. We present the upcoming challenges and potential solutions for personalised medical technology which is currently being developed at the Biomedical Diagnostics Institute (BDI) in Dublin, Ireland. This chapter will focus on microfluidic assays for cell-based analyses and will demonstrate the efficacy of novel cell capturing techniques with particular emphasis on the detection of ESR1 in breast cancer cells.

2. Microscale technology

Since its origins in the 1980s, microfluidics has evolved into an exciting branch of biomedical engineering. The growing interest in microfluidics is largely due to its potential to revolutionise conventional laboratory handling, processing and bioanalytical techniques. A major advantage is their miniaturisation, enabling nano- and picolitre volumes to be processed. In the conventional laboratory setting micro- to millilitre volumes are routinely handled; however, by significantly reducing this volume, reagent consumption, assay time and the related costs are significantly reduced.

An important feature of microfluidic technology lies in the design of the microfluidic channels. Owing to their small dimensions, fluid flows in a strictly laminar i.e., essentially without turbulence. Mixing under laminar flow conditions is governed by mere diffusion of molecules across the phase interface (Hessel *et al.*, 2005). The laminar character in microchannels can be harnessed for fluid control within, e.g. for fine adjustments of concentrations of molecules or cells over spatial and temporal microenvironments. As a consequence, new cellular applications are made possible with the unprecedented capability of closely mimicking *in vivo* conditions whereby cells are exposed to well-defined chemical gradients and changing microenvironments (Englert, 2009; Yu, 2005). These new and exciting capabilities become valuable to personalised medicine, both, from the point of view of basic research in cancer biology as well as for drug efficacy studies (Kang *et al.*, 2008). The process of adaptation of cancer cells to altered microenvironments *in vivo*, in particular to hypoxic conditions, is still not fully understood. Microfluidics can provide a more in-depth insight into cell responses under these conditions mimicking specific microenvironments on chip (Polinkovsky *et al.*, 2009). Microfluidic devices could therefore enable the study of combined effects of altered microenvironments and anticancer drugs on tumour cells and help to understand why anticancer drugs lose effectiveness in solid tumours over time (Minchinton & Tannock, 2006).

High level of parallelisation in microfluidic systems is another important feature which allows the investigation of a large number of experimental conditions at the same time, thereby reducing time and costs compared to conventional laboratory settings. The benefits of parallelisation in concert with the miniaturisation make microfluidic devices an excellent tool for high throughput analyses. This is a fundamental advantage for disciplines such as genomics and proteomics as they rely on large-scale analysis of genes and proteins. High throughput techniques provide also a sound foundation for personalised medical research, as large numbers of tests at various conditions are required when studying the effects of drugs. Microscale devices, also known as Lab-on-a-Chip, can integrate several laboratory unit operations (LUOs) on just one miniaturised platform. The high degree of integration of independent LUOs using microfluidics has the potential to revolutionise personalised healthcare medicine through drug discovery (Dittrich & Manz, 2006) and point-of-care diagnostics (Yager *et al.*, 2006).

Finally, but not of less importance, many novel fabrication methods are continuously being developed. Microfluidic devices are often made of polymers using mass production processes such as injection moulding and hot embossing which are optimised for microscale dimensions (Voldman *et al.*, 1999). These microfabrication methods allow the devices to be produced in large volume and at low cost, which can potentially impact on global health, providing the opportunity to fabricate portable and disposable point-of-care devices for diagnostics applicable in poorly equipped environments.

3. Biomedical applications

Microscale technologies have significantly contributed to numerous biomedical applications over the past two decades. Encouraging advances brought by genomics and proteomics are helping to better understand complex molecular mechanisms of diseases. However, there is a growing need to translate results from genomic and proteomic research studies into clinical practice. This can be achieved by breaking barriers across disciplines and integrating various microscale technologies. Molecular profiling technologies are therefore adopting the microfluidic approach to solve challenges not amenable to conventional laboratory methods (Wlodkowic & Cooper, 2010).

The sequencing of the human genome has immensely increased our knowledge on human health and disease. Genome-wide analyses can now be performed with microfluidic devices for on-chip DNA amplification, electrophoresis and DNA hybridisation on microarrays (Yeo *et al.*, 2011). Incorporating microfluidic technology not only improves conventional methods by reducing diffusion distances and assay times (Wang *et al.*, 2003), but it may also significantly enhance assay sensitivities (Liu & Rauch, 2003). The most recent advances in microfluidics allow patient specific genetic analyses, such as whole-genome haplotyping from a single cell (Fan *et al.*, 2011). Although many of the genomics platforms for the analysis of nucleic acids are still at research stages, some are particularly far advanced and ready for clinical application.

Microfluidics based proteomics is by far more challenging compared to on-chip genomics (Yeo *et al.*, 2011). Proteins consist of polymers comprising 20 different L-α-amino acids and require a three dimensional globular structure to retain their function and activity. In addition, purified protein quantities are often limited due to the lack of simple methods for amplifying proteins similar to the powerful polymerase chain reaction (PCR) technique for nucleic acids. Despite the challenges with protein-based microfluidic devices, several applications for protein analysis have been developed including protein microarrays (Alvarez *et al.*, 2008; Avseenko *et al.*, 2002), chip-mass spectroscopy interfaces (Lazar *et al.*, 2006) protein crystallization (Du *et al.*, 2009) and most recently devices for monitoring of temporal expression events in immune cells within a clinical setting (Kotz *et al.*, 2010).

The microfluidic approach to genomics and proteomics has the potential to help molecular profiling technologies to reach the maturity required for tests in clinical practice. It may pave the way towards the development of novel medical devices which utilise minute quantities of patient sample to analyse DNA and protein signatures in high throughout systems. Furthermore, these novel bioassays may potentially allow preliminary self-screening or even basic treatment by front-line nursing staff, reducing the burden on practitioners and hospitals.

4. Novel approaches for cell trapping on a microfluidic chip

Microfluidic devices offer a unique opportunity to investigate individual cells derived from patients' samples. Subsets of cell populations involved in pathological processes can be monitored and a personalised medical approach can be tailored individually to the patient's needs. Although many different microfluidic cell trapping techniques are currently available, they frequently encounter problems such as low cell capture efficiencies, cell impairment through non-physiological shear stresses and limited measures of on-chip molecular analyses.

Immobilisation and contact–free cell trapping are the two main cell capture methods which are routinely used in microfluidics (Johann, 2006). Both techniques provide unique advantages with regard to the capturing of individual cells. Cell immobilisation utilises chemical and/or hydrodynamic approaches to trap cells efficiently. The chemical approach is based on antibody-protein interactions, whereby cells are immobilised onto surfaces which are micro-patterned with antibodies directed against specific proteins expressed on the surface of the cell (Anderson *et al.*, 2004). The micro-patterning techniques provide high spatial resolution of immobilised cells and allow monitoring of individual cells in response to soluble stimuli. The hydrodynamic approach for immobilisation-based cell trapping relies on three dimensional surface topography microstructures to sieve cells from fluid flow in a microfluidic cavity. Mechanical barriers such as walls or micropores are utilised to retain the cells at rest next to a moving fluid (Khademhosseini *et al.*, 2005). One of the main advantages of hydrodynamic trapping is its rapid cell immobilisation compared with chemical trapping methods as well as the often simple and inexpensive design.

In contrast to cell immobilisation, contact-free cell trapping uses magnetic, acoustic, dielectrophoretic and optical capture techniques to separate and handle cells (Johann, 2006). The contact-free techniques allow versatile and flexible cell handling, enabling cell positioning, holding, sorting and release with high accuracy and high selectivity (Werner *et al.*, 2011). A possible disadvantage of the contact-free techniques is that cells are maintained in suspension which prevents adherent cells to grow in cell culture, thereby limiting contact-free trapping to bioanalytical applications. In addition, cells are exposed to certain electromagnetic or mechanical forces and to slightly increased temperatures which may have an undesirable effect on the analysed clinical specimen.

In the following section, we describe two novel hydrodynamic trapping methods which employ a sedimentation approach to capture micrometer-sized beads and cells. The first method allows the capture of beads within a microscale V-cup array based on a centrifugally driven sedimentation. The second method utilises gravitational sedimentation to capture cells within a microfluidic trench structure. Both methods facilitate particle capture with exceptionally high efficiencies and minimal exposure to hydrodynamic shear stress. We show on-chip molecular analysis of the breast cancer related oestrogen receptor ESR1 in cell lines as an example for potential personalised medicine applications.

4.1 Bead capture and analysis on a centrifugal microfluidic chip

Although various methods are available for actuating small volumes of liquids in microfluidic devices, the centrifugal microfluidics "lab-on-a-disc" approach offers a unique platform well suitable for high-performance point-of-care testing. In addition to forces present in most microfluidic systems such as capillarity, the actuation principle utilises rotationally induced inertial forces such as the centrifugal, Coriolis and Euler forces to move fluids and particles. Under the impact of the centrifugal force, fluids are propelled from the centre of rotation to the outer rim of the chip by an "artificial gravity" encountered in the rotating system. The centrifugal force scales with the square of the rotational frequency and is proportional to the distance from the centre of rotation as well as the radial length of the liquid plug. This allows controlling of flow velocities of liquids within the chip by using different rotational frequencies.

A major advantage of this approach is that it enables the design of systems consisting of an integrated drive unit, i.e., a motor with a self-contained disposable chip which is advantageous when dealing with clinical samples such as blood. Furthermore, the centrifugal pumping is widely independent of the physical properties of the liquids such as viscosity, conductivity, surface tension and pH. This feature is especially interesting for biological applications where samples with a broad range of viscosities and pH values need to be processed. Another unique feature of the centrifugal platform is that sample preparation steps such as separation of plasma from whole blood can be readily implemented by virtue of the density difference between cells and plasma. A comprehensive portfolio of LUOs such as valving, mixing and metering has already been demonstrated, as well as their integration into full-fledged sample-to-answer systems. For reviews of centrifugal microfluidic platforms see Ducrée, 2007 and Madou, 2006.

The particle trapping method presented here utilizes V-shaped retention elements often used in pressure driven microfluidic systems (Di Carlo *et al.*, 2006). The centrifugal disc and the particle capture concept are shown in Fig. 1. Briefly, the V-cups are arranged in an array format such that there are no direct radial pathways between sample inlet and the end of the array. During the capturing process, the particles sediment through the array and are trapped when hitting a V-cup structure. Once a cup is occupied a particle, subsequently arriving particles deflect from the bulk and get trapped in subsequent cups. By scale matching the size of the V-cups to the size of the particles as well as the total number of particles introduced with the suspension, the occupancy distribution of particles per cup can be adjusted, even to a sharply peaked single-occupancy distribution.

A major improvement of the centrifugal V-shaped retention scheme is the absence of dynamic flow lines which are inherent to pressure driven systems. The dynamic flow lines within the liquid often drag cells suspended in the flow around the V-shaped structures, thus leading to low capture efficiencies of 20% and lower (Kim, 2011). In contrast, the centrifugal microfluidic device presented here sediments cells under stagnant flow conditions. Thus, suspended particles follow straight (radial) paths, with theoretical capture efficiencies of 100%. In experiments performed using 10-µm silica beads spun at a rotational frequency of 20 Hz, we obtained capture efficiencies greater than 95%. Although there are no dynamic flow lines under stagnant flow conditions, additional effects such as the surplus of particles captured in one V-shaped retention element, other impact factors such as the lateral Coriolis force may deflect the sedimenting particles, reducing the overall capture efficiency.

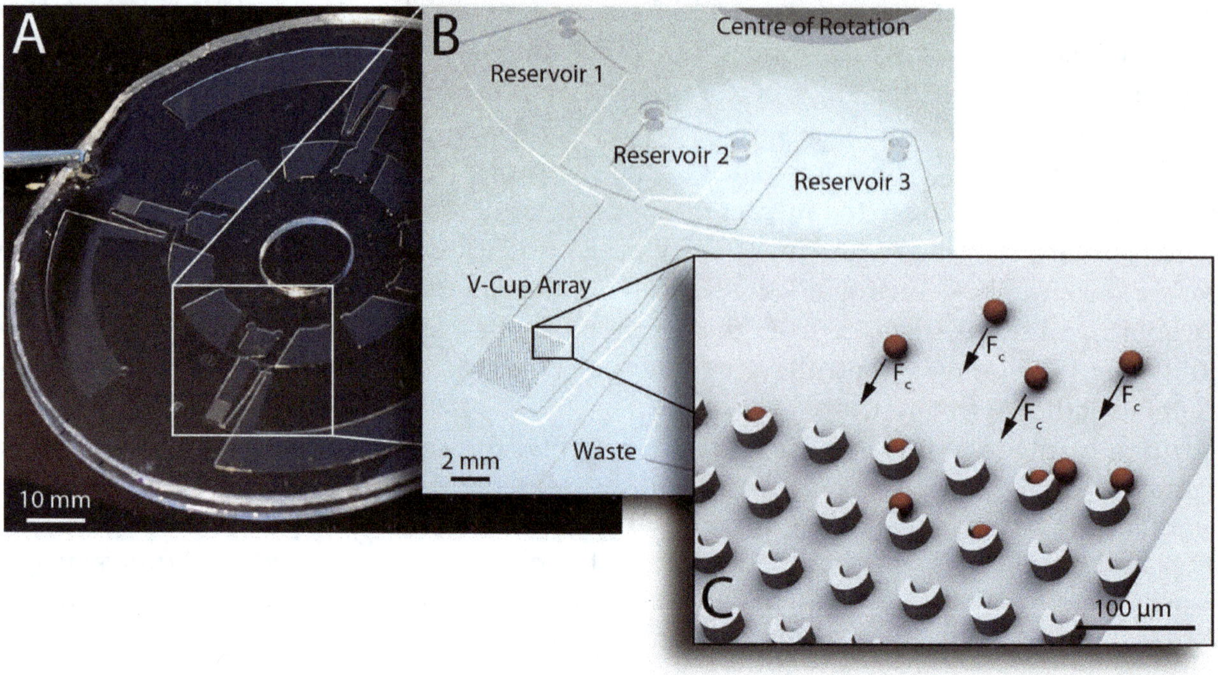

Fig. 1. Microfluidic V-cup array on a centrifugal platform. (A) Disc-shaped chip with four identical bead capture structures. (B) A drawing showing the design of one of four bead capture structures. (C) Magnified view of a V-cup array designed for sedimentation-based particle capture induced by centrifugal forces.

In addition to high capture efficiencies, this centrifugal device provides further benefits when compared with microfluidic bead-bed based immunoassays. In fact, beads introduced by flow towards a geometrical retention barrier tend to assume random aggregation patterns, which provide poorly defined, inhomogeneous flow and assay conditions for each bead. Moreover, in other multilayer arrangements, captured beads are located in individual focal planes making the readout more difficult. In contrast, using this novel device, the location of beads is given by the position of the capture structures, leading to precise flow control in the vicinity of each bead. Furthermore, all beads are located in the same focal plane which facilitates optical readout by a microscope. Experiments were carried out to demonstrate the importance of scale matching between capture element and particles. It has been demonstrated that the occupancy distribution of captured beads in V-cups peaks at single occupancy when the ratio of cup size to bead size is close to unity. We experimentally achieved a single particle occupancy of more than 95% of all occupied V-cups (Burger *et al.*, 2011).

The main feature of the centrifugal chip is the highly efficient capture of cells from clinical samples and subsequent molecular analysis on the chip. On-chip separation of cells allows discriminating between cell types and enables multiplexed immunoassays. In order to demonstrate its ability to separate and pinpoint particles to a specific location on the V-cup array, the device was loaded with a mixture of polystyrene beads coated with either human or mouse IgG antibodies (Fig 2). The mixture of both bead types was trapped in the V-cup array. Individual beads were visualised using Cy5 labelled anti-human IgG (red) and FITC labelled anti-mouse IgG secondary antibodies (green).

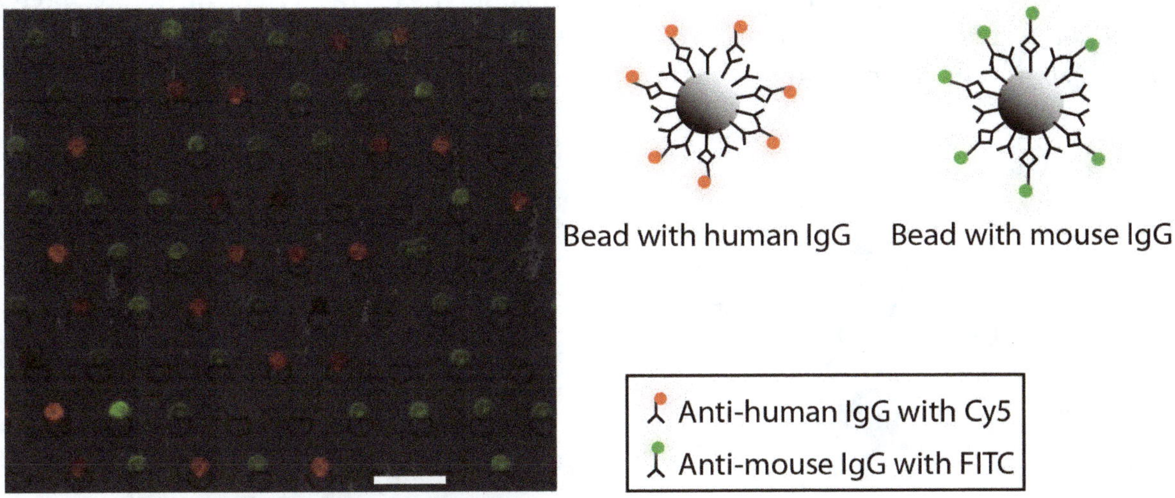

Fig. 2. On-chip immunoassay performed on the centrifugal platform. (A) Beads coated with human or mouse IgG antibodies were separated on the V-cup array and visualised using Cy5 labelled anti-human IgG and FITC labelled anti-mouse IgG secondary antibodies. The figure shows superimposed bright field, Cy5 fluorescent and FITC fluorescent images. Scale bar is 100 µm.

4.2 Cell capture and molecular analysis on a novel microfluidic trench chip

The second micro-particle capture approach which we recently developed utilises gravitational sedimentation in conjunction with a microfluidic trench structure for efficient cell capture and subsequent molecular analyses. The device was fabricated using standard soft lithography methods and consists of a network of microfluidic channels leading to a cell capture chamber. The design utilizes a microfluidic trench structure with characteristic dimensions (220 µm deep, 100 µm x 400 µm cross section) as a region of minimal flow for hydrodynamic cell capture (Fig. 3). Cells are loaded onto the microfluidic chip and dragged with the flow through the microfluidic channels into the capture chamber where the cells are effectively trapped. The widened section of the flow channel reduces the flow velocity, providing sufficient time for cells to irreversibly sediment into the trench. This is a highly efficient, merely sedimentation-based cell capture method, whereby experiments with HeLa and MCF7 cells show capture efficiencies close to 100% at flow velocities of 20 $\mu m\ s^{-1}$ (Dimov *et al.*, 2011).

Cell loading onto the chip and flow velocities within the microfluidic channels are controlled by fluid levels within a pipette tip at the inlet of the chip. The pipette tip serves as an open liquid column generating hydrostatic pressure within the microfluidic channels. Flow velocities within the microfluidic channels and the trench structure were simulated using a computational fluid dynamics (CFD) approach (Fig. 3). The CFD simulation revealed decreasing flow velocities towards the base of the trench. Flow velocities at the bottom of the trench were calculated to be three orders of magnitude lower than in the channel above. Cells entering the low velocity region were therefore effectively retained at the base of the trench. Importantly, the minute flow velocities at the base of the trench significantly reduce shear stresses exerted on cells. Such shear-protected regions provide an advantage over other microfluidic cell retention methods, in particular in biomedical applications. Fluid shear stresses may considerably modify the state of captured cells and introduce a bias into microfluidic bioassays. Minimising shear stress exposure may have a positive effect on microfluidic cell culture and opens up a route to analyse highly sensitive cells such as stem cells directly on this platform.

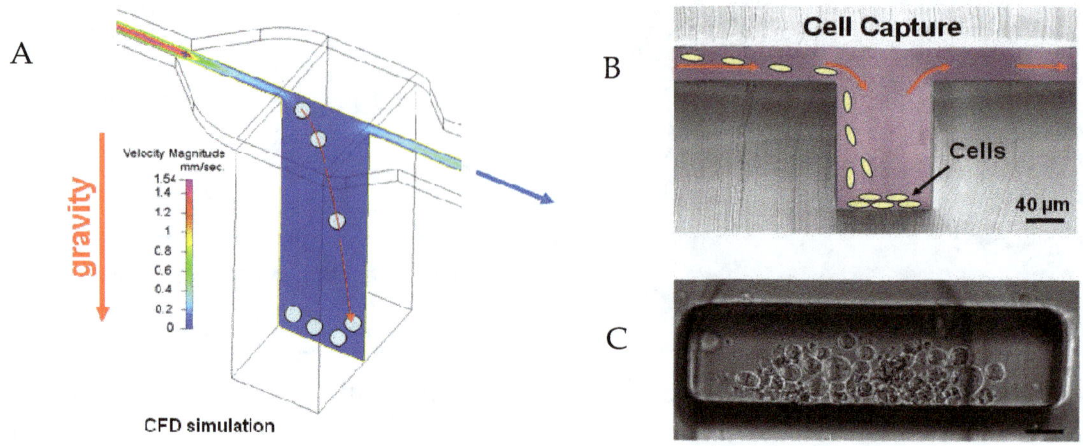

Fig. 3. Microfluidic trench structure: design and working principle. (A) CFD simulation of flow velocities within the trench structure. (B) Cells are captured based on the sedimentation of cells to the bottom of a microscale trench (side view). (C) Photograph of HeLa cells captured within the microfluidic trench structure (top view).

An important feature of the microfluidic trench device is its capability to perform several different bioassays in parallel (Kijanka *et al.*, 2009). Its key characteristic is a simple loading of liquids onto the chip, hence enabling rapid replacement of reagents within the trench for multi-step bioassays. Here we demonstrate an immunoassay performed directly on the chip. Cells and reagents were loaded onto the chip. The reagents were allowed to interact with captured cells through diffusive mixing within the trench structure. Finally, cell staining was visualised using a fluorescent microscope (Fig. 4).

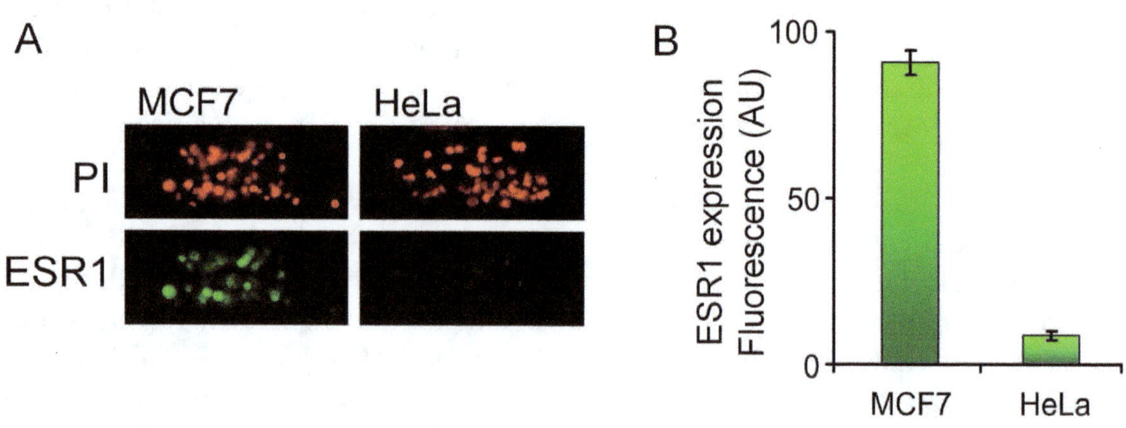

Fig. 4. On-chip immunoassay performed on the microfluidic trench platform. (A) MCF7 and HeLa cells were captured within the microfluidic trench structure. Cells were stained with propidium iodide (PI) to mark nuclei of all cells (red) and with anti-oestrogen receptor antibodies (ESR1) to visualise ESR1 expression (green). (B) MCF7 cells show specific nuclear staining for oestrogen receptor ESR1.

To determine the ESR1 levels in mammalian cells, cervical cancer cells (HeLa) and breast cancer cells (MCF7) were captured on the chip (Fig.4). Cells resting within the trench structure were exposed to a multi-step immunostaining protocol. Initially, cells were fixed with a 4% formaldehyde solution and permeabilised with ice cold acetone. These permeabilised cells were then treated with a 4% skimmed milk (Marvel) blocking solution to avoid non-specific binding. Both cells types were then incubated with a mouse anti-ESR1 antibody and corresponding anti-mouse secondary antibody labelled with the Alexa488 fluorophore. Since we expected a nuclear expression of ESR1, cells were counter-stained with propidium iodide (PI), a fluorophore with a specific red staining at cell nuclei. As shown in Fig. 4, both cell types were successfully immobilised in the microfluidic device and the immunostaining was performed. The counter-stain with PI revealed the location of nuclei within the cells (red). However, only the MCF7 cells, and not HeLa cells showed ESR1 expression when treated with specific, fluorescently labelled antibodies (green). The results show the ability of the device to perform complex molecular protocols directly on the chip. In this immunostaining experiment we could detect breast cancer related oestrogen receptor ESR1 in the breast cancer cell line MCF7 and the absence of this receptor in cervical cancer cell line HeLa.

5. Conclusion

Personalised medicine is gaining significant momentum in the medical field as a means to tailor patient care, based on a unique molecular signature. The application of novel methods to assess patient samples through minimally invasive technology will emerge as key tool in the diagnosis and monitoring of disease in the future. Low-cost, mass produced microfluidic devices have the capability to process patient samples in a highly efficient manner and enable the detection of markers of disease through the manipulation of cells under controlled microfluidic conditions. These technologies provide a suitable platform for the investigation of cells both on a genomic and proteomic level.

Current interdisciplinary research efforts focus on faster, accurate, reliable, and reproducible microfluidic tests applicable to clinical settings. In this chapter we described two novel approaches for cell capture and subsequent molecular analysis in a microfluidic chip. Both microfluidic devices demonstrate high particle capture efficiencies with the potential for application in diagnostic bead based immunoassays. Minimising shear stress exposure maintains the physiological integrity of cells within these microfluidic devices, thus helping to recreate *in vivo* conditions on chip. As personalised medicine emerges as the key approach to monitor and treat disease in the future, the accessibility and cost-effectiveness of these personalised tests will be critical for its success.

6. Acknowledgements

This material is based on works supported by the Science Foundation Ireland under Grants Nos. 05/CE3/B754 & 10/CE/B1821 and the Irish Cancer Society Research Fellowship Award CRF10KIJ.

7. References

Alvarez, M.; Friend, J.R. & Yeo, L.Y. (2008). Surface vibration induced spatial ordering of periodic polymer patterns on a substrate. *Langmuir*, Vol. 24, No. 19, (October 2008), pp. 10629-10632, ISSN 0743-7463

Anderson, D.G.; Levenberg, S. & Langer, R. (2004). Nanoliter-scale synthesis of arrayed biomaterials and application to human embryonic stem cells. *Nat Biotechnol*, Vol. 22, (June 2005), pp 863–866, doi:10.1038/nbt981

Avseenko, N.V.; Morozova, T.Y.; Ataullakhanov, F.I. & Morozov, V.N. (2002). Immunoassay with multicomponent protein microarrays fabricated by electrospray deposition. *Analytical Chemistry*, Vol. 74, No. 5, (March 2002), pp. 927-933, ISSN 0003-2700

Burger, R.; Reith, P.; Kijanka, G.; Akujobi, V.; Abgrall, P. & Ducrée, J. (2011). Array Based Capture, Distribution, Counting and Assaying of Individual Beads on a Centrifugal Microfluidic Platform. *Lab on a Chip*, Submitted 7th of June 2011

Di Carlo, D.; Wu, L.Y. & Lee, L.P. (2006). Dynamic single cell culture array. *Lab on a Chip*, Vol. 6, No. 11, (September 2006), pp. 1445-1449, ISSN 1473-0197

Dimov, I.K.; Kijanka, G.; Park, Y.; Ducrée, J.; Kang, T. & Lee, L.P. (2011). Integrated microfluidic array plate (iMAP) for cellular and molecular analysis. *Lab on a Chip*, Advanced Article on web, (June 2011), DOI: 10.1039/C1LC20105K

Dittrich, P.S. & Manz, A. (2006). Lab-on-a-chip: microfluidics in drug discovery. *Nature Reviews Drug Discovery*, Vol. 5, No. 3, (March 2006), pp. 210-218, ISSN 1474-1776

Du, W.B.; Li, L.; Nichols, K.P. & Ismagilov, R.F. (2009). SlipChip. *Lab On A Chip*, Vol. 9, No. 16, (August 2009), pp. 2286-2292, ISSN 1473-0197

Ducrée, J.; Haeberle, S.; Lutz, S.; Pausch, S.; von Stetten, F. & Zengerle R. (2007). The centrifugal microfluidic Bio-Disk platform. *Journal of Micromechanics and Microengineering*, Vol. 17, No. 7, (July 2007), pp. S103-S115, ISSN 0960-1317

Eicheler, H. (2010). The challenge of changing health. *Pathways: the changing science, business and experience of health*, p. 12, Scientific American, New York, USA

Englert, D.L.; Manson,M.D. & Jayaraman, A. (2009). Flow-Based Microfluidic Device for Quantifying Bacterial Chemotaxis in Stable, Competing Gradients. *Applied and Environmental Microbiology*, Vol. 75, No. 13 (July 2009), pp. 4557–4564, doi:10.1128/AEM.02952-08

Fan, H.C.; Wang, J.; Potanina, A. & Quake, S.R. (2011). Whole-genome molecular haplotyping of single cells. *Nature Biotechnology*, Vol. 29, No. 1, (January 2011), pp. 51–57, ISSN 1087-0156

Hessel, V.; Löwe, H. & Schönfeld, F. (2005). Micromixers - a review on passive and active mixing principles. *Chemical Engineering Science*, Vol. 60, No. 8-9, (April-May 2005), pp. 2479-2501, ISSN 0009-2509

Johann, R.M. (2006). Cell trapping in microfluidic chips. *Analytical and Bioanalytical Chemistry*, Vol. 385, No. 3, (June 2006), pp. 408-412, ISSN 1618-2642

Kang, L.; Chung, B.G.; Langer, R. & Khademhosseini, A. (2008). Microfluidics for drug discovery and development: From target selection to product lifecycle management. *Drug Discovery Today*, Vol 13, No 1/2 (January 2008), pp. 1-13, doi:10.1016/j.drudis.2007.10.003

Khademhosseini, A.; Yeh, J.; Eng, G.; Karp, J.; Kaji, H.; Borenstein, J.; Farokhzad, O.C. & Langer, R. (2005). Cell docking inside microwells within reversibly sealed microfluidic channels for fabricating multiphenotype cell arrays. *Lab on a Chip*, Vol. 12, No. 5, (October 2005), pp. 1380–1386, DOI: 10.1039/B508096G

Kijanka, G.; Dimov, I.K.; Lee, L.P. & Ducrée, J. (2009). A fully integrated cell-based cytotoxicity, gene and protein expression analysis platform. In Tae Song Kim and Yoon-Sik Lee, editors, Proceedings of the 13th International Conference on Miniaturized Systems for Chemistry and Life Sciences, µTAS2009, Jeju, Korea (November 2009), pp. 691-693

Kim, M.C.; Isenberg, B.C.; Sutin, J.; Meller, A.; Wong, J.Y. & Klapperich, C.M. (2011). Programmed trapping of individual bacteria using micrometre-size sieves. *Lab On A Chip*, Vol. 11, No. 6, (March 2011), pp. 1089-1095, ISSN 1473-0197

Kotz, K.T.; Xiao, W.; Miller-Graziano, C.; Qian, W.; Russom, A.; Warner, E.A.; Moldawer, L.L.; De, A.; Bankey, P.E.; Petritis, B.O.; Camp II, D.G.; Rosenbach, A.E.; Goverman, J.; Fagan, S.P.; Brownstein, B.H.; Irimia, D.; Xu, W.; Wilhelmy, J.; Mindrinos, M.N.; Smith, R.D.; Davis, R.W.; Tompkins, R.G.; Toner, M. & the Inflammation and the Host Response to Injury Collaborative Research Program (2010). Clinical microfluidics for neutrophil genomics and proteomics. *Nature Medicine*, Vol. 16, No. 9, (September 2010), pp. 1042–1047 ISSN 1078-8956

Lazar, I.M.; Grym, J. & Foret, F. (2006). Microfabricated devices: A new sample introduction approach to mass spectrometry. *Mass spectrometry Reviews*, Vol. 25, No. 4, (July-August 2006), pp. 573-594, ISSN 0277-7037

Liu, Y.J. & Rauch, C.B. (2003). DNA probe attachment on plastic surfaces and microfluidic hybridization array channel devices with sample oscillation. *Analytical Biochemistry*, Vol. 317, No. 1, (June 2003), pp. 76-84, ISSN 0003-2697

Madou, M.; Zoval, J.; Jia, G.; Kido, H.; Kim, J. & Kim, N. (2006). Lab on a CD. *Annual Review of Biomedical Engineering*, Vol. 8, (August 2006), pp. 601-628, ISSN 1523-9829

Minchinton, A.I. & Tannock, I.F. (2006). Drug penetration in solid tumours. *Nature Reviews Cancer*, Vol.6, No.8, (August 2006), pp.583-592, ISSN 1474-175X

Polinkovsky, M.; Gutierrez, E.; Levchenko, A. & Groisman, A. (2009). Fine temporal control of the medium gas content and acidity and on-chip generation of series of oxygen concentrations for cell cultures. *Lab On A Chip*, Vol. 9, No. 8 (April 2009), pp. 1073-1084, ISSN 1473-0197

Voldman, J.; Gray, M. L. & Schmidt, M. A. (1999). Microfabrication in biology and medicine. *Annual Review of Biomedical Engineering*, Vol. 1, (August 1999), pp. 401-425, ISSN 1523-9829

Wang, Y.; Vaidya, B.; Farquar, H.D.; Stryjewski, W.; Hammer, R.P.; McCarley, R.L.; Soper, S.A.; Cheng, Y.W. & Barany, F. (2003). Microarrays assembled in microfluidic chips fabricated from poly(methyl methacrylate) for the detection of low-abundant DNA mutations. *Analytical Chemistry*, Vol. 75, No. 5, (March 2003), pp. 1130-1140, ISSN 0003-2700

Werner, M., Merenda, F.; Piguet, J.; Salathé R. & Vogel, H. (2011). Microfluidic array cytometer based on refractive optical tweezers for parallel trapping, imaging and sorting of individual cells. *Lab on a Chip*, Vol. 14, No. 11, (June 2011), pp. 2432–2439, DOI: 10.1039/C1LC20181F

Wlodkowic, D. & Cooper, J.M. (2010). Tumors on chips: oncology meets microfluidics. *Current Opinion in Chemical Biology*, Vol. 14, No. 5 (October 2010), pp. 556-567, doi:10.1016/j.cbpa.2010.08.016

Yager, P.; Edwards, T.; Fu, E.; Helton, K.; Nelson, K.; Tam, M.R. & Weigl, B.H. (2006). Microfluidic diagnostic technologies for global public health. *Nature*, Vol. 442, No. 7101, (July 2006), pp. 412-418, ISSN 0028-0836

Yeo, L.Y.; Chang, H.; Chan, P.P.Y. & Friend, J.R. (2011). Microfluidic Devices for Bioapplications. *Small*, Vol. 7, No. 1, (January 2011), pp. 12-48, ISSN 1613-6810

Yu, H.; Meyvantsson, I.; Shkel, I.A. & Beebe, D.J. (2005). Diffusion dependent cell behavior in microenvironments. *Lab on a Chip*, Vol 10, No. 5, (October 2005), pp. 1089–1095, DOI: 10.1039/b504403k

5

Integrating the Electronic Health Record into Education: Models, Issues and Considerations for Training Biomedical Engineers

Elizabeth Borycki, Andre Kushniruk, Mu-Hsing Kuo and Brian Armstrong
School of Health Information Science, University of Victoria,
Victoria, British Columbia
Canada

1. Introduction

The use of Electronic Health Record (EHR) systems is increasing worldwide. Electronic health records (EHRs) are electronic repositories of a patient's health information and their encounters with the health care system over a lifetime (Shortliffe & Cimino, 2006). Internationally, there has been a push to implement such systems worldwide. However, adoption rates of EHRs continue to remain low in North America, and biomedical engineers are encountering many challenges associated with integrating EHRs into health care work settings. This is especially the case when medical devices and other healthcare equipment (e.g. cardiac monitors, smart beds and intravenous pumps) are integrated into EHRs. To improve adoption rates and student ability to seamlessly introduce this technology, there is need to provide greater EHR experience and exposure to the problems associated with EHR use and to solve some of the real-world EHR related challenges by developing creative solutions. Our recent work in the area of health IT and health professional educational curricula (i.e. in medicine, nursing, allied health and health/biomedical informatics) demonstrates that there is a need for biomedical engineers to learn about several areas at the intersection of medical device usage by health professionals and EHRs: (1) healthcare systems analysis and design, (2) usability of health care information systems, (3) interoperability of EHRs and (4) implementation of differing configurations of medical devices and EHRs to support clinical work. The purpose of this paper will be to describe our experiences to date in using an EHR portal in the classroom setting to teach individuals about these key aspects of EHR design and implementation in hospital settings (where biomedical engineers are typically employed). In the next section of this paper we define and describe how we have introduced EHRs into education, using a novel Web portal. Following this, we describe how we have integrated exposure to differing EHRs in the classroom setting to a range of students (i.e. from medical students to health informatics students).

As noted above, the use of Electronic Health Record (EHR) systems in hospitals is increasing. Information technology, health and biomedical engineering professionals are encountering a variety of complex problems in integrating EHRs into healthcare work settings. For example, integrating EHRs, medical devices and health care equipment can be a difficult undertaking. To improve student ability to effectively design, develop, implement and work with EHRs there is need to provide students with experiences that expose them to challenges typically encountered in hospital settings (using a wide range of examples of real-world EHRs, tools and problems). Our recent work in the area of health IT and health professional educational curricula (including medicine, nursing and health informatics) has revealed that typical educational programs (e.g. health informatics, medicine, computer science and engineering) often provide only limited exposure to EHRs (Borycki et al., 2009; Kushniruk et al., 2009).

2. The need for EHRs in biomedical engineering education

Graduates of biomedical engineering programs are being expected to deal with the design, implementation and customization of EHRs and medical devices in hospital settings. Therefore, it is important that future biomedical engineering graduates have training and experience with a full range of EHRs. Work on competencies related to EHRs indicates that graduates of biomedical engineering programs should understand interoperability issues, basic data standards, user interface design issues, and have an understanding of the impact of EHRs upon healthcare workflow and practice (Canada's Health Informatics Association, 2009). Additional areas of skill and knowledge needed include: the ability to assess usability issues, understand risk management, assess software safety, effectively test and procure HIS, understand security and privacy issues, and understand analytic methods for evaluating and improving EHR implementation/customization (Borycki et al., 2009; Borycki et al., 2011; Joe et al., 2011; Kushniruk et al., 2009). Providing an in-depth understanding of these topics requires a basic understanding of EHRs, including hands-on access and exposure to a variety of EHRs to assess their potential to improve healthcare and to learn about the current issues and challenges associated with their use. This also involves developing an understanding of the issues associated with the design, development, interoperability, implementation and customization associated with the integration of EHRs and medical devices. However, due to practical limitations, such as cost, the need for trained biomedical engineering professionals, and the complexity of work involved in setting up this technology locally (within educational settings), biomedical engineering student access to working examples of such systems has been limited (Borycki et al., 2009; Borycki et al., 2011). It must be noted that this is also the case for computer science, medical, nursing and health informatics professional students (as they are also expected to be able to work with full EHRs) upon graduation (Borycki et al., 2009; Joe et al., 2011).

3. The University of Victoria EHR portal

To address the need for ubiquitous, remote and easy access to a repository of EHRs and related technology, the authors have worked on developing a Web accessible portal known as the University of Victoria Electronic Health Record (EHR) Portal. The portal provides students from many differing health care disciplines with access to several electronic records or electronic repositories where a patient's health information or encounters with the healthcare system can be stored virtually (Borycki et al., 2009). The portal houses several types of EHRs including electronic medical records (EMRs), electronic patient records (EPRs) and personal health records (PHRs). EMRs are electronic health records used in the physician's office. EPRs are electronic health records that are used by health professionals such as physicians and nurses in the management of a patient's health care in a hospital. PHRs are electronic health records that patients store information (on the World Wide Web, on their home computer or on a mobile device) about their own personal health status or a family members' health status (e.g. child, parent or grand parent). PHRs are maintained by an individual but may be used by health professionals to obtain additional information about the patient's health status. The University of Victoria EHR Portal has several of these EHRs (e.g., Digital Anthrologix® - an EMR, OpenVista® - an EPR, OpenMRS – an EPR, Indivo – a PHR and a range of other systems) (Borycki et al., 2009; Borycki et al., 2011; Kushniruk et al., 2009). One of the motivations for the portal's development was to leverage the investment - creating a repository of systems by housing them on a Web-based platform that can be accessed locally, nationally and internationally for use in the education of biomedical engineers and other health professionals such as physicians and health informatics professionals (Borycki et al., 2011).

As a result, this unique, web-based portal allows students to access and interact with a set of representative EHRs over the WWW. To date, the portal, which links to several EMRs, EPRs and PHRs, has been used by several hundred students from different locations across Canada. The portal also provides practicing health and technology professionals with opportunities for continuing education. So that they are able to learn about how EHRs work and their impacts upon the health practice and workflow (Borycki et al., 2009; Borycki et al., 2011). Furthermore, we have been able to develop several approaches to integrating EHRs into student education so that there are opportunities to learn about differing solutions to healthcare problems that have prevented full adoption and integration of these systems (e.g. problems related to issues such as interoperability, usability, testing for safety and integration of systems into health professional individual and group workflow). The portal has been used successfully in the classroom, in the laboratory and with distance education students to give hands-on exposure to a variety of EHRs in several locations across Canada (Borycki et al., 2009).

To illustrate access to the portal, Figure 1 shows the screen that students see if they access the portal via the WWW (in Figure 1 the student has clicked on the icon for starting up an instance of the OpenVista® EHR system). The remote desktop that the student logs onto is located on servers in Victoria, Canada (that can be accessed worldwide) and allows each student private read and write access to a range of EHRs, including EMRs, PHRs and EPRs (represented as icons). In Figure 2, the student has entered OpenVista® and is examining a fictitious or dummy patient record. Fictitious or dummy patient records are used to avoid privacy and confidentiality issues associated with the use of real patient data. There are also a number of other benefits associated with using this approach. Fictitious patient data can be used to generate a wide variety and complexity of cases that can be used to illustrate the features and functions of EHRs as well as their limitations in supporting health professional work. Lastly, fictitious patient cases allow students to make errors typical of students learning an EHR. In a virtual EHR environment this allows for errors to occur without their being a direct impact on patients (e.g. if a medical order is submitted then it is not associated with a real patient) (Borycki et al., 2009; Borycki et al., 2011).

In Figure 3, the student is viewing a display of a fictitious patient's vital signs. By instructing students to explore all the tabs and all the main features and functions of systems such as OpenVista, the functionality and design of a full EHR can be conveyed. This includes the functionality essential to working EHRs such as the following: (a) ability of EHRs to provide an integrated and comprehensive view of patient data (e.g. as shown in Figure 1), (b) the ability of EHRs to provide decision support capabilities, such as patient alerts and reminders, (c) links to online educational resources such as drug databases, and (d) communication support for transferring and receiving information about patients, their conditions, their laboratory values etc.

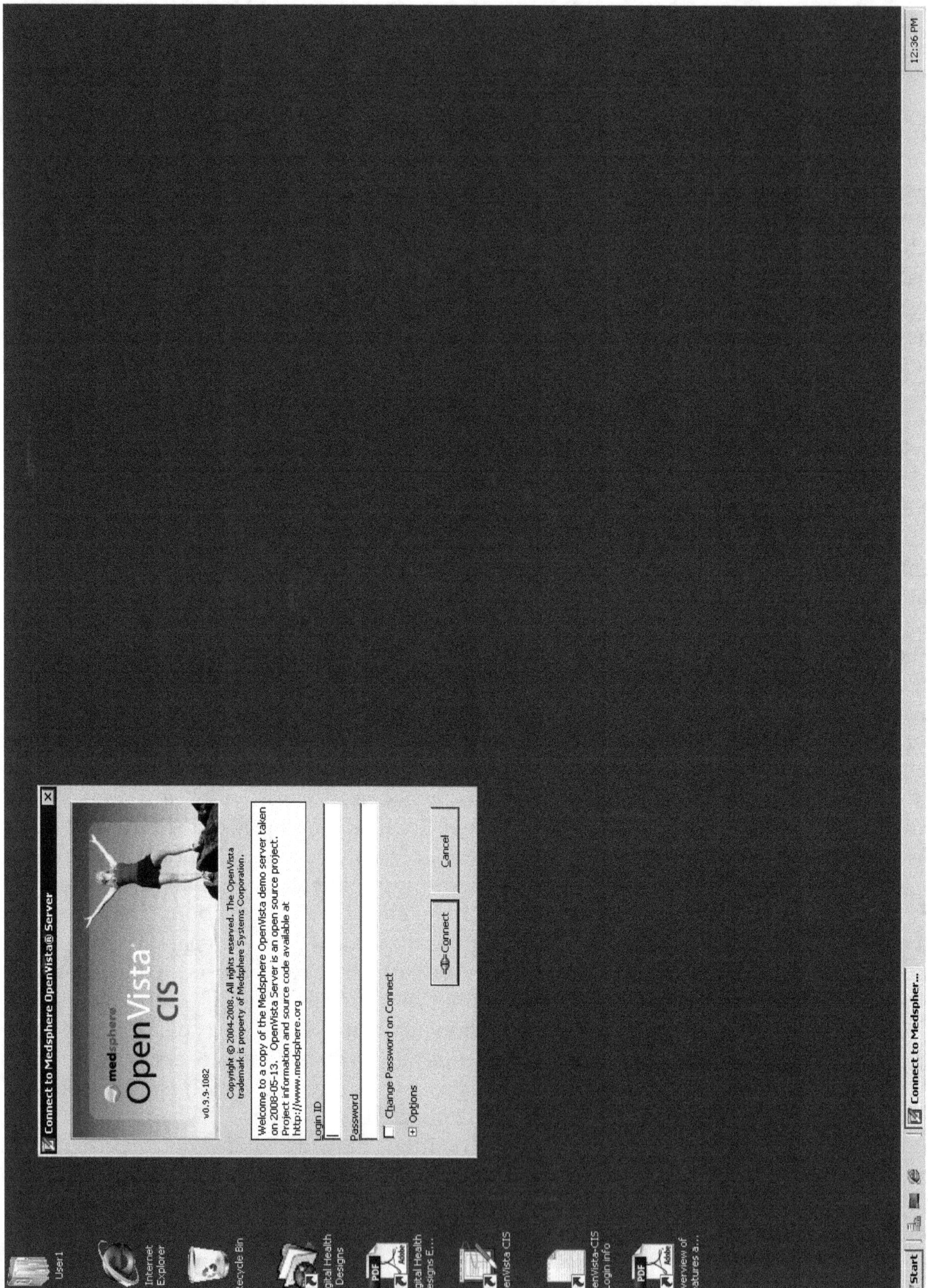

Fig. 1. Remote desktop of the UVic-EHR Portal, as seen by a student logging into the OpenVista® system remotely.

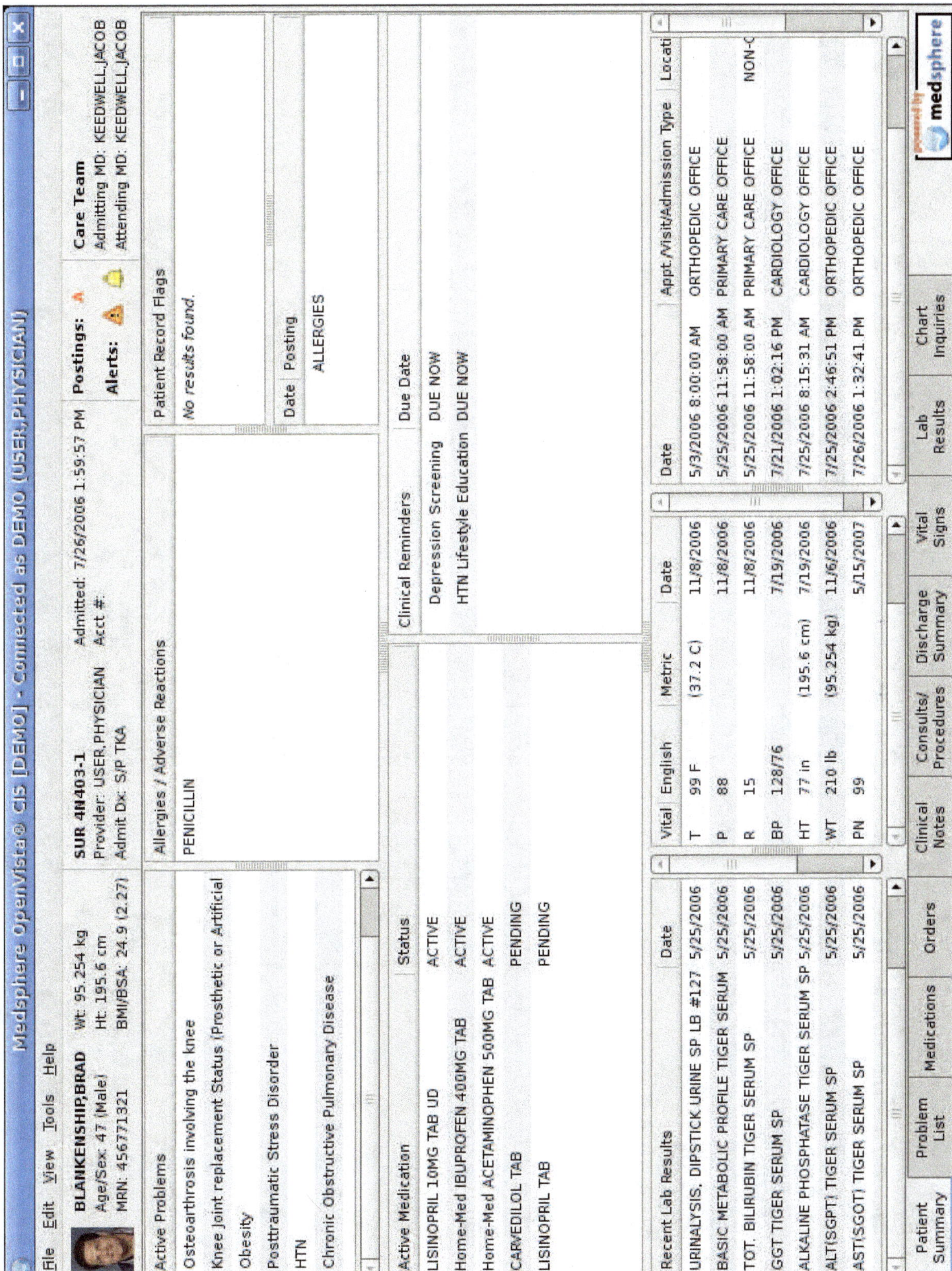

Fig. 2. Student view of a fictitious patient record displayed in OpenVista®.

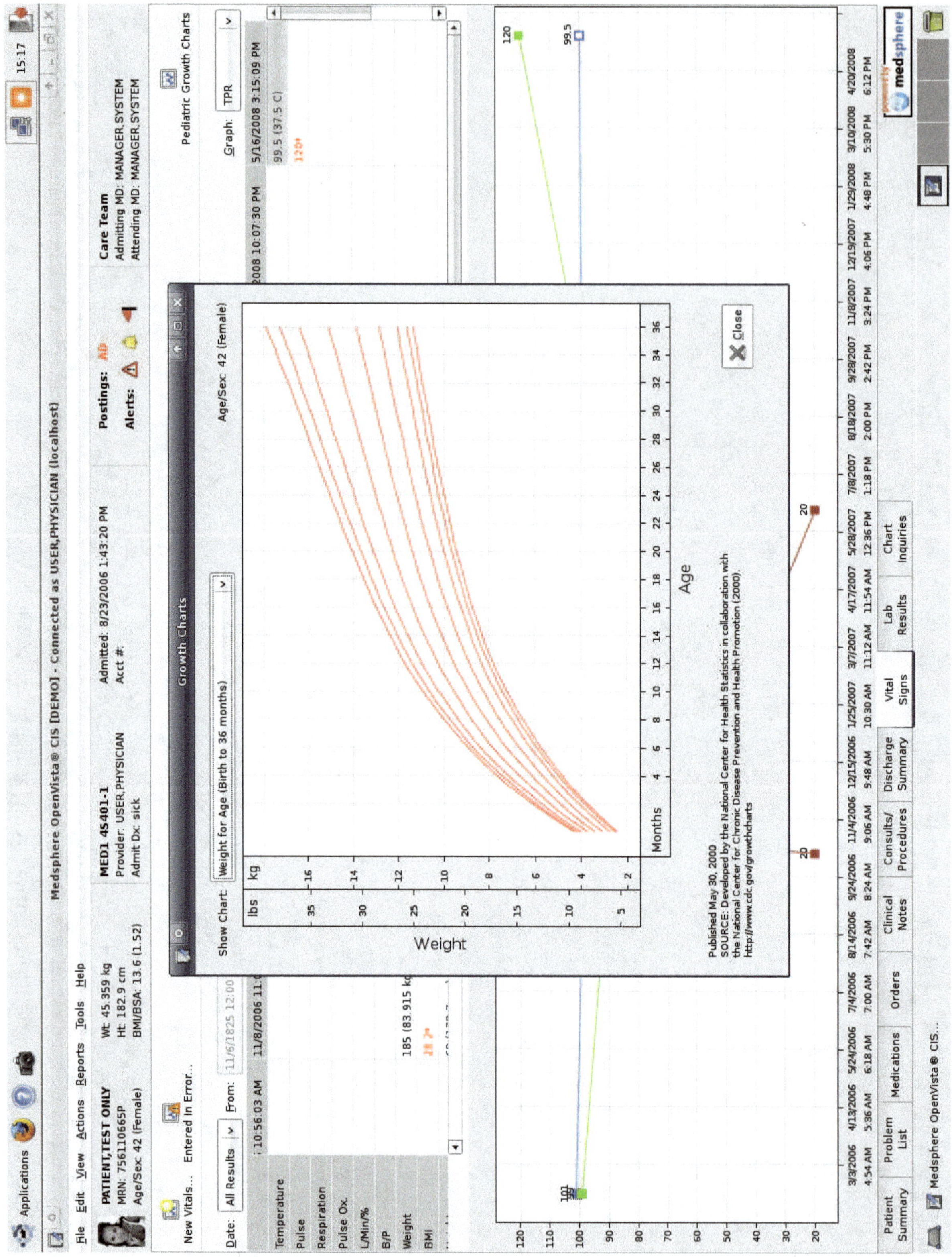

Fig. 3. Student view of a fictitious patient's vital signs displayed in OpenVista®.

In summary we have developed a portal that allows for ubiquitous access to working EHRs over the WWW. The portal has been used by students to learn about EHRs and some of the challenges and issues associated with their design, development, implementation and customization to health care settings such as physician offices and hospitals. The portal provides access to varying types of EHRs including EMRs, EPRs and PHRs so that students can have a full range of exposures to differing types of EHRs. This access is invaluable in courses where students need to explore the look and feel as well as functionality of working EHR systems, as will be described. In addition, EHR system components and systems developed by students (in courses) can be developed and hosted on the portal (as will be described) to allow for testing and deployment of project work in a realistic Web-based environment. In the next section of this paper we will discuss some of the uses of the EHR portal (including its integration in biomedical engineering education - especially where biomedical engineers must learn about EHRs).

4. Application of the EHR portal in biomedical engineering education

There are a number of current and emerging applications and models for integrating the EHR into biomedical engineering education. In our work this has included the incorporation of the EHR portal (as described above) to provide hands-on access to working EHRs and EHR system components (Borycki et al., 2009; Kushniruk et al., 2009) The applications described below are embedded within an integrated curricula focused on integrating informatics skills with understanding of user needs and healthcare requirements (as described by Kushniruk et al., 2006). The curriculum includes courses at both the undergraduate and graduate levels.

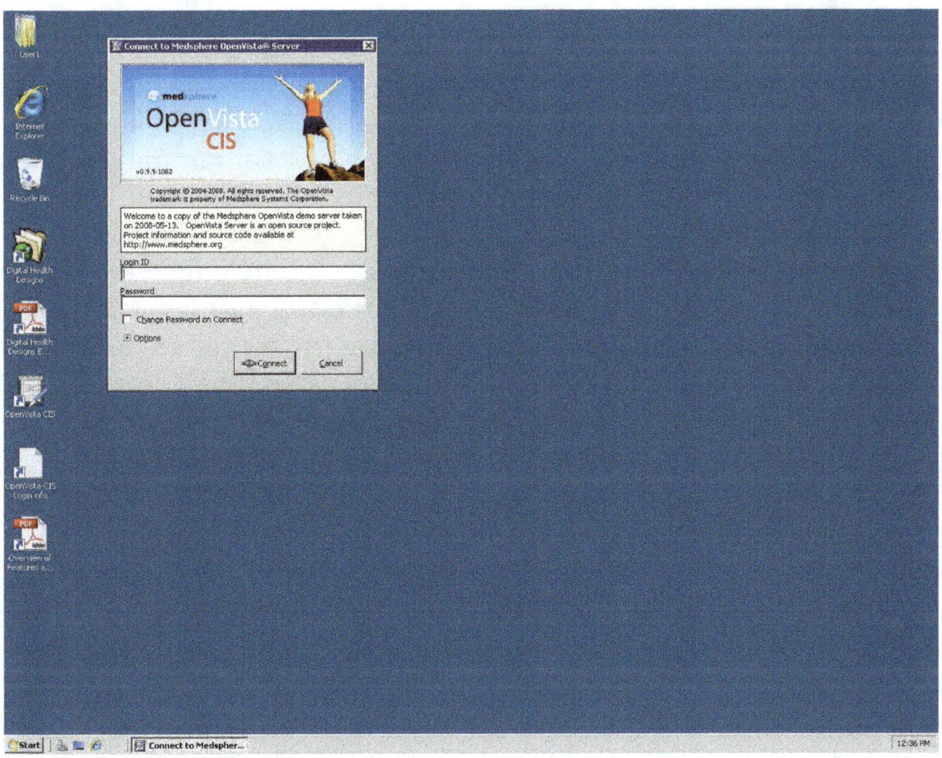

Fig. 4. Remote desktop of the UVic-EHR Portal, as seen by a student logging into the OpenVista®.

4.1 Healthcare systems analysis and design

As described above currently there are many issues facing the effective and widespread deployment of EHR technology in healthcare. There are many examples of failed EHR projects and implementations throughout the world. Reasons for such failure are varied but issues around the selection and application of inappropriate methods and approaches to healthcare system analysis and development have been implicated in many of these failures (Kushniruk, 2002). Biomedical engineering students who will become future designers and developers of these systems require improved training in more effective systems analysis and design, particularly in the context of healthcare. This training must go beyond the standard textbook knowledge contained in the generic software engineering literature as the challenges of designing and implementing healthcare systems have proven to be more difficult than in other traditional business areas. In addition, a focus on the whole System Development Life Cycle (SDLC), including consideration of methods and techniques that have proven to work most effectively in the domain of healthcare, is needed. In particular, healthcare information systems have often been criticized for not meeting the needs of their varied users (e.g. physicians, nurses, pharmacists, and allied health professionals) and their varied work contexts (e.g. emergency care, chronic care etc.). To address this and to allow students to see a range of possible functions and features of systems, we have used the University of Victoria EHR Portal to allow students to compare and contrast different types of EHRs. Thus, one way of applying the portal has been to have students access and assess EHRs as part of courses related to healthcare information system analysis and design. The instructions given to students typically have involved asking them to assess one or more EHRs in terms of identifying the following: (a) user interface design features (b) system features, (c) product advantages and disadvantages and (d) potential technical and user problems.

In addition, at the University of Victoria we have used the University of Victoria EHR Educational Portal to teach principles of systems analysis and design in an advanced fourth year undergraduate course (HINF 450 - "Systems Analysis and Design in Healthcare"). The intent of the course is teach object-oriented design approaches and students are required to develop working EHR modules (using UML and Java programming). The availability of open source EHRs on the portal offers the opportunity for students to assess existing system designs and to design and create working modules that can interface with existing open source software, reinforcing their programming and software engineering skills. In addition, the course focuses on training students in application of rapid prototyping and iterative refinement of systems based on iterative user testing. Allowing students to create modules early in the course, host their solutions and test them, can create a working test bed for them to improve their skills both in requirements gathering and system design.

4.2 Usability of health care information systems

Issues related to the poor usability of many healthcare information systems (in particular vendor based EHRs) is becoming increasingly recognized as a key factor in the failure of many efforts to implement EHRs and related technology (Kushniruk, et al., 1996; Kushniruk et al., 2005; Patel et al., 2000). Indeed complex socio-technical factors related to better understanding user needs, system usability and ensuring the usefulness of information provided to users have come to the fore in efforts to improve healthcare IT (Kushniruk and Patel, 2004). During several offerings of core courses in the undergraduate bachelor's degree program in health informatics at the University of Victoria, the portal has been used to provide students in health informatics (HI) with opportunities to explore EHRs from a range of formal analytical perspectives, from the technical to the cognitive and socio-technical. For example, in a third year undergraduate course entitled "Human, Social and Organizational Aspects of Healthcare Information Systems" several hundred students have been asked to critically analyze different EHRs currently available on the portal using evaluation methods from the field of usability engineering (e.g. using methods such as heuristic inspection, cognitive walkthrough as well as usability testing approaches). For example, given access to an EHR student work may involve having students conduct usability inspections of the system to identify: (a) violations of standard usability heuristics (b) usability problems (c) areas where the user interface and interaction should be improved (d)"usability catastrophes" that must be fixed to ensure proper system interaction and safety. Additionally, students are typically asked to design studies involving the video analysis of representative users interacting with the system under study and development. This has involved students creating full study protocols where a subject pool is identified, study materials designed, study procedures defined and also analysis methods indicated. The approach to this has involved teaching students about carrying out low-cost rapid usability testing (Kushniruk & Borycki, 2006), where subjects' computer screens are recorded, along with all user physical interactions and verbalizations. A focus of some of the courses where this has been introduced has been on training students to understand how usability problems may be highly related to safety issues and introduction of medical error (Kushniruk et al., 2005). This is termed technology-induced error. In courses students have had the opportunity to assess and evaluate the safety of EHR software and the implications of integrating EHRs with other medical devices such as IV pumps and smart beds on nurse and physician cognitive load, workflow and subsequent error rates (Borycki et al., 2008; Kushniruk et al., 2006). These learning experiences involving EHRs then formed the basis for student projects (see Carvalho et al., 2008).

In a number of iterations of this course, real systems were either accessed remotely by students (or systems hosted on the portal were accessed). Feedback, in the form of consulting reports developed by small groups of students, is typically presented to the system developers. Using this approach, students in the course have been involved in improving the usability of a number of Web-based EHR systems, allowing for experiential learning involving real systems. The portal thus has allowed students to compare and contrast different EHR user interface styles and designs and gain experience in evaluating differing EHRs in terms of both usability and safety, through both individual and group project work.

4.3 Interoperability of EHRs

There are many benefits associated with the use of Electronic Health Records (EHRs). According to IEEE, interoperability refers to "*the ability of two or more systems or components to exchange information and to use the information that has been exchanged*" (IEEE, 1991). Health data interoperability is an important EHR function as it allows for health data to be transferred electronically from one EHR system to another and from medical devices to the EHR. EHR interoperability has been found to improve the efficiency of healthcare delivery. Research findings have also suggested interoperability can reduce healthcare costs as well as the time taken to access, analyze, and document relevant patient health information by health professionals (Maki and Petterson, 2008).

Unfortunately, many software vendors do not provide EHRs with interoperability functions. Many countries around the world such as Denmark, Taiwan, Canada and the United States have developed or are in the process of developing interoperable EHR systems (iEHRs). For example, Canada Health Infoway working in partnership with federal, provincial and territorial governments is currently working towards implementing a pan-Candian iEHR. Once implemented, it is expected that the new iEHR, will allow healthcare providers (e.g. doctors and nurses) to access and update any Canadian's health record electronically, any time or place (Giokas, 2008). However, there are many challenges associated with iEHR implementation. For example, there are many differing types of EHR users in a typical healthcare system - clinicians, health information management (HIM) professionals, health care administrators, biomedical engineers, medical researchers and data modellers, *etc.* Each type of user uses the same EHR data to perform their work. However, there is considerable variation in the coding methods, terminologies/nomenclatures, software, hardware and medical devices that are used and the definitions that are present between EHR systems and devices. Other challenges include differences in the ways in which users may interpret the same data (e.g. words or medical terms). These challenges still need to be overcome to address issues associated with health data interoperability (Garde et al., 2007).

There are many differing methods that can be used to solve interoperability challenges. Kuo et al. (2011) has categorized a number of models for health system interoperability and they include the: (1) point-to-point oriented model, (2) standard oriented model, and (3) common-gateway model. In the point-to-point oriented model, organizations involved have chosen to use agreed–upon coding terminologies, messaging protocols and business processes. Therefore, health data can only be exchanged among organizations that have contractual agreements in the above mentioned three areas. The US Department of Veterans Affairs and the Department of Defense is a real-world example of an organization that has taken this approach. The US Department of Veterans Affairs (VA) and the Department of Defence (DoD) have built a patient data exchange gateway to exchange patient health information (Bouhaddou et al., 2008). This gateway allows for bi-directional, computable data exchange. It also achieves semantic interoperability. In the standard oriented model for health information exchange, organizations agree to follow a unique standard (terminology and message standard) for health information exchange. The Department of Health Taiwan (DOH-Taiwan) uses this model. The department of health promotes the use of the Taiwan Electronic Medical Record Template (TMT) format. To date the template is used by ten medical centres that collectively are responsible for 10 million outpatient visits a year. The TMT format forms the basis for document-based information standards and the information interoperability infrastructure for the Taiwanese healthcare system (Jian et al. 2007). The common-gateway model employs a messaging broker/bus approach. The model provides a common, standardized point of communication between systems to allow for information sharing. When health organizations exchange information, standard message structures (e.g. HL7 v2.x/v3) are defined to contain the information supplied in requests, responses and submissions by the parties who wish to exchange information. Therefore each health information system needs only to know how to connect to the messaging broker/bus and convert its data to standard message structures - a mutually agreed–upon data structure, coding terminologies and business process is not needed. Health organizations can therefore develop their information systems locally while at the same time reducing costs associated with complex development approaches. The Danish eHealth Portal, sundhed.dk (https://www.sundhed.dk/) uses this approach. Danish citizens can find information about treatments and waiting lists as well as communicate directly with health care providers via the portal. Citizens and health professionals have differing levels of access to the portal. Citizens and health professionals can also access a number of health services including EHRs (Sundhed, 2009).

To help students learn about and understand issues associated with interoperability involving the EHRs a well as the most common models or approaches (as outlined above), student projects have been developed for an undergraduate course entitled "Principles of Health Database Design" at the University of Victoria. As part of coursework students (assigned to groups) were asked to use PHP to design EHRs similar to OpenVista® (after viewing, exploring and assessing several EHRs on the portal). To train students in the basics of developing interoperable healthcare systems, the students were then instructed about how to export and import data across the different systems developed by each group of students. In a simulation system, data was stored in an Oracle or a MySQL database. Groups of students then used PHP and a Document Object Model (DOM) to export the data from Oracle to XML documents. Following this, the XML documents were used to import to other groups' EHR's using a MySQL database. As a consequence, students have developed a better understanding of how health data can be made interoperable among heterogeneous EHRs.

4.4 Implementation of differing configurations of medical devices and EHRs to support clinical work

One of the greatest challenges in effectively implementing EHRs into healthcare practice and settings such as clinics and hospitals has been the need to effectively (and safely) integrate this type of technology with the many other devices and information technologies that exist in healthcare settings. Along these lines, we have been able to use EHRs to teach students about the impact of integrating EHRs with medical devices upon health professional workflow and medical error rates in hospital settings (e.g. medical unit, emergency unit). In regional health authorities across Canada and hospitals worldwide medical devices are being integrated with the EHR (Kushniruk et al., 2006; Koppel et al., 2005 . The EHR is increasingly becoming the one source of information where all patient health information and their encounters with the health care system are being stored (i.e. uploaded to and downloaded from other medical devices). Health professionals (e.g. physicians and nurses) are using information in the EHR that comes from multiple differing devices (Kushniruk et al., 2006). For example, globally, intravenous pumps, smart beds, vital sign monitors, cardiac monitors, tablet computers and mobile phones are being used to collect and upload patient data to the EHR. Similarly, patient data is downloaded from the EHR to mobile tablet devices, mobile phones, mobile workstations and traditional desktop workstations by physicians, nurses and other health professionals for use in patient care related decision making. In every case patient data is being downloaded or uploaded to the EHR from an associated medical device. Initial, research in this area has revealed that medical devices (including mobile and traditional computer workstations), when not adequately integrated with an EHR, can have significant effects upon clinician workflow (Kushniruk, et al., 2006; Borycki et al., 2010) and error rates (Kushniruk et al., 2005; Koppel et al., 2005). This research has also shown that differing constellations of EHRs and medical devices can be tested using clinical simulations (to determine the potential effects of EHR – device integration upon clinician workflow and error rates) prior to the EHR-medical device constellation being implemented in a real-world hospital setting (Borycki et al., 2010). Introducing students to EHRs in the classroom (with hands on exposure opportunities) and providing students with classroom exercises where they can work with and observe the implications of EHR – device integration, helps students to learn about how to effectively procure, implement and customize EHRs- device constellations. Here, students learn how to implement and customize device implementations such that workflow is positively impacted while medical error rates arising from poor interactions with the EHR and its associated medical devices are at the same time reduced. Such work in the classroom also affords students with opportunities to design and evaluate the implications of specific EHR-device constellations on health professionals' workflow and error rates. We have also extended this work to include student discussions regarding procurement and the need for an integrated strategy towards EHR software and device selection and testing as part of the information technology and biomedical engineering department's long term management of EHR software and devices.

5. Discussion

EHR use is becoming increasingly more global as internationally there has been a move towards health information systems (HIS) implementation. As a result, biomedical engineering professionals are encountering a variety of complex problems in integrating EHRs in healthcare settings; for example, software, hardware and medical device interoperability issues. Graduates of educational programs are being expected to deal with the design, implementation and deployment of ever more complex HIS. Yet, biomedical engineering students may have few opportunities to work with more than one HIS before graduating from an undergraduate or a graduate program. This is also the case for many allied health professionals (e.g. physicians and nurses) who have little exposure to HIS before graduating from their educational programs. To address this need the authors worked on developing a number of educational initiatives to better inform students about key issues in EHR design, testing and implementation. Along these lines, we have also developed and employed a Web-based portal that houses a repository of EHRs and related technology for use in classroom instruction of health professionals who use EHRs. The authors have previously deployed portal EHRs for use in health professional educational programs (e.g. physician, nurse and health informatics training and education). This chapter represents a new advance in that it describes how portal EHRs can be integrated into and used for teaching biomedical engineering students. Portal EHRs have been used in a variety of ways to teach students about best practices in HIS design, development and implementation and to develop specialized knowledge that can be used to advance the design of HIS into the future. By providing students with practical hands-on experience (targeted at key areas where healthcare IT has been known to be problematic) it is hoped that upon graduation biomedical engineering students will be better prepared to meet the great challenges of implementing information technology in healthcare.

6. References

Armstrong, B., Kushniruk, A., Borycki, E. (2009). Solutions for deploying multi-architecture EHRs on a single EHR educational portal. *Studies in Health Technology and Informatics, 150*,167-71.

Armstrong, B., Kushniruk, A., Joe, R., Borycki, E. (2009). Technical and architectural issues in deploying electronic health records (EHRs) over the WWW. *Studies in Health Technology and Informatics,* Vol. 143:93-8.

Borycki, E. M., Kushniruk, A. (2005). Identifying and preventing technology-induced error using simulations: Application of usability engineering techniques. *Electronic Healthcare/Healthcare Quarterly, 8*, 99-106.*

Borycki, E., Joe, R., Armstrong, B., Bellwood, P., Campbell, R. (2011). Educating health professionals about the electronic health record (EHR): Removing the barriers to adoption through improved understanding. *Knowledge Management and E-Learning: An International Journal, 3*(1), 51-62.

Borycki, E. M., Kushniruk, A. W., Joe, R., Armstrong, B. et. al.. (2009). The University of Victoria Interdisciplinary EHR Educational Portal. *Studies in Health Technology and Informatics*. Vol. 143. 49-54.

Borycki, E. M., Kushniruk, A. W., Kuwata, S., Watanabe, H. (2009). Simulations to assess medication administration systems (pp. 144-159). In B. Staudinger, V. Hoess & Herwig Ostermann (Eds.). *Nursing and Clinical Informatics: Socio-Technical Approaches*. Hershey, Pennsylvania: IGI Global.

Borycki, E. M., Kushniruk, A. W. (2008). Where do technology-induced errors come from? Towards a model for conceptualizing and diagnosing errors caused by technology (pp. 148-166). In A. W. Kushniruk and E. M. Borycki (Eds.). *Human, Social, and Organizational Aspects of Health Information Systems*. Hershey, Pennsylvania: Idea Group.

Bouhaddou, O., Warnekar, P., Parrish, F., Do, N., Mandel, J., Kilbourne, J. and Lincoln, M.J. (2008) 'Exchange of Computable Patient Data between the Department of Veterans Affairs (VA) and the Department of Defense (DoD): Terminology Mediation Strategy', *Journal of the American Medical Informatics Association*, Vol. 15, No. 2, p.174-183.

Canada's Health Informatics Association. Health informatics professional core competencies: Version 2.0. 2009.

Carvalho, C. J., Borycki, E. M., Kushniruk, A. (2009). Ensuring the safety of health information systems: Using heuristics for patient safety. *Healthcare Quarterly*, Vol. 12, 49-54.

Garde, S., Knaup, P., Hovenga, E.J.S. and Heard, S. (2007) 'Towards Semantic Interoperability for Electronic Health Records - Domain Knowledge Governance for openEHR Archetypes', *Methods of Information Medicine*, Vol. 46, p.332-343.

Giokas, D. (2008) 'EHRS Blueprint: An Interoperable Framework. Canada Health Infoway', Retrieved March 14, 2011 from http://www.omg.org/news/meetings/workshops/HC-2008/15-06_Giokas.pdf

HL7book. (2009). 'A basic overview of Clinical Document Architecture', Retrieved Feb. 10, 2011, from Hl7book web site: http://hl7book.net/index.php?title=CDA

IEEE. (1991) 'IEEE standard computer dictionary- A compilation of IEEE standard computer glossaries', IEEE Std. 610.

Jian, W.S., Hsu, C.Y., Hao, T.H., Wen, H.C., Hsu, M.H., Lee, Y.L., Li, Y.C. and Chang, P. (2007) 'Building a portable data and information interoperability infrastructure - framework for a standard Taiwan Electronic Medical Record Template', *Computer Methods and Programs in Biomedicine*, Vol.88, No. 2, p.102-111.

Joe, R. S., Otto, A., Borycki, E. (2011). Designing an electronic medical case simulator for health professional education. *Knowledge Management and E-Learning: An International Journal*. 3(1), 63-71.

Joe, R. S., Kushniruk, A. W., Borycki, E. M., Armstrong, B., Otto, T., Ho, K. (2009). Bringing electronic patient records into health professional education: Software architecture and implementation. *Studies in Health Technology and Informatics, 150,* 888-92.

Kushniruk, A.W., Kaufman, D.R., Patel, V.L., Levesque, Y., Lottin, P. (1996). Assessment of a computerized patient record system: A cognitive approach to evaluating an emerging medical technology. *M.D. Computing*, 13(5), 406-415.

Kushniruk, A.W. (2002). Evaluation in the design of health information systems: Applications of approaches emerging from systems engineering. *Computers in Biology and Medicine*, 32(3), 141-149.

Kushniruk, A. W., Borycki, E. M. (2006). Low-cost rapid usability engineering: Designing and customizing usable health information systems. *Electronic Healthcare/Healthcare Quarterly, 5*(2), 98-102.

Kushniruk, A., Borycki, E., Armstrong, B., Joe, R., Otto, T. (2009). Bringing electronic patient records into health professional education: Towards an integrative framework. *Studies in Health Technology and Informatics, 150*, 883-7.

Kushniruk, A.W., Borycki, E. M., Kuwata, S., Kannry, J. (2006). Predicting changes in workflow resulting from healthcare information systems: Ensuring the safety of healthcare. *Healthcare Quarterly, 9*, 78-82.

Kushniruk, A.W., Borycki, E. M., Kuwata, S., Watanabe, H. (2008). Using a low-cost simulation approach for assessing the impact of a medication administration system on workflow. *Studies in Health Technology and Informatics. 136*, 567-72.

Kushniruk, A., Lau, F., Borycki, E., Protti, D. (2006). The School of Health Information Science at the University of Victoria: Towards an integrated model for health informatics education and research. Yearbook of Medical Informatics, 15-165.

Kushniruk, A. W., Patel, V.L. (2004). Cognitive and usability engineering approaches to the evaluation of clinical information systems. *Journal of Biomedical Informatics,* 37(1), 56-57.

Kushniruk, A.W., Triola, M., Borycki, E.M., Stein, B., Kannry, J. (2005). Technology induced error and usability: The relationship between usability problems and prescription errors when using a handheld application. *International Journal of Medical Informatics, 74*(7-8), 519-526.

Kuo, M.H., Kushniruk A. and Borycki, E. (2011). 'A Comparison of National Health Data Interoperability Approaches in Taiwan, Denmark and Canada', *Healthcare Quarterly*, 2011. (to appear)

Lenza, R., Beyera, M. and Kuhnb, K.A. (2007) 'Semantic integration in healthcare networks', *International Journal of Medical Informatics*, Vol. 76, p.201–207.

Maki S.E. and Petterson, B.P. (2008) *Using the Electronic Health Record in the Healthcare Provider Practice*, Bonnie Petterson.

Merrill, M. (2009) 'RFID to track patient files at Cleveland Clinic', Retrieved March 15, 2011 from http://www.healthcareitnews.com/news/rfid-track-patient-files-cleveland-clinic

Patel, V.L., Kushniruk, A.W., Yang, S., Yale, J.F. (2000). Impact of a computer-based patient record system on data collection, knowledge organization and reasoning. *Journal of the American Medical Informatics Association*, 7(6), 569-585.

Shortliffe EH, Cimino JJ, Eds. Biomedical Informatics: Computer Applications in Heath Care and Biomedicine. Springer, New york, 2006.

Sundhed. (2009) 'Danish Health Portal', Retrieved on Feb 14, 2011 from https://www.sundhed.dk/Profil.aspx?id=11062.105.1258

6

Biomedical Time Series Processing and Analysis Methods: The Case of Empirical Mode Decomposition

Alexandros Karagiannis[1],
Philip Constantinou[1] and Demosthenes Vouyioukas[2]
[1]*National Technical University of Athens, School of Electrical and Computer Engineering, Mobile RadioCommunication Laboratory*
[2]*University of the Aegean, Department of Information and Communication Systems Engineering*
Greece

1. Introduction

1.1 Typical measurement systems chain

Computational processing and analysis of biomedical signals applied on the time series follow a chain of finite number of processes. Typical schemes front process is the acquisition of signal via the sensory subsystem. Next steps in the acquisition processing and analysis chain include buffers and preamplifiers, the filtering stage, the analog-digital conversion part, the removal of possible artifacts, the event detection and the analysis and feature extraction. Figure 1 depicts this process.

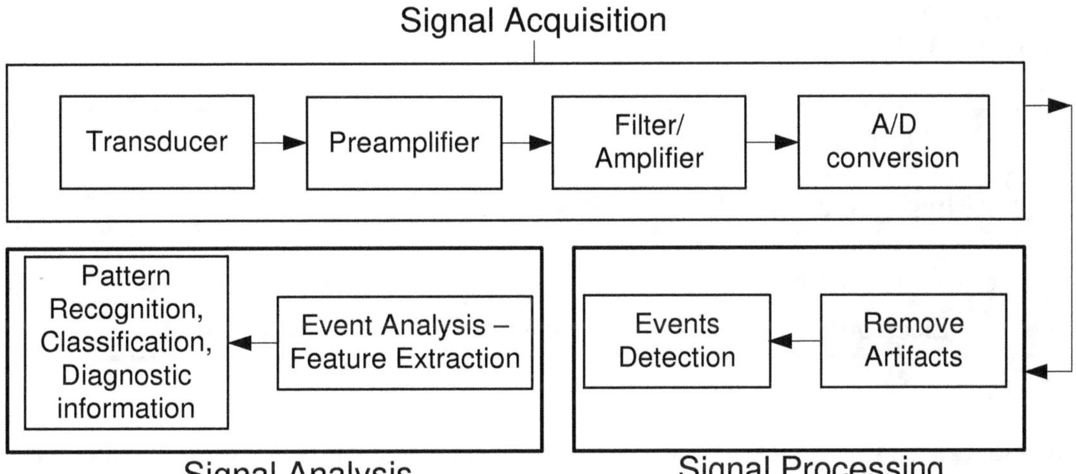

Fig. 1. Chain of processes from the acquisition of a biomedical signal to the analysis stage

Biomedical signal measurement, parameter identification and characterization initiate by the acquisition of diagnostic data in the form of image or time series that carry valuable

information related to underlying physical processes. The analog signal usually requires to be amplified and bandpass or lowpass filtered. Since most signal processing is easier to implement using digital methods, the analog signal is converted to digital format using an analog-to-digital converter. Once converted, the signal is often stored, or buffered, in memory.
Digital signal processing algorithms applied on the digitized signal are mainly categorized as artifact removal processing methods and events detection methods. The last stage of this a typical measurement system refers to digital signal analysis with a higher level of sophistication techniques that extract features out of the digital signal or make a pattern recognition and classification in order to deliver useful diagnostic information.
A transducer is a device that converts energy from one form to another. In signal processing applications, the purpose of energy conversion is to gather information, not to transform energy. Usually, the output of a biomedical transducer is a voltage (or current) whose amplitude is proportional to the measured energy. The energy that is converted by the transducer may be generated by the physical process itself or produced by an external source. Many physiological processes produce energy that can be detected directly. For example, cardiac internal pressures are usually measured using a pressure transducer placed on the tip of catheter introduced into the appropriate chamber of the heart.
Whilst the most extensive signal processing is usually performed on digital data using software algorithms, some analog signal processing is usually necessary. Noise is inherent in most measurement systems and it is considered a limiting factor in the performance of a medical instrument. Many signal processing techniques target at the minimization of the variability in the measurement. In biomedical measurements, variability has four different origins: physiological variability; environmental noise or interference; transducer artifact; and electronic noise. The physiological variability is due to the fact that the biomedical signal acquired is affected by biological factors other than those of interest. Environmental noise originates from sources external or internal to the body. A classic example is the measurement of fetal ECG where the desired signal is corrupted by the mother's ECG. Since it is not known a priori the sources of environmental noise, typical noise reduction techniques have partially successful results compared to adaptive techniques which present better behavior in filtering.

Source	Cause
Physiological	Other variables present in the measured variable of interest
Environmental	Other sources of similar energy form
Electronic	Thermal or shot noise

Table 1. Sources of Measurement Variability

Transducer artifact is produced when the transducer responds to energy modalities other than that desired. For example, recordings of electrical potentials using electrodes placed on the skin are sensitive to motion artifact, where the electrodes respond to mechanical movement as well as the desired electrical signal. They are usually compensated by transducer design modifications.
Johnson or thermal noise is produced by resistance sources, and the amount of noise generated is related to the resistance and to the temperature:

$$V_{el} = \sqrt{4kTRB} \tag{1}$$

where R is the resistance in Ohms, T is the temperature in degrees Kelvin, k is Boltzman's constant ($k = 1.38 * 10^{-23}$ J/°K) and B is the bandwidth, or range of frequencies, that is allowed to pass through the measurement system.

It is a common assumption that electronic noise is spread evenly over the entire frequency range of interest. However it is common to describe relative noise as the noise that would occur if the bandwidth were 1.0 Hz. Such relative noise specification can be identified by the unusual units required: volts/√Hz or amps/√Hz.

When multiple noise sources are present, as is often the case, their voltage or current contributions to the total noise add as the square root of the sum of the squares, assuming that the individual noise sources are independent. For voltages

$$V_T = (\sqrt{V_1^2 + V_2^2 + ... + V_N^2})^{1/2} \tag{2}$$

where $V_1, V_2, ..., V_N$ are the voltages caused by any source of noise.

The relative amount of signal and noise present in the time series acquired by means of measurement systems is quantified by signal to noise ratio, SNR. Both signal and noise are measured in RMS values (root mean squared). SNR is expressed in dB (decidels) where

$$SNR = 20\log(\frac{Signal}{Noise}) \tag{3}$$

Various types of filters are incorporated according to the frequency range of interest in measurement systems. Lowpass filters allow low frequencies to pass with minimum attenuation whilst higher frequencies are attenuated. Conversely, highpass filters pass high frequencies, but attenuate low frequencies. Bandpass filters reject frequencies above and below a passband region. Bandstop filter passes frequencies on either side of a range of attenuated frequencies. The bandwidth of a filter is defined by the range of frequencies that are not attenuated.

The last analog element in a typical measurement system is the analog-to-digital converter (ADC). In the process of analog-to-digital conversion an analog or continuous waveform, x(t), is converted into a discrete waveform, x(n), a function of real numbers that are defined only at discrete integers, n. Slicing the signal into discrete points in time is termed time sampling or simply sampling. Time slicing samples the continuous waveform, x(t), at discrete prints in time, nTs, where Ts is the sample interval. Since the binary output of the ADC is a discrete integer whilst the analog signal has a continuous range of values, analog-to-digital conversion also requires the analog signal to be sliced into discrete levels, a process termed quantization.

The speed of analog to digital conversion is specified in terms of samples per second, or conversion time. For example, an ADC with a conversion time of 10 μsec should, logically, be able to operate at up to 100000 samples per second (or simply 100 kHz). Typical conversion rates run up to 500 kHz for moderate cost converters, but off-the-shelf converters can be obtained with rates up to several MHz. Lower conversion rates are usually acceptable for biological signals.

Most of biomedical signals are low energy signals and their acquisition takes place in the presence of noise and other signals originating from underlying systems that interfere with the original one. Noise is characterized by certain statistical properties that facilitate the estimation of Signal to Noise ratio.

Biomedical data analysis aims at the determination of parameters required for models development of the underlying system and its validation. Problems usually encountered at the processing stage are related to the small length of sampled time series or the lack of stationarity and non linearity of the process that produces the signals.

1.2 Difficulties in acquisition and biomedical signal analysis

The proximity of the sensory subsystem to the physical phenomenon, biomedical signal's dynamic nature as well as the interconnections and interactions of multiple physical systems are set difficulties in acquisition and biomedical signal processing and analysis. The impact of measurement equipment and different sources of artifacts and noise in biomedical signals such as electrocardiogram are considered in the determination of properties that affect the processing stage.

1.3 Sensor proximity

Most of physiological systems are located deep inside the human body and this sets a difficulty in biosignal acquisition and measurement. A typical case is electrocardiogram which is acquired by means of electrodes in the level of chest. The measured signal is a projection of a moving 3D cardiac electric vector at a level defined by the electrodes. If the purpose of the electrocardiogram acquisition is related to the monitoring of cardiac rhythm then this signal provides sufficient information. However, if the purpose is the atrium electric activity monitoring the processing and analysis of this signal is difficult.

Proximity to the physiological system that produces biosignals is usually accomplished by means of invasive methods which require certain conditions for the patients and the available equipment.

1.4 Signal variability

Physiological systems are dynamic systems controlled by numerous variables. Biomedical signals represent the dynamic nature of the underlying physiological systems. These processes as well as the variables have a deterministic or random (stochastic) nature and in some cases they are periodic.

A normal electrocardiogram may present a normal cardiac rhythm with easily identifiable and detectable complexes. A normal electrocardiogram could be characterized as deterministic and periodic signal; however a patient's circulatory system may have significant time variability both in the form of the complexes and the cardiac rhythm.

The dynamic nature of biological systems results in the stochastic and non stationary nature of biomedical signals. Statistical parameters such as average value and variance as well as the spectral density are time variant. In this case, a common approach is the signal analysis in wide time windows in order to include all the possible conditions of the underlying biological systems.

1.5 Interconnections and Interactions between physiological systems

Various physiological systems of the human body are not independent; on the contrary they are interconnected and interact. Some of the interactions cause physiological variable compensation, feedback loops or even affect other physiological systems. These operations in the level of physiological systems interactions should be considered as well in monitoring, processing and biomedical signal analysis.

1.6 Measurement equipment and measurement procedures

The front end of a measurement system which is the transducer subsystem and the connection with the rest of the measurement equipment affects the performance of the measurement system and may cause significant changes in signal's characteristics.

1.7 Artifacts and interference

When electrocardiogram is acquired it is required the immobility of the body in order to minimize the interference from other signals such as electromyogram. Even the respiratory signal can cause interference to the electrocardiogram.

Artifacts in acquired biomedical signal and interference from other physiological systems raise the need for biomedical signal processing techniques in order to deal with these phenomena.

1.8 Measurement equipment sensitivity

Monitoring of biomedical signals in the range of a few microvolts or millivolits which are produced by physiological systems demands the use of equipment with increased levels of sensitivity as well as low levels of noise. Shielded cables are used in order to minimize the electromagnetic interference from other medical equipment or any other sources of electromagnetic fields.

2. Spectral and statistical properties of biomedical signals

In scientific study, noise can come in many ways: it could be part of the natural processes generated by local and intermittent instabilities and sub-grid phenomena; it could be part of the concurrent phenomena in the environment where the investigations were conducted; and it could also be part of the sensors and recording systems. A generic model for the acquired signal is described by formula 4:

$$x(t) = s(t) + n(t) \tag{4}$$

where x(t) represents the acquired data, s(t) is the true signal and n(t) is noise. Once noise contaminates data, data processing techniques are employed to remove it.

For the obvious cases, when the processes are linear and noise have distinct time or frequency scales different from those of the true signal, Fourier filters can be employed to separate noise from the signal. Historically, Fourier based techniques are the most widely used.

The problem of separating noise and signal is complicated and difficult when there is no knowledge of the noise level in the data. Knowing the characteristics of the noise is an essential first step.

Most of the biosignals are characterized by the small levels of their energy as well as the existence of various types of noise during the acquisition. Any signal of no interest rather than the true signal is characterized as artifact, interference or noise. The existence of noise deteriorates the performance of a measurement system and the processing and analysis stages.

The amplitude of a deterministic signal can be calculated by a closed form mathematical formula or predicted if the amplitude of previous samples is considered. All the other signals are characterized as random signals. Kendal and Challis [1] , [2] proposed a test for the determination of the randomness of a signal which is based on the number of signal's extremas.

2.1 Noise

The term random noise refers to the interference of a biosignal caused by a random process. Considering a random variable η with probability density function $p_\eta(\eta)$, the average value μ_η of the random process η is defined as

$$\mu_\eta = \mathrm{E}[\eta] = \int_{-\infty}^{+\infty} \eta p_\eta(\eta) d\eta \tag{5}$$

where E[.] is the expected value of random variable η.
Mean square value of random process is defined as

$$\mathrm{E}[\eta^2] = \int_{-\infty}^{+\infty} \eta^2 p_\eta(\eta) d\eta \tag{6}$$

and the variance of the process is defined as

$$\sigma_\eta^2 = \mathrm{E}[(\eta - \mu_\eta)^2] = \int_{-\infty}^{+\infty} (\eta - \mu_\eta)^2 p_\eta(\eta) d\eta \tag{7}$$

The square root of the variance provides the standard deviation σ_η of the process.

$$\sigma_\eta^2 = \mathrm{E}[\eta^2] - \mu_\eta^2 \tag{8}$$

The average value of a stochastic process $\eta(t)$ represents the DC component of the signal; the mean square value represents the mean energy of the signal and the mean square root of the variance represents the RMS value. These statistical parameters are the essential components in the SNR estimation.

2.2 Ensemble averages

When the probability density function of a random process is not known then it is common practice to estimate the statistical expected value of the process via the averages computed at sample sets of the process.
The estimation of average defined in t_1 is

$$\mu_x(t) = \lim_{M \to \infty} \frac{1}{M} \sum_{k=1}^{M} x_k(t_1) \tag{9}$$

The autocorrelation function $\varphi_{xx}(t_1, t_1+\tau)$ of a random process is defined

$$\varphi_{xx}(t_1, t_1 + \tau) = \mathrm{E}[x(t_1)x(t_1 + \tau)] = \int_{-\infty}^{+\infty} x(t_1)x(t_1 + \tau) p_x(x) dx \tag{10}$$

2.3 Non stationary biomedical time series

Biomedical data analysis aims at the determination of parameters which are required for the development of models for the underlying physiological processes and the validation of those models. The problems encountered in the analysis of biomedical time series are due to the total data length, the non stationarity of the time series and the non linearity of the underlying physiological processes. The first two problems are related. Biomedical time series which are short in terms of time duration could be shorter than the longer time scale of a stationary process and to be characterized in this way as a non stationary process.

Fourier spectral analysis is a general method for the energy distribution of signal's frequency components. It has dominated in the data analysis and has been applied in almost all the biomedical time series acquired. However Fourier transform is applicable under certain conditions that set limitations. Linearity and strict periodicity as well as the strict stationary process are some of the conditions that should be satisfied in order to apply Fourier transform and interpret in a correct way the physical meaning of the results.

The stationarity requirement is not particular to the Fourier spectral analysis; it is a general one for most of the available data analysis methods. According to the traditional definition, a time series, x(t), is stationary in the wide sense, if, for all t

$$\begin{aligned} &E[\,|\,x(t)^2\,|\,] < \infty \\ &E[x(t)] = \mu_x \\ &Cov(x(t_1), x(t_2)) = Cov(x(t_1+\tau), x(t_2+\tau)) = Cov(t_1 - t_2) \end{aligned} \tag{11}$$

in which E(.) is the expected value defined as the ensemble average of the quantity, and C(.) is the covariance function. Stationarity in the wide sense is also known as weak stationarity, covariance stationarity or second-order stationarity.

Few of the biomedical data sets, from either natural phenomena or artificial sources, can satisfy the definition of stationarity. Other than stationarity, Fourier spectral analysis also requires linearity. Although many natural phenomena can be approximated by linear systems, they also have the tendency to be nonlinear. For the above reasons, the available data are usually of finite duration, non-stationary and from systems that are frequently nonlinear, either intrinsically or through interactions with the imperfect probes or numerical schemes. Under these conditions, Fourier spectral analysis is of limited use [3]. The uncritical use of Fourier spectral analysis and the adoption of the stationary and linear assumptions may give misleading results.

3. Biomedical signal processing and analysis methods

Many waveforms—particularly those of biological origin-are not stationary, and change substantially in their properties over time. For example, the EEG signal changes considerably depending on various internal states of the subject. A wide range of approaches have been developed in order to extract both time and frequency information from a waveform. Basically they can be divided into two groups: time-frequency methods and time-scale methods. The latter are better known as Wavelet analysis.

3.1 The spectrogram

The first time-frequency methods were based on the straightforward approach of slicing the waveform of interest into a number of short segments and performing the analysis on each of these segments, usually using the standard Fourier transform [4]. A window function is applied to a segment of data, effectively isolating that segment from the overall waveform, and the Fourier transform is applied to that segment. This is termed the spectrogram or "short-term Fourier transform" (STFT).

Since it relies on the traditional Fourier spectral analysis, one has to assume the data to be piecewise stationary. This assumption is not always justified in non-stationary data. Furthermore, there are also practical difficulties in applying the method: in order to localize an event in time, the window width must be narrow, but, on the other hand, the frequency resolution requires longer time series.

3.2 Wigner-Ville distribution

A number of approaches have been developed to overcome some of the shortcomings of the spectrogram. The first of these was the Wigner-Ville distribution. It is a special case of a wide variety of similar transformations known under the heading of Cohen's class of distributions.

The Wigner-Ville, and in fact all of Cohen's class of distributions, use a variation of the autocorrelation function where time remains in the result. This is achieved by comparing the waveform with itself for all possible lags, but instead of integrating over time.

The Wigner-Ville distribution is sometimes also referred to as the Heisenberg wavelet. By definition, it is the Fourier transform of the central covariance function. For any time series, x(t), we can define the central variance as

$$C_c(\tau,t) = x(t-\frac{\tau}{2})x^*(t+\frac{\tau}{2}) \tag{12}$$

Then the Wigner-Ville distribution is

$$V(\omega,t) = \int_{-\infty}^{+\infty} C_c(\tau,t)e^{-i\omega\tau}d\tau \tag{13}$$

The classic method of computing the power spectrum was to take the Fourier transform of the standard autocorrelation function. The Wigner-Ville distribution echoes this approach by taking the Fourier transform of the instantaneous autocorrelation function, but only along the τ (i.e., lag) dimension. The result is a function of both frequency and time.

3.3 Evolutionary spectrum

The evolutionary spectrum was proposed by Priestley [5]. The basic idea is to extend the classic Fourier spectral analysis to a more generalized basis: from sine or cosine to a family of orthogonal functions $\varphi(\omega,t)$ indexed by time, t, and defined for all real ω, the frequency. Any real random variable, x(t), can be expressed as

$$x(t) = \int_{-\infty}^{+\infty} \varphi(\omega,t)dA(\omega,t) \tag{14}$$

in which $dA(\omega,t)$, the Stieltjes function for the amplitude, is related to the spectrum as

$$E(|dA(\omega,t)|^2) = d\mu(\omega,t) = S(\omega,t)d\omega \tag{15}$$

where $\mu(\omega,t)$ is the spectrum, and $S(\omega,t)$ is the spectral density at a specific time t, also designated as the evolutionary spectrum.

4. Empirical mode decomposition

A recently proposed method, the Hilbert-Huang Transform (HHT) [3], satisfies the condition of adaptation employed in nonlinear - nonstationary time series processing. HHT consists of EMD and Hilbert Spectral Analysis (HSA) [6]. The lack of mathematical foundation and analytical expressions sets difficulty in the theoretical study of the method. Nevertheless there has been an exhaustive validation in an empirical fashion especially in the time-frequency representations [7].

Empirical Mode Decomposition (EMD) lies in the core of HHT method decomposing nonstationary time series originating from nonlinear systems in an adaptive fashion without predefined basis function. An intrinsic mode function (IMF) set is produced through an iterative process which is related to the underlying physical process.

Unlike wavelet processing, Hilbert-Huang transform decomposes a signal by direct extraction of the local energy associated with the time scales of the signal. This feature reveals the applicability of HHT in both nonstationary time series and signals originating from nonlinear biological systems.

Literature references' variety reveals the extensive range of EMD applications in several areas of the biomedical engineering field. Particularly there are publications concerning the application of EMD in the study of Heart Rate Variability (HRV) [8], analysis of respiratory mechanomyographic signals [9], ECG enhancement artifact and baseline wander correction [10], R-peak detection [11], Crackle sound analysis in lung sounds [12] and enhancement of cardiotocograph signals [13]. The method is employed for filtering electromyographic (EMG) signals in order to perform attenuation of the incorporated background activity [14]. Numerous research papers have been published concerning applications of EMD in biomedical signals and especially towards the direction of optimizing traditional techniques of acquisition and processing of signals such as Doppler ultrasound for the removal of artifacts [15], the analysis of complex time series such as human heartbeat interval [16], the identification of noise components in ECG time series [17] and the denoising of respiratory signals [18].

Lack of solid theoretical foundation concerning empirical mode decomposition constitutes the basis for a series of problems regarding the adaptive nature of the method as well as the selection of an efficient interpolation technique. Identification of nonlinear characteristics of the physical process and optimum threshold selection for the implementation of the algorithm set challenges for further research on EMD method.

The empirical mode decomposition does not require any known basis function and is considered a fully data driven mechanism suited for nonlinear processes and nonstationary signals.

Each component extracted (IMF) is defined as a function with

- Equal number of extrema and zero crossings (or at most differed by one)
- The envelopes (defined by all the local maxima and minima) are symmetric with respect to zero. This implies that the mean value of each IMF is zero.

Given a signal x(t), the algorithm of the EMD can be summarized as follows :

1. Locate local maxima and minima of $d_0(t)=x(t)$.

2. Interpolate between the maxima and connect them by a cubic spline curve. The same applies for the minima in order to obtain the upper and lower envelopes $e_u(t)$ and $e_l(t)$, respectively.
3. Compute the mean of the envelopes:

$$m(t) = \frac{e_u(t) + e_l(t)}{2} \tag{16}$$

4. Extract the detail $d_1(t)= d_0(t)-m(t)$ (sifting process)
5. Iterate steps 1-4 on the residual until the detail signal $d_k(t)$ can be considered an IMF (satisfy the two conditions): $c_1(t) = d_k(t)$
6. Iterate steps 1-5 on the residual $r_n(t)=x(t)- c_n(t)$ in order to obtain all the IMFs $c_1(t)$,.., $c_N(t)$ of the signal. The result of the EMD process produces N IMFs ($c_1(t)$, $c_2(t)$,…$c_N(t)$) and a residual signal ($r_N(t)$) :

$$x(t) = \sum_{n=1}^{N} c_n(t) + r_N(t) \tag{17}$$

In step 5, in order to terminate the sifting process it is commonly used a criterion which is the sum of difference

$$SD = \sum_{t=0}^{T} \frac{| d_{k-1}(t) - d_k(t) |^2}{d_{k-1}^2(t)} \tag{18}$$

When SD is smaller than a threshold, the first IMF is obtained and this procedure iterates till all the IMFs are obtained. In this case, the residual is either a constant, or a monotonic slope or a function with only one extremum.
Implementation of the aforementioned sifting process termination criterion along with the conditions that should be satisfied in order to acquire an IMF result in a set of check points in the algorithm (Eq. 19, 20, 21).

$$\sum \left\{ \frac{\text{MA}}{EA} > Threshold_1 \right\}_{boolean} < TOLERANCE \tag{19}$$

$$\frac{MA}{EA} < Threshold_2 \tag{20}$$

$$| \sum \text{zeros-} \sum \text{extrema} \; | <= 1 \tag{21}$$

where MA is the absolute value of m(t) and EA is given by the equation 22.

$$EA = \left| \frac{e_u(t) - e_l(t)}{2} \right| \tag{22}$$

Control of the progress of the algorithm and the IMF extraction process is determined by equations 19-22 and termination as well as the number of IMFs are related to the selection of threshold values. Different values result in different set of IMFs and significant computation effect on the whole process of the EMD algorithm especially at the level of the number of iterations required. Optimum threshold values are still under investigation in the research field concerning the method as well as in the effect on the set of IMFs and the relation of certain IMFs with the underlying physical process [19].

Each component extracted (IMF) is defined as a function with equal number of extrema and zero crossings (or at most differed by one) with its envelopes (defined by all the local maxima and minima) being symmetric with respect to zero.

The application of the EMD method results in the production of N IMFs and a residue signal. The first IMFs extracted are the lower order IMFs which captures the fast oscillation modes while the last IMFs produced are the higher order IMFs which represent the slow oscillation modes. The residue reveals the general trend of the time series.

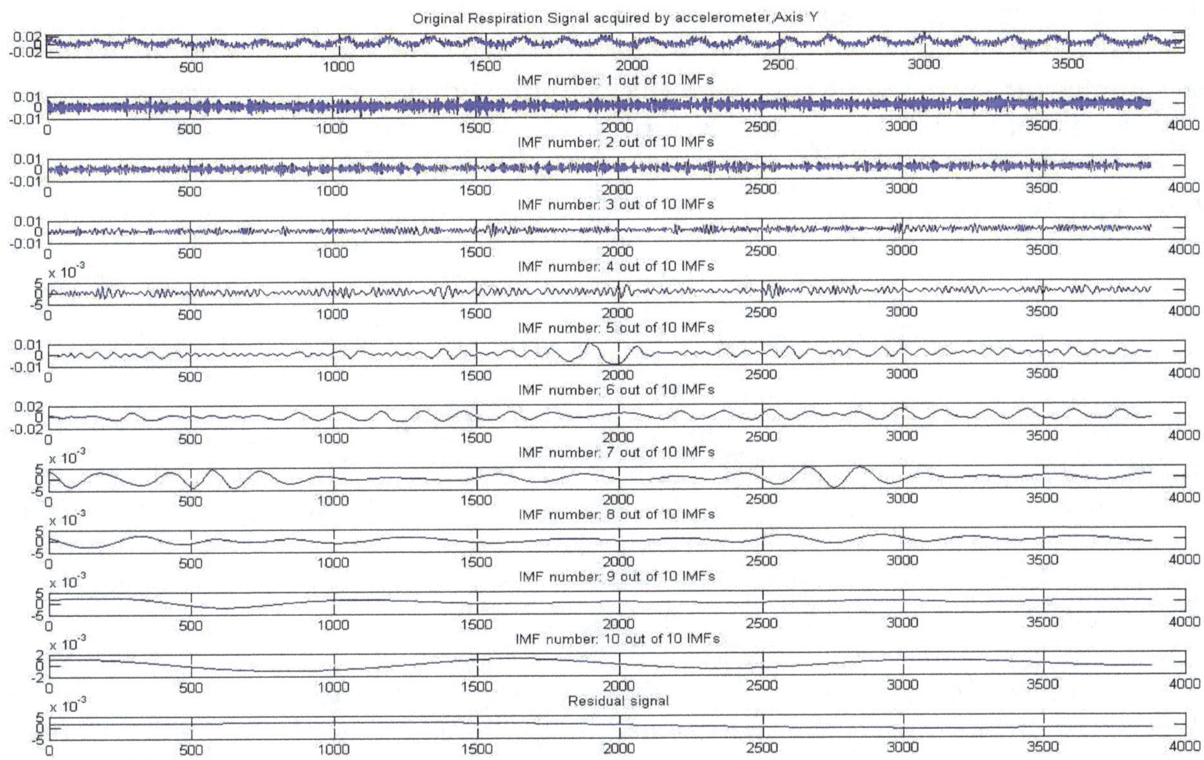

Fig. 2. Experimental respiratory signal processed with Empirical Mode Decomposition. At the upper plot is depicted the original signal Axis Y of a dual axis accelerometer which is sampled in both axes by a mote of a Wireless Sensor Network [18].

5. Statistical significance of IMFs

Intuitively, a subset of IMF set produced after the application of EMD on biomedical ECG time series is related to the signal originating from the physical process. Although high correlation values between the noise corrupted time series with specific IMFs may occur, there is a difficulty in defining a physical meaning and identifying those IMFs that carry information related to the underlying process.

The lack of EMD mathematical formulation and theoretical basis complicates the process of selecting the IMFs that may confidently be separated from the ones that are mainly attributed to noise. Flandrin et al [21] studied fractional Gaussian noise and suggested that

EMD acts as a dyadic filter. Wu and Huang [20] confirmed Flandrin's findings by studying White Gaussian Noise in time series processed with EMD. Wu and Huang empirically discovered a linear relationship between mean period and time series energy density expressed in log-log scale.

Study of noise statistical characteristics initiates the computation of the IMF's energy distribution function. The establishment of energy distribution spread function for various percentiles according to literature conclusions mentioned in this section constitutes an indirect way to quantify IMFs with strong noise components thus defines their statistical significance.

Each IMF probability function is approximately normally distributed, which is expected from the central limit theorem. This finding implies that energy density of IMFs should have a chi-square distribution (x^2).

Determination of the IMF mean period is accomplished by counting the number of extrema (local maxima-minima) or the number of zero crossings. The application results on typical 6000 samples MIT-BIH record 100 [23] for both unfiltered and Savitzky-Golay filtered time series are summarized in tables 2 and 3 respectively. Mean period is expressed in time units (sec) by taking into consideration the number of local maxima and the frequency sampling of the time series [22].

Energy Density of the nth IMF is calculated by mathematical expression 23.

$$E_n = \frac{1}{N}\sum_{j=1}^{N}[c_n(j)]^2 \tag{23}$$

Energy distribution and spread function constitute the basis for the development of a test in order to determine the IMFs statistical significance. The algorithm implemented is described below assuming that biomedical ECG time series are corrupted by White Gaussian Noise:

1. Decompose the noisy time series into IMFs via EMD.
2. Utilize the statistical characteristics of White Gaussian Noise in the time series to calculate energy spread function of various percentiles.
3. Select the confidence interval (95%, 99%) to determine upper and lower spread lines.
4. Compare the energy density of the IMFs with the spread function.

IMF energies that lie outside the area defined by the spread lines, determine the statistical significance of each one. The application results are depicted in figure 3 for a MIT-BIH ECG record 100 time series of 6000 samples length processed with Savitzky-Golay method. As far as step 2 of the algorithm concerns, a detailed approach is described in [20] with analytical formula expression for the determination of spread lines at various percentiles.

Statistical significance test indicates a way to separate information from noise in noise corrupted time series. Nevertheless, partial time series reconstruction by proper selection of the IMFs outside the spread lines area reveals that noisy components still exist in reconstructed time series. The interpretation of an IMF subset physical meaning by means of instantaneous frequencies, a typical characteristic of IMFs revealed when treated with Hilbert Transform, is based on the assumption that instantaneous frequencies related to the underlying process are spread in the whole IMF set. Combining this observation with the addition of white Gaussian noise and the application of the algorithm that takes into advantage the statistical characteristics of WGN one draws the conclusion that the algorithm proposed is lossy in terms of physical meaning in the reconstructed time series. A loss of information related to the underlying process is caused due to exclusion of an IMF subset.

This observation reveals a trade off situation in the level of partial signal reconstruction between the amount of information related to the physical process in the reconstructed time series and the noise level. Inclusion of wider IMF subset in the reconstruction process also increases noise levels and deteriorates SNR in the reconstructed time series.
Reconstruction process results of the proposed algorithm are presented in [17] for a MIT-BIH ECG record time series of 6000 samples length which is EMD processed and the algorithm of IMFs statistical significance is applied. Cross correlation value of 0.7 is achieved only by including the statistically significant IMFs.

IMF	1	2	3	4	5	6	7	8	9	10	11	12	13	14	15	16
# extrema	1764	943	691	537	430	351	265	211	212	112	85	44	22	8	5	1
Mean Period (sec)	0.003	0.006	0.009	0.011	0.014	0.017	0.023	0.028	0.028	0.054	0.071	0.136	0.273	0.750	1.200	6.001

Table 2. IMFs mean period of 6000 samples unfiltered MIT-BIH ECG record 100

IMF	1	2	3	4	5	6	7	8	9	10	11	12	13
# extrema	1123	735	456	349	283	245	125	94	64	38	21	7	1
Mean Period (sec)	0.005	0.008	0.013	0.017	0.021	0.025	0.048	0.064	0.094	0.158	0.286	0.857	6.001

Table 3. IMFs mean period of 6000 samples Savitzky-Golay filtered MIT-BIH ECG record 100

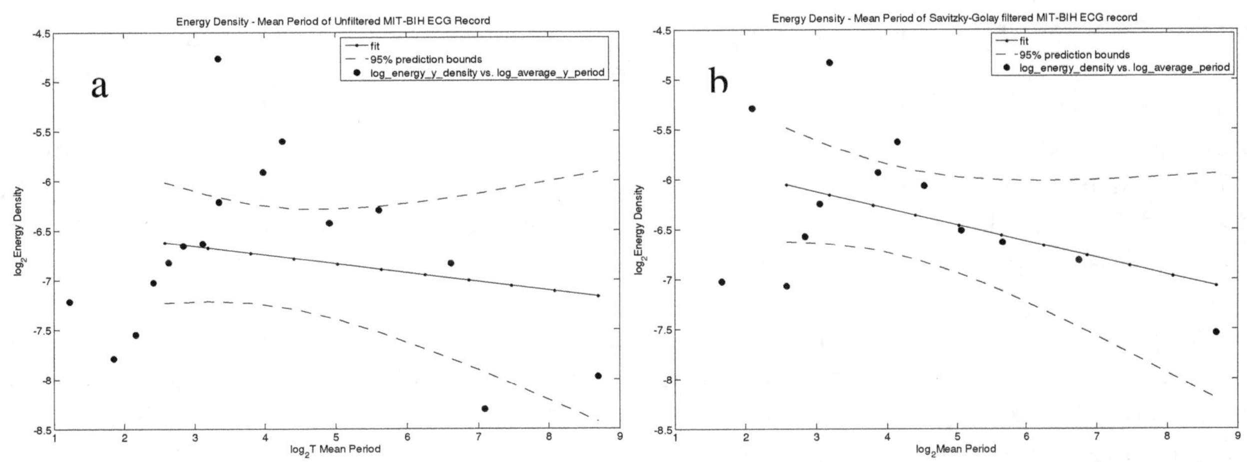

Fig. 3. IMF Energy Density of MIT-BIH ECG record 100 of 6000 samples as a function of the Mean Period. Fitting of the experimental results exhibits a linear relationship for log-log scale of IMF's Energy Density and Mean Period at 95% confidence interval.

6. Noise assisted data processing with empirical mode decomposition

Time series are considered to be IMFs if they satisfy two conditions concerning the number of zero crossings and extrema (equal or at most differ by one) and the required symmetry of the envelopes with respect to zero. A complete description of the EMD algorithm is included in [3].

The majority of data analysis techniques aim at the removal of noise in order to facilitate the following stages of the processing-analysis chain. However, in certain cases, noise is added to the time series to assist the detection of weak signals and delineate the underlying process. A common technique in the category of Noise Assisted Data Analysis (NADA) methods is pre-whitening. Adding noise to time series is an assistive way for the investigation of analysis method sensitivity. Furthermore the superimposition of noise samples following specific distribution functions in time series facilitates the study of EMD performance in processing of typical noise corrupted biomedical signals.

In the framework of NADA applications on biomedical signals, the addition of White Gaussian Noise (WGN) boosts the tendency of time series to develop extrema. EMD sensitivity in extrema detection is related to the interpolation technique. In the current implementation, cubic spline curve is selected as the interpolation technique; still there are multiple arguments in literature for different interpolation schemes.

The proposed methodology is depicted in figure 4. Simulated biomedical signals, in this case electrocardiogram (ECG), are contaminated with WGN in a controlled way. The study of EMD performance is accomplished by comparative evaluation of the method results in respect of three aspects. First, EMD performance is studied by investigating the statistical significance of an IMF set. Secondly, computation time of the method's application on biomedical signals is measured in both possible routes depicted in methodology diagram and thirdly the size of the IMF set is monitored.

The preprocessing stage is carefully selected after an exhaustive literature review and represents three different filtering techniques in order to tackle with various artifacts present in ECG time series. Namely, it constitutes a preparative stage, which changes the spectral characteristics of the time series in a predefined way.

Mainly there are two modes of operation in electrocardiography, the monitor mode and diagnostic mode. Highpass and lowpass filters are incorporated in monitor mode with cutoff frequencies in the range of 0.5-1Hz and 40Hz respectively. The selection of the aforementioned cutoff frequencies is justified by the accomplishment of artifact limitation in routine cardiac rhythm monitoring (Baseline Wander reduction, power line suppression). In diagnostic mode, lowpass filter cutoff frequency range is wider from 40Hz to 150Hz whereas for highpass filter cutoff frequency is usually set at 0.05Hz (for accurate ST segment recording).

Apparently noise assisted data analysis methods coexistence with noise reduction techniques set two antagonistic factors. The target for the addition of white Gaussian noise is threefold. It simulates a typical real world biomedical signal case whereas the superimposition of noise samples increase the number of extrema developed in the time series in order to evaluate EMD application results due to the high sensitivity of the method in extrema detection. Finally, the study of the IMF set statistical significance is facilitated taking under consideration the noise samples distribution function as well as the statistical properties of the noisy time series.

Preprocessing stage implemented as various filtering techniques is commonly incorporated in typical biomedical signal processing chain. Apart from the trivial case of taking into account these techniques to process ECG time series, preprocessing stage is introduced prior to the application of EMD method in order to comparatively evaluate the performance of the mixed scheme in terms of size of IMF set and its statistical significance as well as the total computation time. Each technique deals with specific types of artifacts in ECG time series and a significant part of initial noise level is still present in the time series processed via EMD.

The flowchart of the proposed methodology is applied on both simulated and real record ECG time series and the branch outputs are compared in order to evaluate the pre-processing stage and the effect in EMD performance.

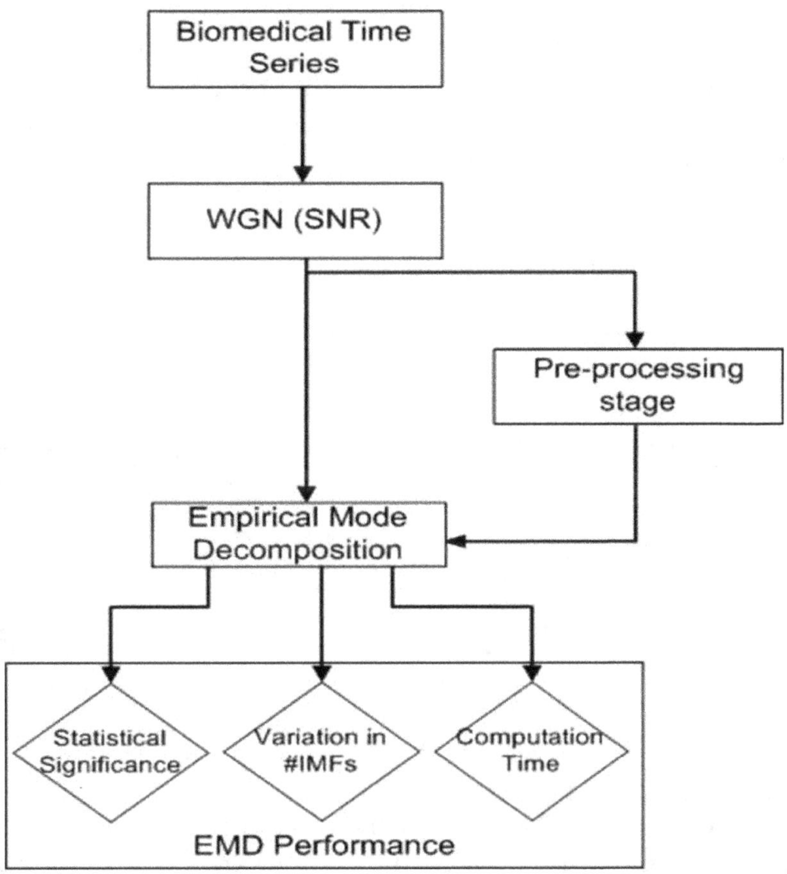

Fig. 4. Methodology process for the performance study of EMD applied on ECG time series

Results of the proposed methodology are provided in [22] and [17] with more details concerning the pre-processing stage which is implemented as typical filters and the way this stage affects the output of the empirical mode decomposition application on the simulated and real biomedical time series. Empirical mode decomposition performance is checked in terms of statistical significance of the IMF set produced, the variation of the IMF set length as a function of time series length and SNR and the computation time.

Some results are included in this chapter and depicted in figure 5.

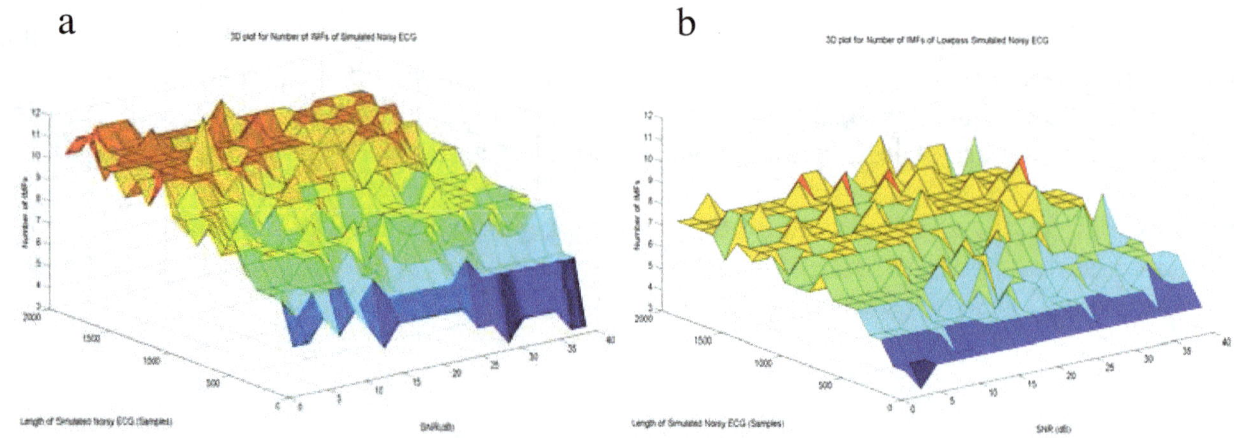

Fig. 5. a. 3D plots of the number of IMFs as a function of the SNR and the length of a simulated White Gaussian Noise corrupted ECG time series without the application of preprocessing stage (a) and with application of a lowpass filter (b), See [22].

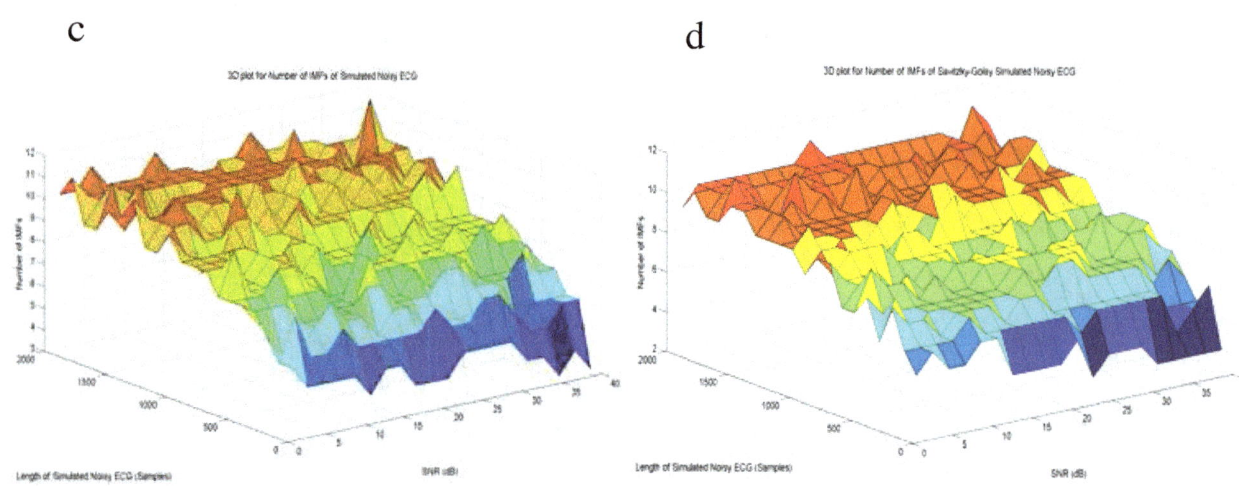

Fig. 5. b. 3D plots of the number of IMFs as a function of the SNR and the length of a simulated White Gaussian Noise corrupted ECG time series without the application of preprocessing stage (c) and with application of the Savitzky-Golay filter (d), See [22].

Savitzky-Golay method is considered mainly for its wide acceptance in ECG processing and especially for the ability of the filter to preserve the peaks with minimal distortion. Minor effects are expected on the peaky nature of the noise corrupted ECG time series. As a result, the variation in the number of extracted IMFs after the application of EMD on Savitzky-Golay filtered ECG time series is relatively small.

The effect on the peaky nature of time series processed with lowpass filters results in the reduction of the IMF set size. Various cut-off frequencies attenuate in a different way high frequency content. Number of extrema is decreased in the lowpass filtered time series however distribution of peaks in the time series is dependent on the frequency components distorted by the different cut-off frequencies.

7. Computation time considerations for empirical mode decomposition

Considering the characteristics of EMD algorithm a straight forward way for computation time estimation takes into account the size of IMF set as well as the number of iterations required in order to produce this set. This goes down to implementation issues concerning the EMD algorithm and the thresholds used in termination criterion as well as the maximum number of iterations allowed.

Multiple lengths of noise corrupted simulated ECG time series of various SNR levels are studied. For demonstration reasons the minimum and maximum number of samples (1000, 8000) are depicted in figure 6 along with the computation time of unfiltered EMD processed time series.

Computation time of EMD processed ECG time series is depicted in figure 6 for comparison reasons. In both graphs EMD performance in terms of computation time is worst compared to the corresponding performance of ECG time series preprocessed with the suitable filter. Overall, EMD performance of LP_1 highlights the important role of suitable preprocessing stage selection [22].

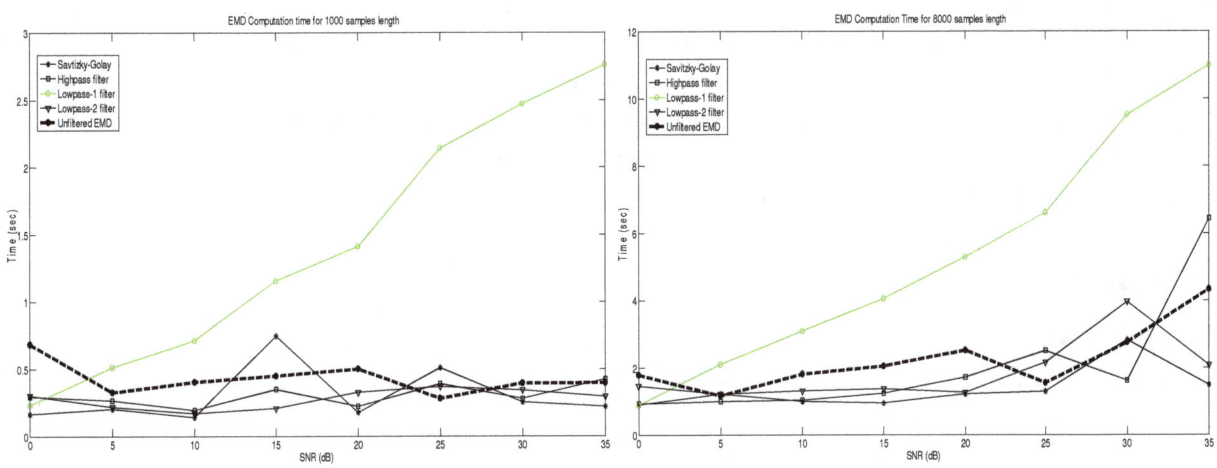

Fig. 6. Comparison results of EMD Computation Time for 1000 and 8000 samples of Simulated ECG time series

8. Conclusions - discussion

In practice, in noisy time series it is difficult to separate confidently information from noise. The implemented algorithm deduces a 95% bound for the white Gaussian noise in ECG time series. The core idea is based on the assumption that energy density of an IMF exceeds a noise bound if it represents statistically significant information.

Preprocessing stage affects the spectral characteristics of the input signal and any distortions of the time series' statistical and spectral contents have an effect in EMD performance. Based on the inherent properties of the time series to be processed, one may select an appropriate preprocessing stage in order to achieve smaller number of IMFs and minimization of computation time without changing in a significant degree the physical content of IMFs.

Total computation time is an essential aspect that should be taken under consideration when implementing EMD algorithm on resource constrained systems. It is concluded that time series length, number of extrema and total number of iterations are significant parameter determining total computation time.

Simulation campaigns remain the only way to study EMD performance and various issues related to the method due to the lack of analytical expression and solid theoretical ground.

EMD implementation takes into account the termination criterion, a significant parameter to be optimized in order to avoid numerous iterations for the extraction of IMFs. Research effort is still to be undertaken to investigate in what degree tight restrictions in number of iterations drain the physical content of IMFs. An optimization procedure for both termination criterion and number of iterations is an open issue in this field.

Considering ECG time series of low SNR levels, noise is prevalent resulting in smoother spline curves and generally faster extraction due to smaller number of iterations. In high SNR, a tendency is observed towards the increase of computation time raising the issue of the optimum magnitude of noise to be added in the signal in NADA methods.

Empirical mode decomposition is a widely used method which has been applied on multiple biomedical signals for the processing and analysis. Focus is given on both application issues as well as the properties of the method and the formulation of a mathematical basis. Since this issue is addressed the only option remains the simulation and numerical experiments. It has been proved that empirical mode decomposition has various advantages compared to other methods which are employed in biomedical signal processing such as wavelets, Fourier analysis, etc. Research interest about the method is rapidly growing as it is represented by the number of related publications.

9. References

[1] Kendall M. Time-Series. Charles Griffin, London,UK,2nd edition,1976

[2] Papoulis A. Probability, Random Variables and Stochastic Processes. McGraw-Hill, New York, NY, 1965

H. H. Liu, 1998: The empirical mode decomposition method and the Hilbert spectrum for non-stationary time series analysis, Proc. Roy. Soc. London, 454A, 903-995.

[4] Semmlow J.L., Biosignal and Biomedical Image Processing, Signal Processing and Communications Series, Mercel Dekker, NY, 2004

[5] Priestley, M. B. 1965 Evolutionary spectra and non-stationary processes. J. R. Statist. Soc. B27, 204{237.

[6] S. Hahn: Hilbert Transforms in Signal Processing. Artech House, 442pp, 1995

[7] N.E Huang, M.C Wu, S.R Long, S.S.P Shen, W. Qu, P. Gloersen, K.L Fan, A confidence limit for the empirical mode decomposition and Hilbert spectral analysis. Proc. R. Soc. A 459, 2317–2345 pp. doi:10.1098/rspa.2003.1123, 2003

[8] J. C. Echeverría, J. A. Crowe, M. S. Woolfson and B. R. Hayes-Gill, Application of empirical mode decomposition to heart rate variability analysis. Med. Biol. Eng. Comput. Volume 39, Number 4, 471-479pp, DOI: 10.1007/BF02345370, 2001

[9] Abel Torres, José A. Fiz, Raimon Jané, Juan B. Galdiz, Joaquim Gea, Josep Morera, Application of the Empirical Mode Decomposition method to the Analysis of Respiratory Mechanomyographic Signals, Proceedings of the 29th Annual International Conference of the IEEE EMBS Cité Internationale, Lyon, France

[10] M. Blanco-Velasco, B. Weng, KE Barner, ECG signal denoising and baseline wander correction based on the empirical mode decomposition. Comput. Biol Med; 38(1):1-13pp 2008 Jan

[11] AJ Nimunkar, WJ Tompkins. R-peak detection and signal averaging for simulated stress ECG using EMD. Conf Proc IEEE Eng Med Biol Soc. 2007; 1261-1264pp, 2007

[12] S. Charleston-Villalobos, R. Gonzalez-Camarena, G. Chi-Lem,; T. Aljama-Corrales, Crackle Sounds Analysis by Empirical Mode Decomposition. Engineering in Medicine and Biology Magazine, IEEE Vol. 26, Issue 1, Page(s):40 – 47pp, Jan.-Feb. 2007

[13] B.N. Krupa, M.A. Mohd Ali, E.Zahedi. The application of empirical mode decomposition for the enhancement of cardiotocograph signals. Physiol. Meas. 30, 729-743pp, 2009

[14] A. O. Andrade, V. Nasuto, P. Kyberd, C. M. Sweeney-Reed, F.R. V. Kanijn, EMG signal filtering based on Empirical Mode Decomposition, Biomedical Signal Processing and Control, Volume 1, Issue 1, 44-55 pp, DOI: 10.1016/j.bspc.2006.03.003, January 2006

[15] Y. Zhang, Y Gao, L Wang, J Chen, X Shi. The removal of wall components in Doppler ultrasound signals by using the empirical mode decomposition algorithm, IEEE Trans Biomed Eng. Sep; 54(9):1631-1642 pp, 2007

[16] Yeh JR, Sun WZ, Shieh JS, Huang NE Intrinsic mode analysis of human heartbeat time series, Ann Biomed Eng. 2010 Apr;38(4):1337-1344 pp. Epub 2010 Jan 30

[17] Karagiannis A., Constantinou, P., Noise components identification in biomedical signals based on Empirical Mode Decomposition, 9th International Conference on Information Technology and Applications in Biomedicine, ITAB 2009. 10.1109/ITAB.2009.5394300, 2009

[18] Karagiannis A., Loizou L., Constantinou, P., Experimental respiratory signal analysis based on Empirical Mode Decomposition, First International Symposium on Applied Sciences on Biomedical and Communication Technologies,. ISABEL 2008. 10.1109/ISABEL.2008.4712581, 2008

[19] Karagiannis, A.; Constantinou, P.; , "Investigating performance of Empirical Mode Decomposition application on electrocardiogam," Biomedical Engineering Conference (CIBEC), 2010 5th Cairo International , vol., no., pp.1-4, 16-18 Dec. 2010 doi: 10.1109/CIBEC.2010.5716048

[20] Z. Wu, N.E. Huang: A study of the characteristics of white noise using the empirical mode decomposition method. Proc. R. Soc. London, Ser. A, 460, 1597-1611 pp, 2004

[21] P.Flandrin, G. Rilling, P. Goncalves, Empirical Mode Decomposition as a filter bank. IEEE Signal Process Letter, 11, 112-114 pp, 2004.

[22] Karagiannis, A.; Constantinou, P.; "Noise-Assisted Data Processing With Empirical Mode Decomposition in Biomedical Signals," Information Technology in Biomedicine, IEEE Transactions on, vol.15, no.1, pp.11-18, Jan. 2011 doi: 10.1109/TITB.2010.2091648

[23] http://www.physionet.org/physiobank/database/mitdb

7

Spatial Unmasking of Speech Based on Near-Field Distance Cues

Craig Jin[1], Virginia Best[2], Gaven Lin[2] and Simon Carlile[2]
[1]*School of Electrical and Information Engineering, The University of Sydney, Sydney NSW*
[2]*School of Medical Sciences and Bosch Institute, The University of Sydney, Sydney NSW Australia*

1. Introduction

These days it is recognised that for bilateral hearing loss there is generally benefit in fitting two hearing aids, one for each ear (see Byrne, 1980 and Feuerstein, 1992 for clinical studies, see Byrne *et al.*, 1992, Durlach *et al.*, 1981, and Zurek, 1981 for laboratory studies). Bilateral fitting is now standard practice for children with bilateral loss and as of 2005 bilateral fittings account for approximately 75% of all fittings (Libby, 2007). Nonetheless, it is only within the last half-decade that it has become possible to transfer audio signals between bilaterally-fitted hearing aids (Moore, 2007). This is primarily attributed to the technological advances in integrated circuit design, longer lasting batteries and also wireless inter-communication between the two hearing aids, e.g., using near-field magnetic induction (NFMI) communication. The possibility to exchange audio signals between bilaterally-fitted aids opens the door to new types of binaural signal processing algorithms to assist hearing-impaired listeners separate sounds of interest from background noise. In this chapter, we consider whether or not the manipulation of near-field distance cues may provide a viable binaural signal processing algorithm for hearing aids. More specifically, this chapter describes three experiments that explore the spatial unmasking of speech based on near-field distance cues.

In a typical cocktail party setting, listeners are faced with the challenging task of extracting information by sifting through a mixture of multiple talkers overlapping in frequency and time. This challenge arises as a result of interference in the form of energetic masking, where sounds are rendered inaudible due to frequency overlap, and informational masking, where sounds from different sources are confused with one another (Bronkhorst, 2000; Brungart *et al.*, 2001; Kidd *et al.*, 2008). Despite this, listeners are reasonably adept at parsing complex mixtures and attending to separate auditory events.

One factor that influences speech intelligibility in mixtures is perceived spatial location. Many studies have established that sounds originating from separate locations are easier to distinguish than sounds which are co-located (Hirsh, 1950; Bronkhorst and Plomp, 1988; Ebata, 2003). Separating sounds in space can result in an increase in the signal-to-noise ratio at one ear (the 'better ear'). Moreover, sounds that are spatially separated give rise to differences in binaural cues (interaural time and level differences, ITDs/ILDs) that can improve audibility by reducing energetic masking (Durlach and Colburn, 1978;

Zurek, 1993). Perceived differences in location can also be used as a basis for perceptual streaming, and this has been shown to be a particularly important factor in the segregation of talkers with similar voice characteristics, resulting in a significant reduction of informational masking (Kidd *et al.*, 1998; Freyman *et al.*, 1999; Arbogast *et al.*, 2002; Drennan *et al.*, 2003).

While many studies have established the role of spatial cues in the unmasking of speech mixtures, the majority of these have focused on sources at a fixed, relatively far distance, with spatial separation in the azimuthal plane. Very few studies have examined the perception of speech mixtures in the acoustic 'near field', defined as the region less than one meter from the listener's head. Unlike in the far field, spatial cues at the two ears vary substantially as a function of distance in the near field (Brungart and Rabinowitz, 1999). Listeners can use these cues to estimate the distance of sources in the immediate vicinity (Brungart *et al.*, 1999). A primary distance cue is overall intensity, with near sounds being louder than far sounds. In addition, ILDs increase dramatically with decreasing distance in both high and low frequency regions. Most notably, low-frequency ILDs, which are negligible in the far field, can be as large as 20 dB in the near field (Brungart, 1999; Brungart and Rabinowitz, 1999). In contrast, ITDs in the near field are independent of distance and remain relatively constant. This study investigated whether the increased ILD cues that occur at different distances in this region can provide a basis for improving speech segregation. Understanding the effect of distance cues on speech segregation will also enable a more complete picture of how spatial perception influences behaviour in cocktail party settings.

Two previous studies have shown that spatial separation of sources in the near field can lead to benefits in speech intelligibility. Shinn-Cunningham *et al.* (2001) showed that separating speech and noise in the near field could lead to improvements in speech reception thresholds. When one sound was fixed at one meter and the other was moved in closer to the listener, an improved target to masker ratio (TMR) occurred at one ear. In this case, masking was energetic and performance benefits were well-predicted by improvements in audibility. A study by Brungart and Simpson (2002) showed that separation of two talkers in distance improved accuracy in a speech segregation task. After controlling for better ear effects they found that there was an additional perceptual benefit, particularly when talkers were acoustically similar (the same sex). This suggests that distance cues in the near field may provide a basis for release from informational masking.

The primary aim of the current study was to further investigate the effects of near field distance cues on speech segregation. The first experiment was an extension of the study by Brungart and Simpson (2002). The aim was to measure the benefit of separating two competing talkers in distance, where one was fixed at one meter and the other was moved closer to the head. While Brungart and Simpson examined only the case where the two talkers were equal in level (0-dB TMR) and most easily confused, the current study aimed to discover whether this benefit generalized to a larger range of TMR values. Experiment 2 was identical to Experiment 1, but assessed whether low-frequency (< 2 kHz) spatial cues alone could produce the effects seen in Experiment 1. Experiment 3 investigated the effect of moving a mixture of three talkers (separated in azimuth) closer to the head. It was predicted that this manipulation, which effectively exaggerates the spatial cues, would offer improved segregation of the competing talkers.

2. General methods

2.1 Subjects

Eight subjects (six males and two females, aged between 20 and 32) participated in the experiments. Only one subject had previous experience with auditory experiments involving similar stimuli.

2.2 Virtual auditory space

Individualized head-related transfer functions for the generation of virtual spatialized stimuli were recorded in an anechoic chamber, and details of the procedure can be found elsewhere (Pralong and Carlile, 1994, 1996). In brief, a movable loudspeaker (VIFA-D26TG-35) presented Golay codes from 393 locations on a sphere of radius 1 m around the subject's head. Binaural impulse responses were collected using a blocked-ear approach, with microphones (Sennheiser KE 4-211-2) placed in the subject's ear canals. Recordings were digitized at a sampling rate of 80 kHz, and converted to directional transfer functions (DTFs) by removing location-independent components. The DTFs were bandpass filtered between 300 Hz and 16 kHz, the range in which the measurement system is reliable, but then the energy below 300 Hz was interpolated based on the spherical head model (below) so that fundamental frequency energy in the speech stimuli would not be filtered out.

A distance variation function (DVF) as described by Kan *et al.* (2009) was used to convert the far-field DTFs (1-m distance) to near-field DTFs (0.25- and 0.12-m distances). The DVF approximates the frequency-dependent change in DTF magnitude as a function of distance. It is based on the rigid sphere model of acoustic scattering developed by Rabinowitz *et al.* (1993) and experimentally verified by Duda and Martens (1998). According to this model, the head can be approximated as a rigid sphere of radius a with ears toward the back of the head at 110° from the mid-sagittal plane. If a sinusoidal point source of sound of frequency 'ω' is presented at distance 'r' and angle θ from the centre of the head, the sound pressure 'p' at the ear can be expressed as:

$$p(a,\omega,\theta,r) = -kr\sum_{m=0}^{\infty}(2m+1)\frac{h_m(kr)}{h'_m(ka)}P_m(\cos\theta)e^{-ikr} \tag{1}$$

where h_m is the spherical Hankel function, k is the wave number, and P_m is the Legendre polynomial. DVFs were applied to each subject's individualized DTFs. The head radius, a, for each subject was determined using Kuhn's (1977) equation:

$$\text{ITD} = \frac{3a}{c}\sin\theta_{\text{inc}} \tag{2}$$

where c is the speed of sound in air, θ is the angle of incidence to the head, and ITD is the ITD measured from a pair of DTFs using cross-correlation. Individualized DTFs modified with the DVF in this way were recently verified psychophysically for their ability to give rise to accurate near-field localization estimates (Kan *et al.*, 2009). Fig. 1 shows a set of example DVF gain functions (to be applied to 1-m DTFs) as a function of frequency and distance for three azimuthal locations that were used in the study.

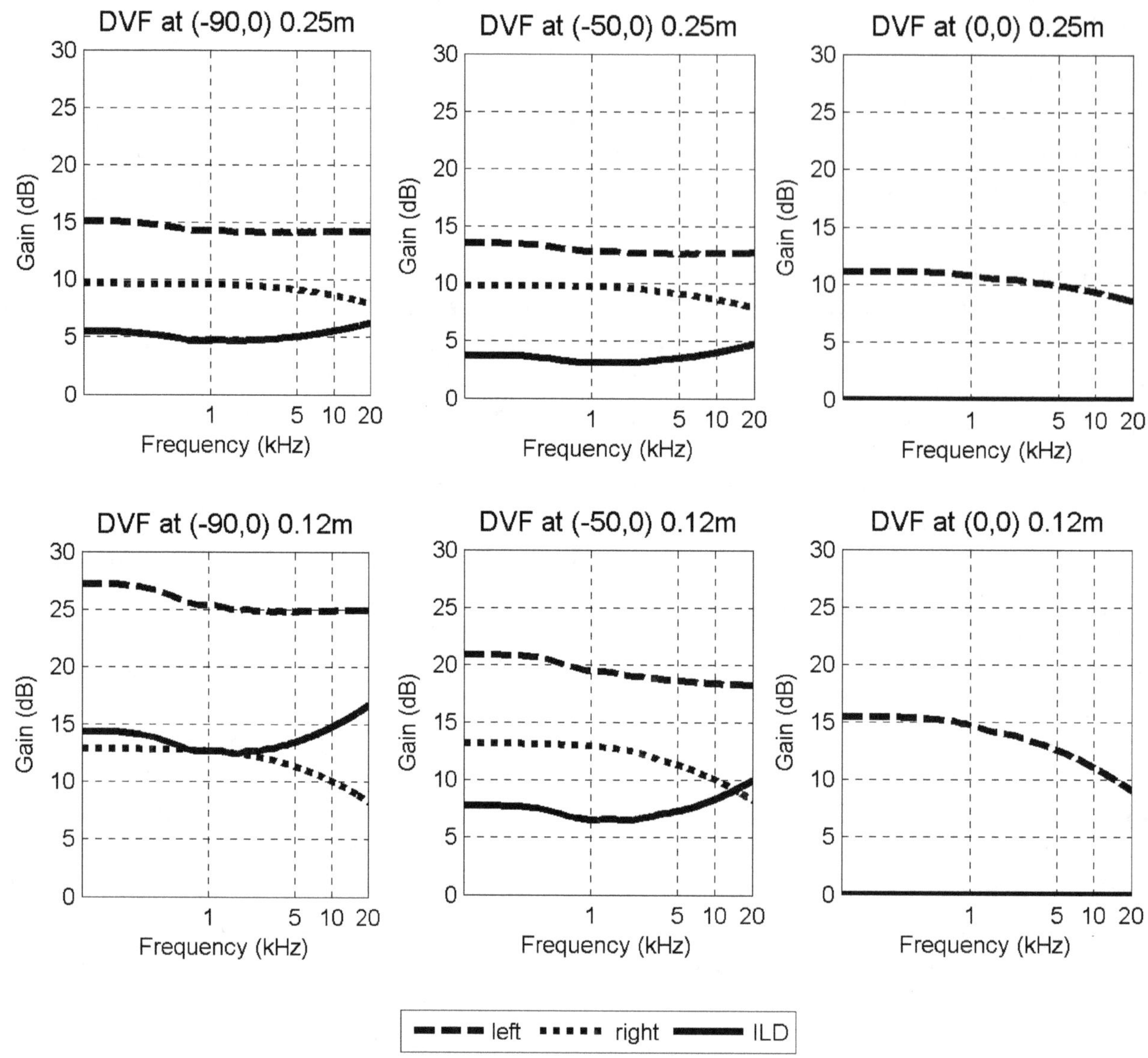

Fig. 1. The DVF for three locations and two near-field distances. The gain in dB is relative to the 1-m far-field case for each azimuth, and is shown for the left and right ears. Shown also is the induced ILD, which increases with increasing laterality (-90°>-50°>0°) and decreasing distance (0.12 m>0.25 m>1 m).

2.3 Speech stimuli

The speech stimuli used for this study were taken from the Coordinate Response Measure (CRM) corpus (Bolia *et al.*, 2000). Each sentence is comprised of a call sign, color and number, spoken in the form "Ready (call sign) go to (color) (number) now". There are a total of 8 possible call signs ("arrow", "baron", "eagle", "hopper", "laker", "ringo", "tiger" and "charlie"), 4 possible colors ("red", "blue", "green" and "white") and 8 possible numbers (1-8). In total, there are 256 possible phrases, which are spoken by a total of 8 different talkers (4 male and 4 female), giving 2048 distinct phrases in the corpus.

In each experimental trial, the sentences were randomly selected without replacement and were chosen such that each sentence in a mixture had a unique talker, call sign, number and color. The same gender was used for each talker in a given trial. The call sign

"Charlie" was always assigned to the target. Sentences were normalized to the same RMS level and resampled from 40 kHz to 48 kHz for playback. The target sentence was then adjusted to achieve the desired TMR before all sentences were filtered through the relevant DTFs (also resampled to 48 kHz) and digitally added. There was no normalization of the stimulus level after the DTF filtering, thus the stimulus level would increase when presented nearer to the head. The stimuli were presented at a comfortable listening level that corresponded to a sensation level of approximately 40 dB for a source directly ahead at a distance of 1 m.

Experiments were conducted in a small audiometric booth. Stimuli were presented via an RME soundcard (48 kHz sampling rate) and delivered using insert earphones (Etymotic Research ER-1[1]). Subjects were seated in front of an LCD monitor, and registered their responses (a color and number combination for the target stimulus) by clicking with a mouse on a custom-made graphical user interface.

2.4 Analysis of results

The listener responses were scored as correct if both the color and number were reported correctly, and percent correct scores (over the 40 repetitions) were plotted as a function of TMR to give raw psychometric functions for each spatial configuration. However, a nominal TMR at the source gives rise to different TMRs at the listener's ears for different spatial configurations (according to the DVF). Thus, a normalization stage was applied to the data to factor out these changes in TMR at the ear. Of particular interest was whether there was still a perceptual benefit of the distance manipulations after taking into account any energetic advantages.

The RMS levels of the target and maskers at each ear were calculated during the experiment for each individual subject under the different spatial configurations. These values were then averaged and used to determine the TMR at the better ear for each condition. This better-ear TMR represented a consistent shift from the nominal TMR, and thus the psychometric functions could be re-plotted as a function of better-ear TMR by a simple shift along the TMR axis. The average normalization shifts for each condition are shown in Tables 1 and 2. A single mean value was appropriate (rather than individual normalization values for each listener) because the values varied very little (range across listeners < 1dB).

The perceptual benefit of separating/moving sources in the near field was defined as the remaining benefit (in percentage points) after taking into account energetic effects. To calculate these benefits, the normalized psychometric functions for the reference conditions were subtracted from the normalized psychometric functions for the various near-field conditions. Values were interpolated using a linear approximation where required.

3. Experiment 1

3.1 Experimental conditions

The spatial configurations used in Experiment 1 were essentially the same as those used by Brungart and Simpson (2002). One target and one masker talker were simulated at -90°

---

[1] Note that the ER-1 earphones reintroduce the ear-canal resonance that is removed by the DTF.

azimuth, directly to the left of the listener. This region was expected to be particularly important in the study of near field perception due to the large ILDs that occur. As illustrated in Fig. 2, there were a total of five different target or masker distances. One talker was always fixed at 1 m while the other was moved closer to the listener in the near field. In some conditions, the masker was fixed at 1 m while the target was presented at 0.25 m or 0.12 m from the head. Conversely, in other conditions, the target was fixed at 1 m while the masker was presented at 0.25 m or 0.12 m from the head. In the co-located condition, both talkers were located at 1 m. Five different TMR values were tested for each spatial configuration (see Table 1), resulting in a total of 25 unique conditions. Two 20-trial blocks for each condition were completed by each listener resulting in a total of 2x20x25=1000 trials per listener. The spatial configuration and TMR were kept constant within a block, but the ordering of the blocks was randomized.

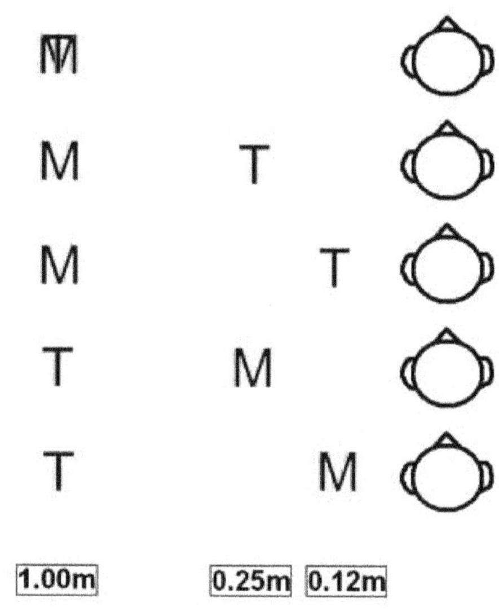

Fig. 2. The five spatial configurations used in Experiments 1 and 2. In one condition, both the target (T) and masker (M) were co-located at 1 m. In "target closer" conditions, the masker was fixed at 1 m while the target was located at 0.25 m or 0.12 m. In "masker closer" conditions, the target was fixed at 1 m while the masker was located at 0.25 m or 0.12 m.

Configuration	TMRs tested (dB)	Normalization shift (dB)
Target 1 m/Masker 1 m	[-30 -20 -10 0 10]	0
Target 0.25 m/Masker 1 m	[-40 -30 -20 -10 0]	+14
Target 0.12 m/Masker 1 m	[-40 -30 -20 -10 0]	+27
Target 1 m/Masker 0.25 m	[-20 -10 0 10 20]	-9
Target 1 m/Masker 0.12 m	[-20 -10 0 10 20]	-13

Table 1. The range of TMR values tested and normalization shifts for each spatial configuration in Experiments 1 and 2. The normalization shifts are the differences in the TMR at the better ear that resulted from variations in target or masker distance (relative to the co-located configuration).

3.2 Results

3.2.1 Masker fixed at 1 m and target near

The left column of Fig. 3 shows results (pooled across the eight listeners) from the conditions in which the masker was fixed at 1 m and the target was moved into the near field. Performance improved (Fig. 3, top left) when the target talker was moved closer (0.12 m>0.25 m>1 m). This trend was observed across all TMRs. Scores also increased with TMR as expected. A two-way repeated-measures ANOVA on the arcsine-transformed data[2] confirmed that there was a significant main effect of both target distance ($F_{2,14}$=266.5, p<.01) and TMR ($F_{3,21}$=58.2, p<.01). There was also a significant interaction ($F_{6,42}$=147.9, p<.01), implying that the effect of target distance differed depending on the TMR.

When the psychometric functions were re-plotted as a function of better-ear TMR, they looked almost identical (Fig. 3, middle left), except at 0-dB TMR. At this point, the co-located performance shows a characteristic plateau that is absent in the separated conditions, and this appears to drive the separation of the functions in this region. Fig. 3 (bottom left) shows the difference (in percentage points) between the separated conditions and the co-located condition as a function of TMR. The advantage is positive for the TMR range between -10 and 10 dB. T-tests confirmed that at 0-dB TMR, the advantages were significant for both the 0.25-m target (mean 23 percentage points, t_7=7.49, p<.01) and the 0.12-m target (mean 26 percentage points, t_7=8.29, p<.01).

3.2.2 Target fixed at 1 m and masker near

The right column of Fig. 3 shows results from the opposite conditions in which the target was fixed at 1 m and the masker was moved into the near field. The raw data (Fig. 3, top right) show that performance decreased as the masker was moved closer to the listener (1 m>0.25 m>0.12 m) for negative TMRs. However at higher TMRs, scores approached 100% for all distances. A two-way repeated-measures ANOVA on the arcsine-transformed data confirmed that there was a significant main effect of masker distance ($F_{2,14}$=37.4, p<.01) and TMR ($F_{3,21}$= 58.2, p<.01). The interaction did not reach significance ($F_{6,42}$=12.9, p=0.07).

When the psychometric functions were re-plotted as a function of better-ear TMR, there was a reversal in their ranking. Once the energetic disadvantage of moving a masker closer was compensated for, mean performance was slightly better when the masker was separated from the target compared to the co-located case. The benefit plots in Fig. 3 (bottom right) show that the spatial advantage was positive at all TMRs, but was particularly pronounced at 0-dB TMR. The advantage at 0-dB TMR was significant for both the 0.25-m masker (mean 26 percentage points, t_7= 7.71, p<.01) and the 0.12-m masker (mean 34 percentage points, t_7=8.44, p<.01). Again this benefit peaks in the region where the psychometric function for the co-located case is relatively flat.

The filled symbols in the middle and bottom rows of Fig. 3 show data from Brungart and Simpson (2002) under the analogous conditions of their study. Mean scores are higher overall in the current study (Fig. 3, middle row), however the benefit of separating talkers in distance is roughly the same across studies (Fig. 3, bottom row).

---

[2] The arcsine transformation converts binomially distributed data to an approximately normal distribution that is more suitable for statistical analysis (Studebaker, 1985).

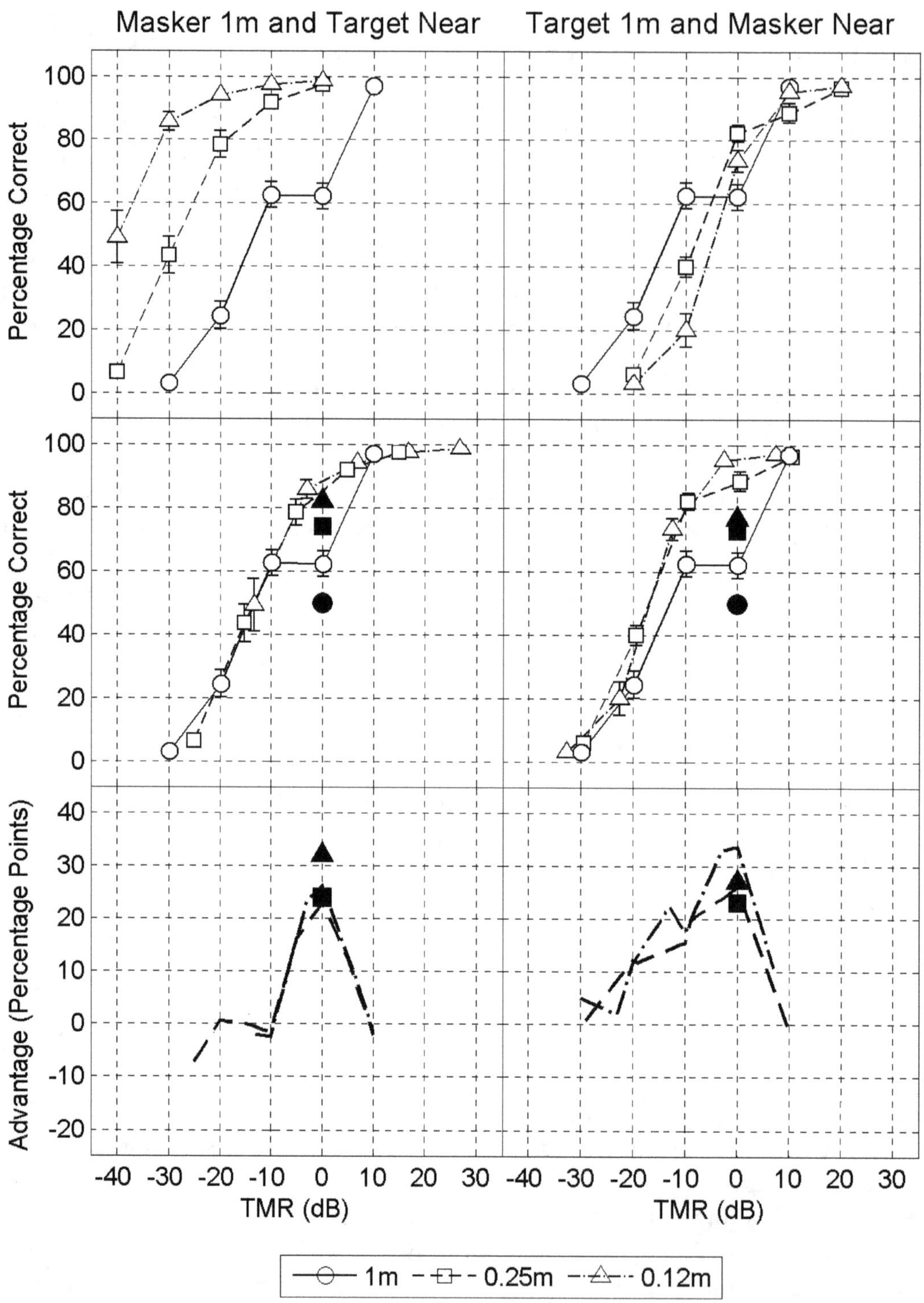

Fig. 3. Mean performance data averaged across all 8 subjects (error bars show standard errors of the means) in Experiment 1. The left panel displays the raw (top) and normalized (middle) data for the conditions where the masker was fixed at 1 m and the target was moved closer to the listener. The right panel displays the raw (top) and normalized (middle) data for the conditions where the target was fixed at 1 m and the masker was moved in closer to the listener. The bottom panels display the benefits of separation in distance, expressed as a difference in percentage points relative to the co-located case. The results obtained by Brungart and Simpson (2002) at 0-dB TMR are indicated by the black symbols.

3.3 Discussion

For a target and masker talker located at a fixed azimuth, target identification improved when the target was moved increasingly nearer to the head (relative to the case where both talkers were co-located at 1 m), but got worse when the masker moved closer. This basic pattern of results was likely driven by energetic effects: the closer source dominates the mixture and this either increases or reduces the effective TMR at the better ear depending on which source is moved.

The remaining benefit of spatial separation after the TMR changes were accounted for was restricted to a better-ear TMR region around 0 dB. This region is approximately where the psychometric function for the co-located case shows a clear plateau, which is no longer present in the separated cases. This plateau has been described previously (Egan *et al.*, 1954; Dirks and Bower, 1969; Brungart *et al.*, 2001), and is thought to represent the fact that listeners have the most difficulty segregating two co-located talkers when they are equal in level (0-dB TMR), but with differences in level listeners can attend to either the quieter or the louder talker. Apparently the perception of separation in distance also alleviates the particular difficulty of equal-level talkers, by providing a dimension along which to focus attention selectively. This finding adds to a growing body of evidence indicating that spatial differences can aid perceptual grouping and selective attention. Interestingly, the effect does not appear to be "all or nothing"; larger separations in distance gave rise to larger perceptual benefits. The lack of a spatial benefit at other TMRs, especially at highly negative TMRs, suggests that the main problem was audibility and not confusion between the target and the masker. Consistent with this idea, in the co-located condition, masker errors made up a larger proportion of the total errors as the TMR approached 0 dB. In Experiment 1, the proportion of masker errors was 38%, 45%, 62%, and 93% at -30, -20, -10, and 0-dB TMR.

Listeners in Experiment 1 performed around 10-20 percentage points better than Brungart and Simpson's (2002) listeners for the same stimulus configurations. This may be simply due to differences in the cohort of listeners, but there are two methodological factors that may have also played a role. Firstly, their study used HRTFs measured from an acoustic mannequin as opposed to individualized filters and thus the spatial percept may have been less realistic and thus less perceptually potent. Secondly, while the two studies used the same type of stimuli, Brungart and Simpson used a low-pass filtered version (upper cut-off of 8 kHz) and we used a broadband version (upper cut-off of 16 kHz). Despite the difference in overall scores, the mean benefit (in percentage points) obtained by separating talkers in distance was equivalent across the two studies.

4. Experiment 2

4.1 Experimental conditions

Experiment 2 was identical to Experiment 1 and used the same set of spatial configurations and TMRs (Fig. 2 and Table 1). The only difference was that the stimuli were all low-pass filtered (before RMS level equalization) at 2 kHz using an equiripple FIR filter with a stopband at 2.5 kHz that is 50 dB down from the passband.

4.2 Results

4.2.1 Masker fixed at 1 m and target near

The left column of Fig. 4 shows results from the conditions in which the masker was fixed at 1 m and the target was moved into the near field for the low-pass filtered stimuli of

Experiment 2. The raw data followed a similar trend to that observed in Experiment 1 (Fig. 4, top left). As the target was moved closer to the listener, performance improved, with best performance in the 0.12-m target case. A two-way repeated-measures ANOVA on the arcsine-transformed data revealed that there was a significant effect of target distance ($F_{2,14}$=332.9, p<.01) and TMR ($F_{3,21}$=120.6, p<.01) and a significant interaction ($F_{6,42}$=5.1, p<.05).

When the psychometric functions were plotted as a function of better-ear TMR, the results for all three distances were very similar (Fig. 4, middle left). After taking into account level changes with distance, there appears to be only a minor additional perceptual benefit of separating the low-pass filtered target and masker in distance. Fig. 4 (bottom left) shows that the advantage of separating the target from the masker was positive only for the small TMR range between -5 and +5 dB. The advantages across TMR were also smaller than those observed in Experiment 1. However, the advantages were still significant for both the 0.25-m target (mean 13 percentage points, t_7=4.20, p<.01) and the 0.12-m target (mean 17 percentage points, t_7=4.88, p<.01).

A three-way ANOVA with factors of bandwidth, distance, and TMR was conducted to compare performance in Experiments 1 and 2 in the target-near configuration (compare Fig. 3 and Fig. 4, top left). The main effect of bandwidth was significant ($F_{1,7}$=8.9, p<.05), indicating that performance was poorer for low-passed stimuli than for broadband stimuli overall. A separate two-way ANOVA on the benefits at 0 dB (compare Fig. 3 and Fig. 4, bottom left) found a significant main effect of distance ($F_{1,7}$=14.5, p<.01) but no significant effect of bandwidth ($F_{1,7}$=3.7, p=.10) and no interaction ($F_{1,7}$=0.7, p=.44).

4.2.2 Target fixed at 1 m and masker near

For the opposite configuration, where the masker was moved in closer (Fig. 4, right column), results were similar to those in Experiment 1. Listeners were less accurate at identifying the target when the masker was moved closer (Fig. 4, top right). A two-way repeated-measures ANOVA on the arcsine-transformed data revealed a significant effect of target distance ($F_{2,14}$=76.4, p<.01) and TMR ($F_{3,21}$=260.2, p<.01) and a significant interaction ($F_{6,42}$=5.1, p<.01).

Normalization of the curves based on better-ear TMR (Fig. 4, middle right) resulted in a reversal of the result, showing that there was indeed a perceptual benefit once the energetic disadvantage of a near masker was accounted for. Normalized scores were higher for maskers at 0.12 m and 0.25 m relative to 1 m, particularly around 0-dB TMR. This is reinforced by the benefit plots (Fig. 4, bottom right) which show that there was a positive advantage across all TMRs. Again, the largest advantage was observed at 0-dB TMR and was statistically significant for both the 0.25-m masker (mean 24 percentage points, t_7=7.31, p<.01) and the 0.12-m masker (mean 32 percentage points, t_7=7.51, p<.01).

A three-way ANOVA comparing the results from Experiments 1 and 2 in the masker-near configuration (compare Fig. 3 and Fig. 4, top right) revealed that performance was poorer for low-passed stimuli than for broadband stimuli overall ($F_{1,7}$=11.7, p<.05). A two-way ANOVA conducted on the benefits at 0 dB (compare Fig. 3 and Fig. 4, bottom right) found a significant main effect of distance ($F_{1,7}$=11.1, p<.05), but no significant effect of bandwidth ($F_{1,7}$=0.2, p=.66) and no interaction ($F_{1,7}$=0.6, p=.47).

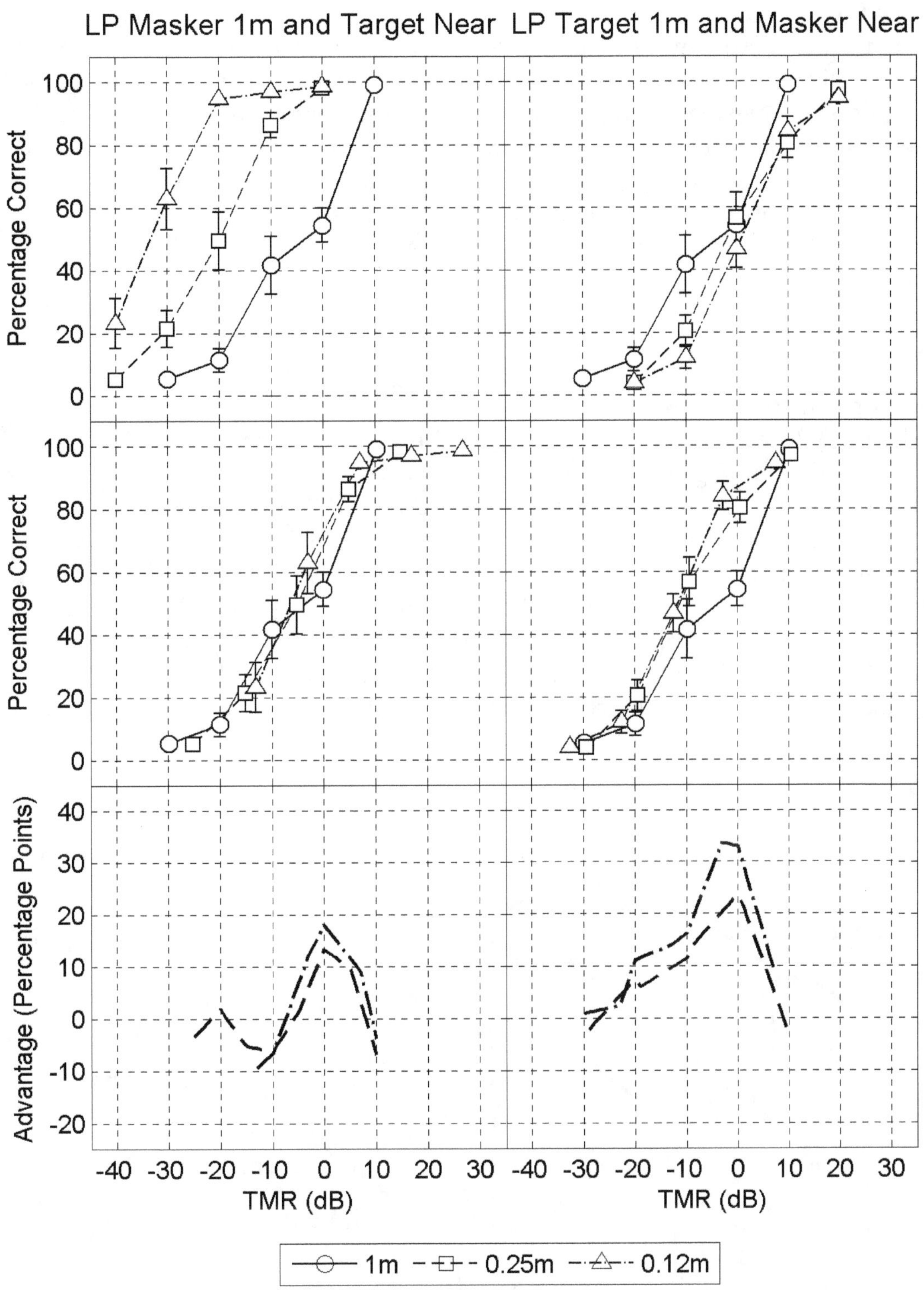

Fig. 4. Mean performance data averaged across all 8 subjects (error bars show standard errors of the means) in Experiment 2. The left panel displays the raw (top) and normalized (middle) data for the conditions where the masker was fixed at 1 m and the target was moved closer to the listener. The right panel displays the raw (top) and normalized (middle) data for the conditions where the target was fixed at 1 m and the masker was moved in closer to the listener. The bottom panels display the benefits of separation in distance, expressed as a difference in percentage points relative to the co-located case.

4.3 Discussion

The results from Experiment 2 in which the speech stimuli were low-pass filtered at 2 kHz were largely similar to those from Experiment 1. Performance across conditions was generally poorer, consistent with a more difficult segregation task, and subjects reported that voices appeared muffled and were more difficult to distinguish from each other in this condition. However, the perceptual benefit of separating talkers in distance condition was for broadband and low-pass filtered stimuli. This demonstrates that the low-frequency ILDs that are unique to this near field region of space are sufficient to provide a benefit for speech segregation.

5. Experiment 3

5.1 Experimental conditions

In Experiment 3, three talkers were used, and they were separated in azimuth at -50°, 0°, and 50° as illustrated in Fig. 5. For a given block, the distance of all talkers was set to either 1 m, 0.25 m or 0.12 m from the listener's head. Six different TMR values were tested for each spatial configuration (see Table 2), resulting in 18 unique conditions. The location of the target within the three-talker array was varied randomly within each block, such that half the trials had the target in the central position and the other half had the target in one of the side positions. Two 40-trial blocks were completed per condition by each listener resulting in a total of 2x40x18=1440 trials per listener. The distance and TMR were kept constant within a block, but the order of blocks was randomized.

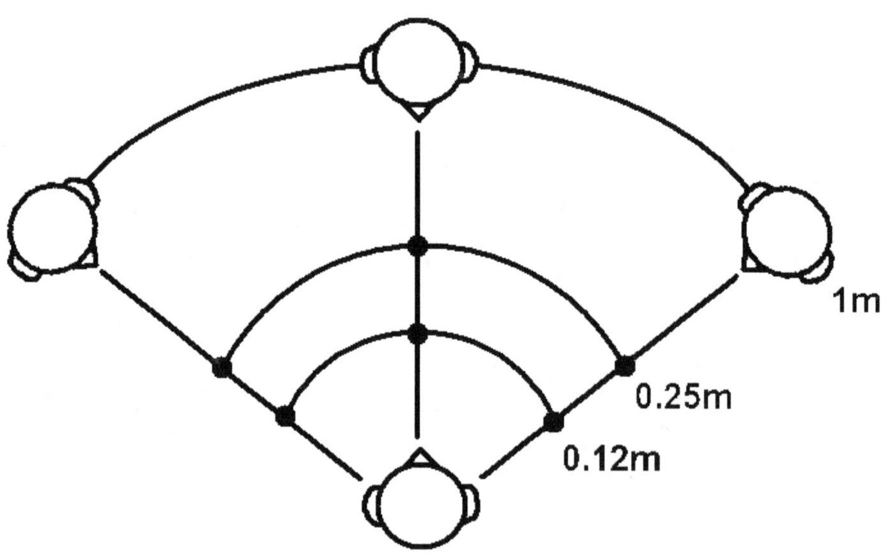

Fig. 5. The spatial configurations used in Experiment 3. Three talkers were spatially separated in azimuth at -50°, 0° and 50°and were either all located at 1 m, 0.25 m or 0.12 m from the listener's head. The location of the target talker was randomly varied (left, middle, right).

Configuration (target position/distance of mixture)		TMRs tested (dB)	Normalization shift (dB)
Central target	1 m	[-20 -15 -10 -5 0 5]	-3
	0.25 m	[-20 -15 -10 -5 0 5]	-5
	0.12 m	[-20 -15 -10 -5 0 5]	-8
Lateral target	1 m	[-20 -15 -10 -5 0 5]	0
	0.25 m	[-20 -15 -10 -5 0 5]	+3
	0.12 m	[-20 -15 -10 -5 0 5]	+6

Table 2. The range of TMR values tested and normalization values for each spatial configuration in Experiment 3. The normalization shifts are the differences in TMR at the better ear that resulted from variations in distance and configuration.

5.2 Results

5.2.1 Centrally positioned target

When the target was directly in front of the listener, with a masker on either side at ±50° azimuth, moving the whole mixture closer to the head had very little effect on raw performance scores (Fig. 6, top left). A two-way repeated-measures ANOVA on the arcsine-transformed data, however, showed that the effect of distance was statistically significant ($F_{2,14}$=7.7, p<.01), as was as the effect of TMR ($F_{5,35}$=159.4, p<.01). The interaction did not reach significance ($F_{10,70}$=1.4, p=0.2).

When the psychometric functions were re-plotted as a function of better-ear TMR, the distance effects were more pronounced (Fig. 6, middle left). This normalization compensates for the fact that the lateral maskers increase more in level than the central target when the mixture approaches the head. Mean performance was better for most TMRs when the mixture was moved into the near field. Fig. 6 (bottom left) shows the difference (in percentage points) between the near field conditions and the 1-m case, illustrating the advantage of moving sources closer to the head. The mean benefits were significant at all TMRs for both distances (p<.05).

5.2.2 Laterally positioned target

Raw results for the condition in which the target was located to the side of the three-talker mixture are shown in Fig. 6 (top right). Performance was better when the mixture was closer to the listener (0.12 m>0.25 m>1 m) particularly for low TMRs (below -5 dB). At higher TMRs, performance for all three distances appears to converge. Performance generally increased with increasing TMR but reached a plateau at around 80%. A two-way repeated-measures ANOVA on the arcsine-transformed data confirmed that there was a main effect of both distance ($F_{2,14}$=24.5, p<.01) and TMR ($F_{5,35}$=104.4, p<.01) and a significant interaction ($F_{10,70}$=17.4, p<.01).

When the psychometric functions were normalized to account for level changes at the better ear, the distinction between the different distances was reduced. An advantage of the near field mixtures over the 1-m mixture was found only at low TMRs (Fig. 6, middle right).

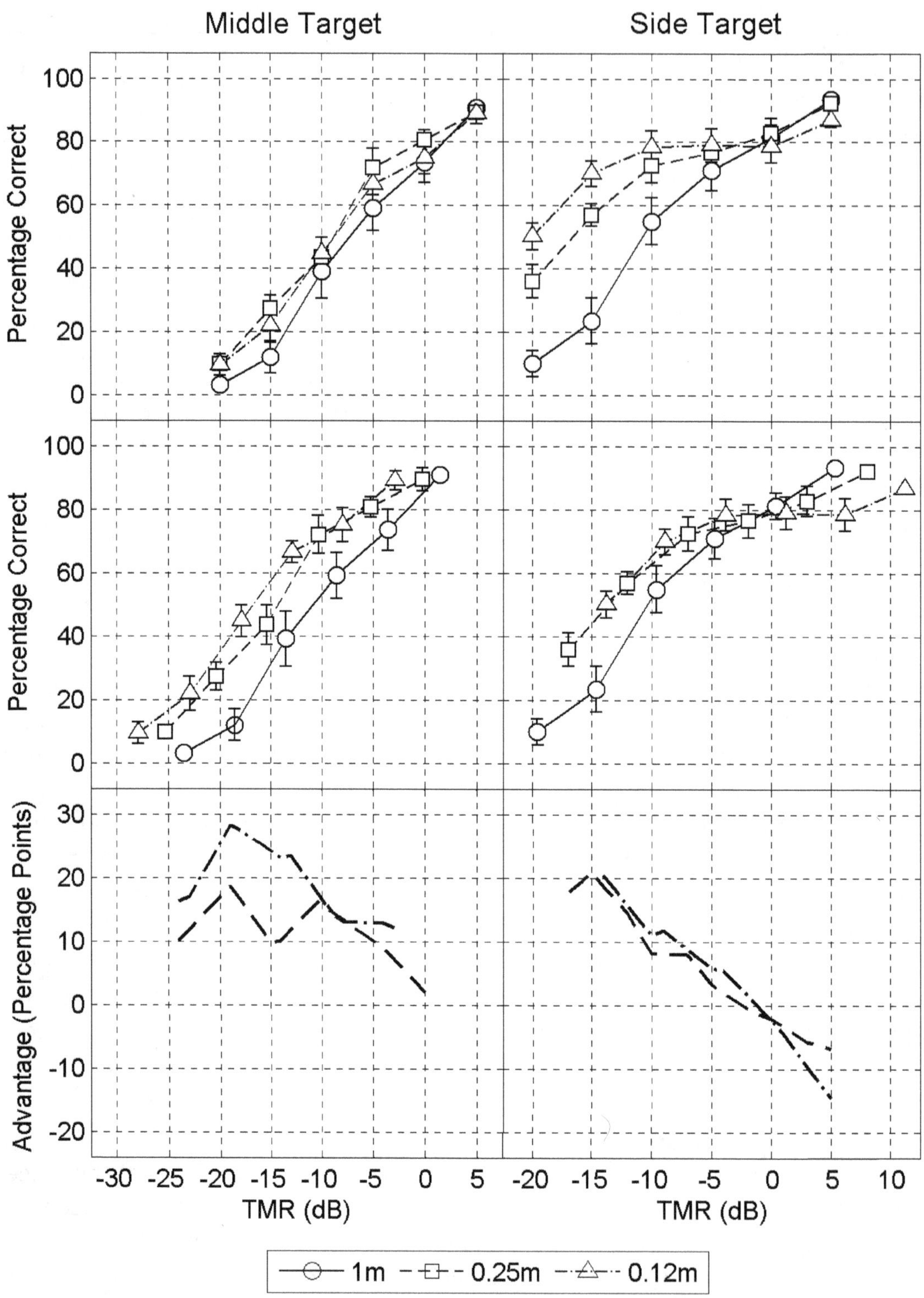

Fig. 6. Mean performance data averaged across all 8 subjects (error bars show standard errors of the means) in Experiment 3. The left panel displays the raw (top) and normalized (middle) data for the conditions where the target was located in the middle of three talkers. The right panel displays the raw (top) and normalized (middle) data for the conditions where the target was located to one side. The bottom panels display the benefits of decreasing the distance of the mixture, expressed as a difference in percentage points relative to the 1-m case.

At higher TMRs, the curves in fact reversed in order. These effects are reiterated in the benefit plots (Fig. 6, bottom right). The advantage was positive at negative TMRs but negative at positive TMRs. The mean benefits were significant at -15-dB TMR ($t_7=4.30$, $p<.01$) for the 0.25-m condition and at -10-dB TMR ($t_7=2.78$, $p<.05$) for the 0.12-m condition. A significant disadvantage was observed at 5-dB TMR for both distances ($p<.05$).

5.3 Discussion

Experiment 3 investigated the effect of moving a mixture of three talkers (separated in azimuth) closer to the head. Given that this manipulation essentially exaggerates the spatial differences between the competing sources, we were interested in whether it might improve segregation of the mixture. The manipulation had different effects depending on the location of the target. When the target was located in the middle, raw performance improved only very slightly with distance. However, this improvement occurred despite a decrease in TMR at the ear (both ears are equivalent given the symmetry) in this configuration (Table 2). In other words, performance improved despite an energetic disadvantage when the mixture was moved closer. Normalized performance thus revealed a perceptual benefit. When the target was located to the side, moving the mixture closer provided increases in better-ear TMR, and raw performance reflected this, but even after normalization there was a perceptual benefit of moving the mixture in closer. We attribute these benefits to an exaggeration of the spatial cues for the sources to the side, giving rise to a greater perceptual distance between the sources. It is not clear to us why this benefit was biased towards the lower TMRs in both cases, although the drop in benefit for high TMRs appears to be related to the flattening of the psychometric functions at high TMRs at the near field distances. It is possible that performance reaches a limit here due to the distracting effect of having three loud sources close to the head.

6. Conclusions

The results from these experiments provide insights into how the increase in ILDs that occurs in the auditory near field can influence the segregation of mixtures of speech. Spatial separation of competing sources in distance, as well as reducing the distance of an entire mixture of sources, led to improvements in terms of the intelligibility of a target source. These improvements were in some cases partly explained by changes in level that increased audibility, but in other cases occurred despite decreases in target audibility. The remaining benefits were attributed to salient spatial cues that aided perceptual streaming and lead to a release from informational masking.

In terms of binaural hearing-aids with the capability of exchanging audio signals, the experimental findings described here with normally-hearing listeners indicate that there may be value in investigating binaural signal processing algorithms that apply near-field sound transformations to sounds that are clearly lateralized. In other words, when the ITD or ILD cues strongly indicate a lateralized sound is present, a near-field sound transformation can be applied which artificially brings the sound perceptually closer to the head. We anticipate further experiments conducted with hearing-impaired listeners to investigate the value of such a binaural hearing-aid algorithm.

7. References

Arbogast, T. L., Mason, C. R., and Kidd, G. (2002). The effect of spatial separation on informational and energetic masking of speech. *Journal of the Acoustical Society of America*, Vol. 112, pp. 2086-2098.

Bolia, R. S., Nelson, W. T., Ericson, M. A., and Simpson, B. D. (2000). A speech corpus for multitalker communications research. *Journal of the Acoustical Society of America*, Vol. 107, pp. 1065-1066.

Bronkhorst, A. W. (2000). The cocktail party phenomenon: A review of research on speech intelligibility in multiple-talker conditions. *Acustica*, Vol. 86, pp. 117-128.

Bronkhorst, A. W., and Plomp, R. (1988). The effect of head-induced interaural time and level differences on speech intelligibility in noise. *Journal of the Acoustical Society of America*, Vol. 83, pp. 1508-1516.

Brungart, D. S. (1999). Auditory localization of nearby sources. III. Stimulus effects. *Journal of the Acoustical Society of America*, Vol. 106, pp. 3589-3602.

Brungart, D. S., Durlach, N. I., and Rabinowitz, W. M. (1999). Auditory localization of nearby sources. II. Localization of a broadband source. *Journal of the Acoustical Society of America*, Vol. 106, pp. 1956-1968.

Brungart, D. S., and Rabinowitz, W. R. (1999). Auditory localization of nearby sources. Head-related transfer functions. *Journal of the Acoustical Society of America*, Vol. 106, pp. 1465-1479.

Brungart, D. S., and Simpson, B. D. (2002). The effects of spatial separation in distance on the informational and energetic masking of a nearby speech signal. *Journal of the Acoustical Society of America*, Vol. 112, pp. 664-676.

Brungart, D. S., Simpson, B. D., Ericson, M. A., and Scott, K. R. (2001). Informational and energetic masking effects in the perception of multiple simultaneous talkers. *Journal of the Acoustical Society of America*, Vol. 110, pp. 2527-2538.

Byrne, D. (1980). Binaural hearing aid fitting: research findings and clinical application, In *Binaural Hearing and Amplification: Vol 2*, E.R. Libby, pp. 1-21, Zenetron Inc., Chicago, IL

Byrne, D., Nobel, W., Lepage, B. W., (1992). Effects of long-term bilateral and unilateral fitting of different hearing aid types on the ability to locate sounds. *J. Am. Acad. Audiology*, Vol. 3, pp. 369-382.

Dirks, D. D., and Bower, D. R. (1969). Masking effects of speech competing messages. *Journal of Speech and Hearing Research*, Vol. 12, pp. 229-245.

Drennan, W. R., Gatehouse, S. G., and Lever, C. (2003). Perceptual segregation of competing speech sounds: The role of spatial location. *Journal of the Acoustical Society of America*, Vol. 114, pp. 2178-2189.

Duda, R. O., and Martens, W. L. (1998). Range dependence of the response of a spherical head model. *Journal of the Acoustical Society of America*, Vol. 104, pp. 3048-3058.

Durlach, N. I., and Colburn, H. S. (1978). Binaural phenomena, In *The Handbook of Perception*, E. C. Carterette and M. P. Friedman, Academic, New York.

Durlach, N. I., Thompson, C. L., and Colburn, H.A. (1981). Binaural interaction in impaired listeners - a review of past research. *Audiology*, Vol. 20, pp. 181-211.

Ebata, M. (2003). Spatial unmasking and attention related to the cocktail party problem. *Acoust. Sci and Tech.* , Vol. 24, pp. 208-219.

Egan, J., Carterette, E., and Thwing, E. (1954). Factors affecting multichannel listening. *Journal of the Acoustical Society of America*, Vol. 26, pp. 774-782.

Feuerstein, J. (1992). Monaural versus binaural hearing: ease of listening, word recognition, and attentional effort. *Ear and Hearing*, Vol. 13,, No. 2, pp. 80-86.

Freyman, R. L., Helfer, K. S., McCall, D. D., and Clifton, R. K. (1999). The role of perceived spatial separation in the unmasking of speech. *Journal of the Acoustical Society of America*, Vol. 106, pp. 3578-3588.

Hirsh, I. J. (1950). The relation between localization and intelligibility. *Journal of the Acoustical Society of America*, Vol. 22, pp. 196-200.

Kan, A., Jin, C., and van Schaik, A. (2009). A psychophysical evaluation of near-field head-related transfer functions synthesized using a distance variation function. *Journal of the Acoustical Society of America*, Vol. 125, pp. 2233-2243.

Kidd, G., Jr., Mason, C. R., Richards, V. M., Gallun, F. J., and Durlach, N. I. (2008). Informational masking, In *Auditory Perception of Sound Sources*, W. A. Yost, A. N. Popper, and R. R. Fay (Springer Handbook of Auditory Research, New York), pp. 143-190.

Kidd, G., Jr., Mason, C. R., Rohtla, T. L., and Deliwala, P. S. (1998). Release from masking due to spatial separation of sources in the identification of nonspeech auditory patterns. *Journal of the Acoustical Society of America*, Vol. 104, pp. 422-431.

Libby, E. R. (2007). The search for the binaural advantage revisited. *The Hearing Review*, Vol. 14, No. 12, pp. 22-31.

Moore, B.C.J. (2007). Binaural sharing of audio signals: Prospective benefits and limitations. *The Hearing Journal*, Vol. 40, No. 11, pp. 46-48.

Pralong, D., and Carlile, S. (1994). Measuring the human head-related transfer functions: A novel method for the construction and calibration of a miniature "in-ear" recording system. *Journal of the Acoustical Society of America*, Vol. 95, pp. 3435-3444.

Pralong, D., and Carlile, S. (1996). The role of individualized headphone calibration for the generation of high fidelity virtual auditory space. *Journal of the Acoustical Society of America*, Vol. 100, pp. 3785-3793.

Rabinowitz, W. M., Maxwell, J., Shao, Y., and Wei, M. (1993). "Sound localization cues for a magnified head: Implications from sound diffraction about a rigid sphere," Presence: Teleoperators and Virtual Environments 2.

Shinn-Cunningham, B. G., Schickler, J., Kopco, N., and Litovsky, R. (2001). "Spatial unmasking of nearby speech sources in a simulated anechoic environment. *Journal of the Acoustical Society of America*, Vol. 110, pp. 1119-1129.

Studebaker, G. A. (1985). A rationalized arcsine transform. *Journal of Speech and Hearing Research*, Vol. 28, pp. 455-462.

Zurek, P. M. (1993). Binaural advantages and directional effects in speech intelligibility, In *Acoustical Factors Affecting Hearing Aid Performance*, G. A. Studebaker and I. Hochberg, pp. 255-276, Allyn and Bacon, Boston.

8

Global Internet Protocol for Ubiquitous Healthcare Monitoring Applications

Dhananjay Singh
Future Internet Team
Division of Fusion and Convergence of Mathematical Sciences, National Institute for mathematical Sciences (NIMS), Daejeon, South Korea

1. Introduction

This chapter encompasses the realm of global healthcare applications monitoring approaches and network selection in IP-based ubiquitous sensor networks. In this chapter we describe the motivation, overview structure of the works, ubiquitous communication techniques and its performance.

The healthcare technology keeps healthcare executives and managers up-to-date about the latest computer-based solutions for improving medical care and making healthcare organizations more efficient. Information Technology (IT) has a unique, news-style approach to implementations at hospitals and other smart home across the country. These installations are profiled because they significantly improve clinical outcomes, reduce costs or raise the efficiency of a healthcare provider or doctor. Recent research has also focused on the development of ubiquitous sensor networks (USN) and pervasive monitoring systems for cardiac patients. IT is the combination of computer and communication technologies. It helps to produce, manipulate, store, communicate, and broadcast changed information. Due to rapid changes in communication technologies, we have new paradigm applications, wireless networks are morphing into IEEE802.15.4–the standard for lowpan (low power personal area networks), which are playing an essential role to realize the envisioned ubiquitous world. Lowpans need to be connecting with other lowpans and with other wired networks in order to maximize the utilization of information and other resources. However, IEEE802.15.4 maximum frame size is 127 octets but UDP and IPv6 have big packet size then no space for health applications data. The PANs consist of various Body Sensor Networks nodes as well as overcome of problems such as network overhead, node discovery and security. When that technology is integrated to IPv6, we have a vast amount of possibilities implementing applications because IP has been used for a long time and technologies related to it already exist because IP-connectivity is spreading to all kinds of applications [1-3].

1.1 Motivation

Since the last century, the number of people of age over 65 has been increasing gradually. For many governments today, this fact is rising as one of the key concerns. The population of this age group is expected to be doubled by the end of 2025. According to the current status, it is estimated that the population of this age group which was 357 million in 1990, will be increased to around 761 million by the year 2025. Since 1990s, the rate of growth in health spending has been two-times greater than the average across OECD (Organization for Economic Co-operation and Development) countries [1], [2]. From Jon Barron in to the Figure 1.1, there is worldwide percentage of elderly person who is 60 and over and all over the world has problem.

1998-2003 growth was 10.2 percent per year (OECD average 4.5 percent) driven mainly by rise in public spending from 37 % in 1990 to 49.4 % in 2003 (OECD average of 72 %) (6 % of GDP in 2003). Several new developments are contributing to the changing face of the South Korea healthcare industry such as aging population and changes in trade policies and regulatory environments [1].

Most of the pharmaceutical companies have increased significantly their R&D expenditure for novel drugs and medications and key driving forces [2]. In fact, R&D spending has drastically increased from 0.3 % of the GDP now to 3 percent. The healthcare field will change as whole since at least: a) role of occupational healthcare will grow, and b) care management chains will change to care management networks. New alternative funding mechanisms arises: self-paid insurances, healthcare paid by employers Demand and supply of privately owned healthcare services will grow, which provides flexible ppp (public-private-partnership) and good balance. Healthcare and wellness services expect activity from citizens, since ensuring the working healthcare system requires broad cooperation in the society [2-3].

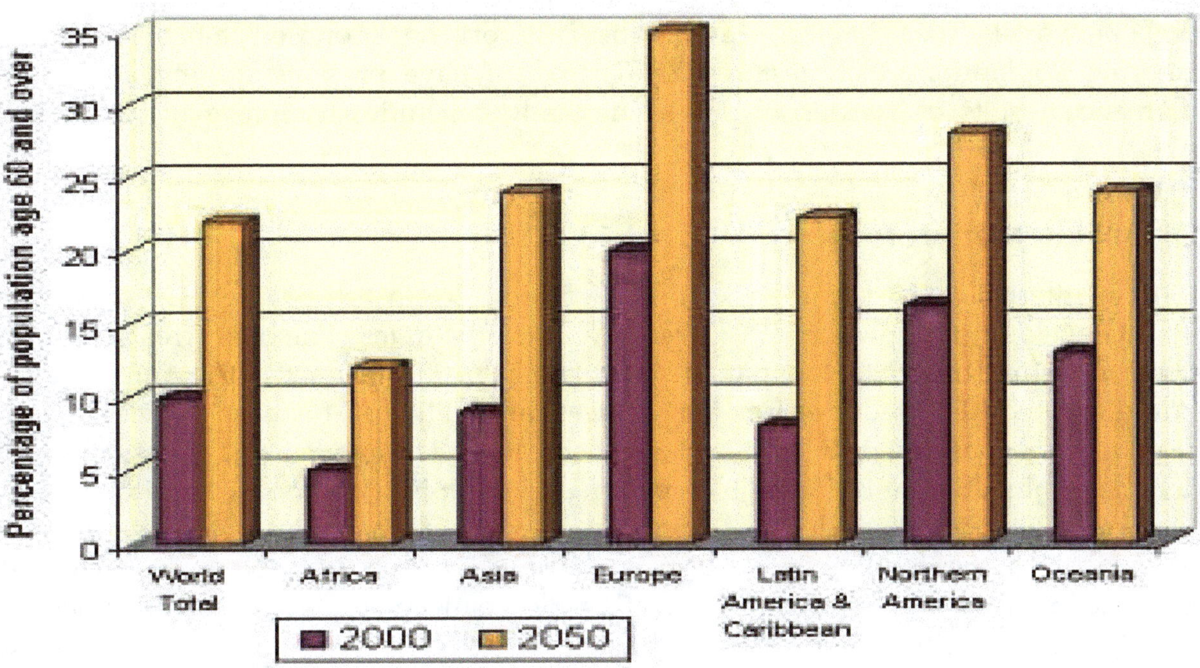

Fig. 1. Percentage of world population age 60 and over.

The healthcare technology keeps healthcare executives and managers up-to-date about the latest computer-based solutions for improving medical care and making healthcare organizations more efficient. Information Technology (IT) has a unique, news-style approach to implementations at hospitals and other smart home across the country. These installations are profiled because they significantly improve clinical outcomes, reduce

costs or raise the efficiency of a healthcare provider or doctor. Recent research has also focused on the development of ubiquitous sensor networks (USN) and pervasive monitoring systems for cardiac patients. A new technology, RFID enabled patient identification and real-time information management in synchronization with a central data base over a wireless connection (according to Alvin) systems are working in global monitoring [4].
There are several international projects use biomedical sensor networks for Body Area Networks. Biomedical sensors, which collect the body signal, need to attach to the patient body. There are many researches such as the Mobile Health System, Code blue etc for example. If user transmits ECG analysis monitoring data on server computer via sensor this can cause the big traffic problem for sensor nodes in a USNs. The USNs has intermittent connectivity and limited resources constraints such as bandwidth and delay. During mobility, it creates big problem, which is due to data centric. In order to overcome this problem, an IP-based ubiquitous sensor network is implemented to improve bandwidth and small delay for multiple layers holding systems [5].

1.2 Chapter organization

This chapter provides novel techniques for globally health monitor system and presented fundamental information related to IEEE802.15.4 standard and discusses the importance of Lowpan networks in the future pervasive paragon to integrate small embedded device with IP-based networks. The chapter has presented two approaches for global healthcare monitoring applications which are SHA (Smart Hospital Area) networks and SA (Smart Home) networks. The chapter presents benefits of the proposed global healthcare monitoring applications their test results. There, we have presents routing and sensor performance results of various IP-USN and finally conclude the information of future aspects.

2. Global internet protocol

The IETF (Internet Engineering Task Force) working group has been presented various drafts to development 6lowpan (IPv6 over Low-Power Wireless Personal Area Networks) it refers IPv6 integrated to Lowpan device. The Fig.1 has depicted the IEEE 802.15.4 standard defined RFD (reduced-function devices) and FFD (full-function devices) type of nodes. We have considered RFD as BMS (Biomedical Sensors) node and FFD as (6lowpan) node. The combination of BMS and 6lowpan makes IP-USNs (IP-Based Ubiquitous Sensor Networks). Whereas BMS nodes are utilized for sensing and transmit MAC layer beacons to 6lowpan in a star topology. The BMS node only interacts with 6lowpan node even though 6lowpan node is able to connect other 6lowpan nodes due to its full functional capability there has IPv6 compression, neighbor discover, mesh routing and BMS packet binding techniques. Lowpan is a network which offers wireless connectivity in applications that have limited computational capacity, power and relaxed throughput. Some typical characteristics of 6LowPAN are: small packet size, support for 16 bit or IEEE 64-bit extended media access control addresses, low bandwidth, two kinds of topologies (mesh and star), low power, low cost and so on. [8] Routing in different kinds of topologies should be implemented in such a way that computation and memory requirements are minimal [7-9].

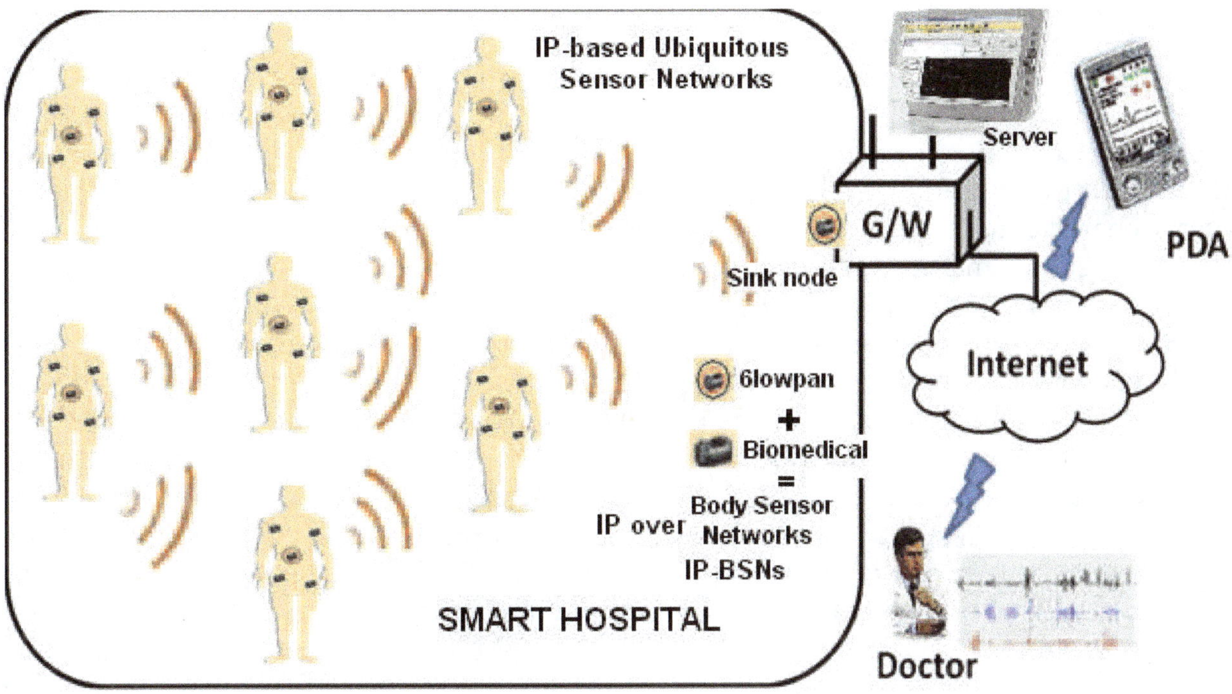

Fig. 2. Ubiquitous Healthcare Monitoring Applications.

The design of routing protocols also highly relies on availability of other information, such as physical location, global ID, etc. A good number of location-aided routing protocols have been proposed, which hold the assumption that each sensor node has the accurate location information. GPS is a simple and direct solution to localization, but it is too costly for sensor networks due to the additional power consumption and high deployment expense. Thus, effective and inexpensive localization techniques have become very important, which is another topic of interest of our research. Global ID is desirable in senor networks so that each sensor can be distinguished from each other. The sensor node has address space for global ID, which will cause to establish communication with IPv6 networks. For operations of some routing protocols, we do need to distinguish sensor nodes to some extent, but a locally unique ID may be enough. Thus, this poses a challenging research opportunity. The health monitoring applications architecture for 6lowpan needs to be scalable and flexible which can handle large number of nodes. At the same time, this architecture must support localization communication in order to increase network capacity. The general USN applications have been designed and realized to provide physical environment monitoring. But, IP-based USN technology has provided mobility and global connectivity. The cognizant of internet on USNs has connects assets in the physical networks to the IP networks. Internet-based USNs architecture has proposed and developed in this chapter. IP-USN tends to be implemented as a separate network for dedicated services in the PANs. An effective smart hospital/ home networks have data aggregation mechanism with limited resources even though connection to infrastructure networks is hardly considered. Current, USNs are far from actualizing a global connectivity. Its considering IEEE802.15.4 for communicate between one USN to another USN but it cannot connect globally and mobility state. The main objective of the chapter has developed architecture to IP over USNs which is integrated with IPv6-based wired networks for global communication between Doctor and patients. In this chapter has considered various applications such as design a new technique of routing protocol, application based MAC frame format, mobility techniques, energy consumption and data delivery ratio and association with one PANs to others [9-14].

2.1 Biomedical sensors and IP-sensor

The IETF working groups has been presented two RFCs 4919 and 4944. Here they presents several characteristics such as low power, low cost, low bandwidth, short range, PAN maintenance, transmission and reception on the physical radio channel, channel access and reliable data transmission port (MAC).

The main role of IP-USNs node is pervasive nature, it allow connectivity with existing IP-based networks. For that there are many challenges for biomedical application based node discovery, network selection method and their packet size. The maximum transmission unit of IPv6 is 1280 octets and IEEE 802.15.4 frame has 127 octets at physical layer. The lowpan network consists of two devices FFD (Full function Devices) and RFD (Reduce Function Devices). The FFD (which is 6lowpan) node supports which is complete implementation of protocol stack and it can operate with Gateway. The RFD (which is normal Biomedical Sensor) node is a simple device with minimum implementation of protocol stack and minimum memory capacity. The Biomedical Sensor (BMS) nodes should communicate only 6lowpan node at a given instance of time. The 6lowpan node should communicate with other 6lowpan node and Biomedical nodes.

IP-USNs node brings up various biomedical sensor devices. The sensor devices are occurrence simultaneously on IP-USNs with complex interactions. In my approach, IP-USNs node has resource allocation and energy conservation techniques which can identify the unique biomedical data. The algorithms have implemented on devices which optimize their performance [9].

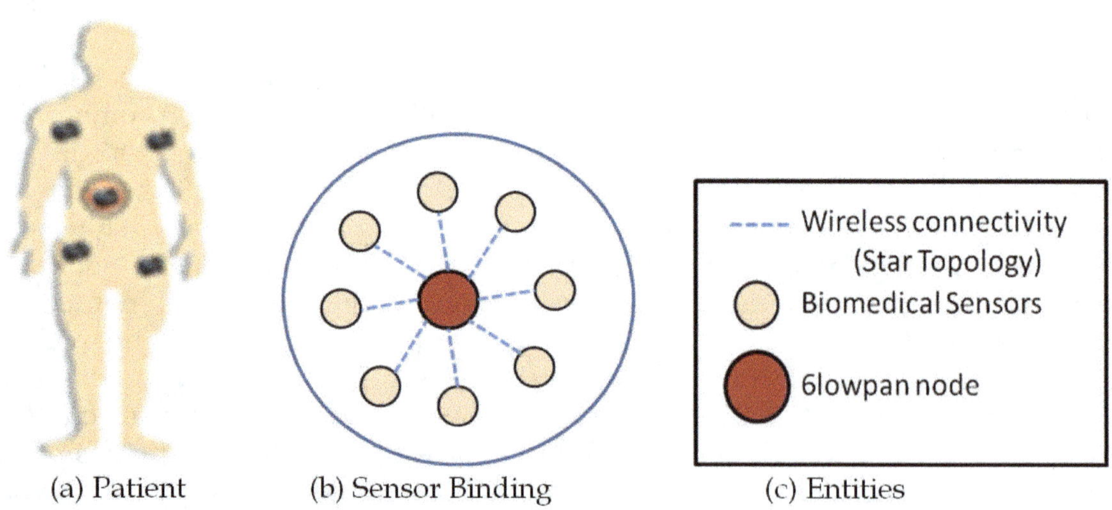

Fig. 3. Biomedical Sensors association with IP-USN.

The Fig.3 has described IP-USNs node which is captured with various biomedical sensors. There are specific gateways associated with IP-USN devices, though routing technique. All IP-USNs nodes have worked its PAN for network utilization with greedy approach of choosing the closest nodes but it has to face lots of challenges.

Case 1. Mobility protocol is balancing between biomedical sensor and IP-USN node in Body Aare Networks.

Case 2. Safely transmit biomedical data from IP-USN node to gateway during patient movement.
Case 3. To optimizes energy latency mobility protocol for different applications with QoS.
Each biomedical sensor node enables to execute a certain tasks which has capability, sense and transmits to IP-USN node. All sensor nodes dense deployments on BAN which should be transmit data in a specific time periods to the IP-USNs. The IP-USNs sensor node transmits all data to the gateway. A gateway initiates the resource solicitation on behalf of an application for a specific gateway via routing. The routing protocol use address centric of the biomedical data packet which used subsequence frame techniques.
The following approaches can help to overcome from above (cases) problems.
Scheme1. The IP-USNs have to choose active IP-USNs node in a mesh network to successfully transmit its data to the gateway, which is based on current novel mobility protocol and remaining battery energy.
Scheme2. The gateway can measure by localization and transmit distance information (by modified gateway packet) of mobile IP-USNs, which is helping choose right path a mobile node.
Scheme3. The gateway broadcast RREQ message to IP-USNs, which is using one or two hop. When IP-USNs node is transmitting data packet then hop (mediator) nodes should be ignored sensing activities and use routing to transmit successfully data to the gateway. This techniques use highly network utilization.

3. Global healthcare monitoring system

The chapter has investigated two scenario for global healthcare monitoring system, SHA (Smart Hospital Area) and SH (Smart Home) The IP-USNs placed on the patient BAN that should be connected to the gateway, which is placed on gateway in a PANs (Personal Area Networks). Each IP-USNs node has its own id and IP-address, Id use the identification of Gateway and IP-address for global connectivity via internet. However, Service Provider directly ping his patient and get globally current status of the patient using internet service provider equipments such as Cell phone, PDA, Note book etc. The system has been evaluated by technical verification, clinical test, user survey and current status of patient. The global monitoring system have a big potential to ease the deployment of new services by getting rid of cumbersome wires and simplify healthcare in hospitals and for home care.
In healthcare environments, delayed or lost information may be a matter of life or death. Thus, we have to use more reliable network topologies. We have used start networks for patient BANs and mesh for IP-USNs networks in PANs. It made of highly constrained nodes (limited power, limited memory, limited CPU) interconnected by a variety of lousy networks. As any IP-USNs has necessarily comprise of biomedical sensors and actuators.
For instance, in a healthcare monitoring system, sensor nodes might detect biomedical data and then send commands to activate the sprinkler system. An IP-USNs network can be seen as small star or mesh networks each consisting of a single node connected to zero or more IP-USNs nodes for healthcare applications.
The following section has been described in details our scenarios and its problems.

3.1 Smart Hospital

The SHA (Smart Hospital Area) has been described the design space of USNs in the context of the 6lowpan working group. The design space is already limited by the unique characteristics of a Lowpan (low-power, short range, low-bit rate) [3].

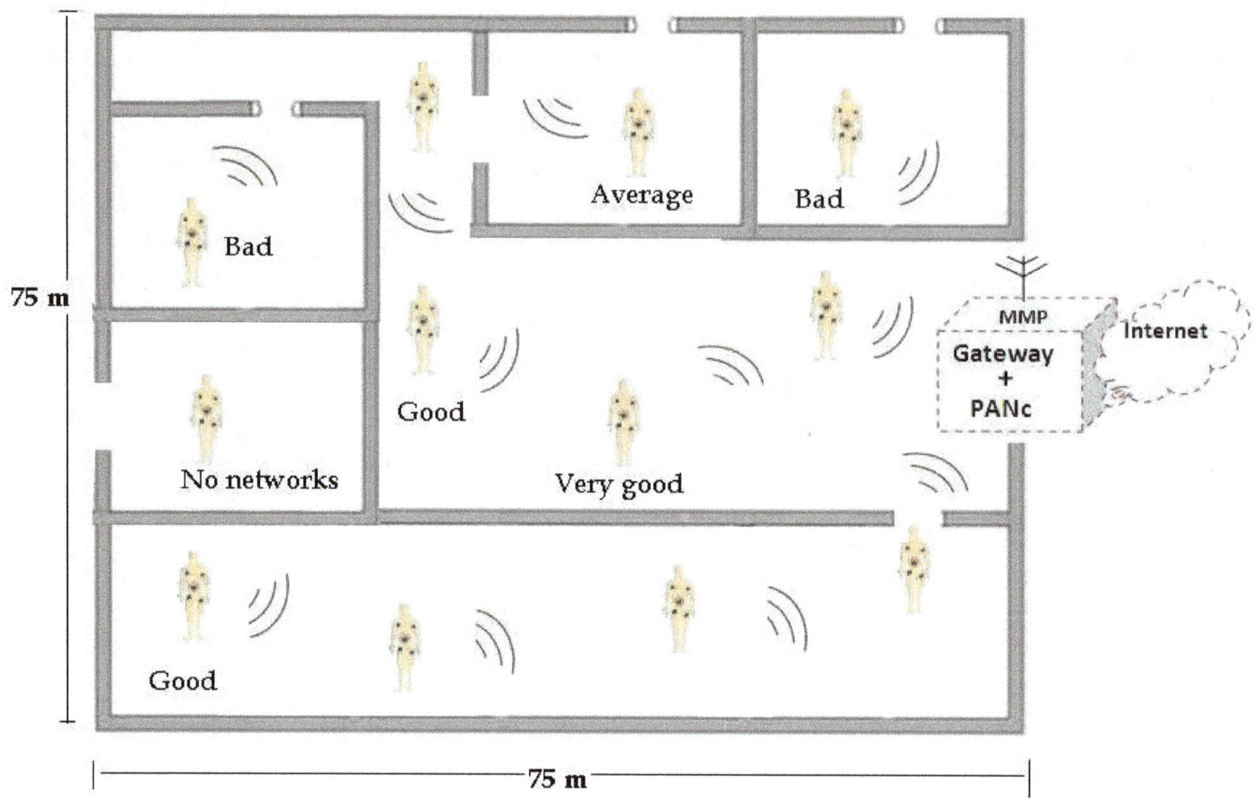

Fig. 4. System Architecture of Hospital Area Networks.

The IP-USNs nodes have to pre-planned deploy in an organized (manually or automatically) manner in SHA. The deployment has an impact on high node density for location to allocate addresses in the networks. The no. of IP-USNs nodes could be less in a PAN- coordinator (6 nodes) to provide the intended network capability and it can moves in the range of PAN coordinator (gateway). The power source of nodes need to be hybrid, whether the nodes are battery-powered or mains-powered, influences the network design. The system has considered that IP-USNs nodes always connected to the Gateway (internet based gateway).

In this system need to be provide data privacy and security. Role based access control is required to be support by proper authentication mechanism and need to be encryption mechanism. The data collection techniques are used point to point, multipoint to point and point to multipoint for traffic. It has plug-and-play configuration during mobility and real-time data acquisition such as in Fig.4, patient IPv6ID-A moves his current position to other into (SHA) PAN-1 then node IPv6ID-A send mobility status to the Gateway and should update its new neighbor's information in its routing table and gateway also update its current position in to the SHA. The point to point connectivity provides efficient data management, reliability and robustness of the networks.

The patient's BANs can be simply configured as a star topology IP-USNs (several biomedical sensors such as ECG, Blood Pressure, Temperature, SpO2 etc. and 6lowpan sensor) for data aggregation and dynamic network during movement of patients. The patient's IP-USNs node uses globally unique IPv6 address for the identification of patients. Thus, the SHA itself does not require globally unique IPv6 address but could be run with link-local IPv6 address. The security used between IP-USNs node and Gateway for reliable and secure data communication.

In this system, patients freely can move inside the SHA and corroborate closely with doctor to sharing biomedical data. In Fig.4 has shown SHA networks there are 5nodes of IP-USNs. Each IP-USNs node has several (Biomedical Sensor) BMS and One 6lowpan node that should be monitored by gateway. IP-USNs retrieves patient's biomedical data and transmit to the PAN-coordinator (gateway).

3.2 Smart Home

The SH (Smart Home) are similar SHA (Smart Hospital Area) which has been described in upper block. This system has fixed gateway in the center of the room and wearable IP-USNs device placed on the patient's BANs. MMP has planted in to middle of the room, this well calculate exact location of the patient during its mobility state. The SH system, use point to point routing and there are no hop node, IP-USNs node directly send data to the gateway. However, the gateway always connected to the internet, and the service provider any time monitors his patient.

3.3 Major challenges

There are several challenges the use of global connectivity. We have given the solution of mobility, biomedical data binding, and IP-USNs node association with gateway as well as we investigate two techniques in SHA.

3.3.1 Handoff techniques

The gateway broadcast a query packet to all IP-USNs nodes (includes approximate receiving signal strength for 1st level) at once and then waits for reply until timer expires. Timer set on the IP-USNs according velocity of signal strength and distance between IP-USNs and gateway. Each level has to define hop distance between IP-USNs and gateway. The gateway broadcast query packet in to mesh topology. IP-USNs received packet within an area then compare the signal strength according to RSS value that node join or establish connection to gateway. Then, IP-USNs send a Query_response (IP-addr.) packet to Gateway that they are joining the coordinator. IP-USNs adjust their transmission power to the coordinator for further communication process.

3.3.2 Patient move one PAN-other-PAN networks

We have presented a technique to detection of a neighboring PAN, identification of the MMP (Micro Mobility protocol). It is a common channel based gating protocol, algorithms to diffuse common interest across collocated PANs, and methods to define and regulate gating scope. The SHA has same region but sharing information of common interest amongst PANs and accessing internet from other PANs. The proposed algorithm has to systematically allow neighboring PANs to communicate with each other by diffusing into each other. The diffusion takes place through gating operation performed by nodes. This resides at the MMP of the two non-interfering PANs. The MMP identification are used common channel based gating mechanism. The mechanism has to diffuse common interest (query/response) across collocated PANs, and regulate gating scope. The PAN association procedure has specified logical channel assignment procedure in IEEE802.15.4 networks that prevents interference amongst overlapping PANs. Relates channel assignment as the bottleneck for diffusion across PANs.

1. //Parameters indicates that the channels are to be scanned and scan time per channel. Active or Passive
2. Network layer issues NLME-NETWORK-DISCOVERY. request [Active Mode] (ScanChannels, ScanDuration)
3. Network layer issues NLME-NETWORK-DISCOVERY.request [Passive Mode]
4. //On the receipt of MLME-SCAN.confirm and NLME-NETWORK-DISCOVERY.confirm
5. Network layer issues MLME-SCAN.request
6. NLME selects a tuple (PANId, LogicalChannel)
7. Such as
8. (PANId, LogicalChannel) New ≠ (PANId, LogicalChannel) Existing⇔ A. V B.
9. Where
10. (PANId)New ≠ (PANId)Existing
11. [(PANId) New = (PANId)Existing ^ (LogicalChannel)New ≠ (LogicalChannel) Existing]

Table 1. Channel Allocation Algorithm

4. Benefit of global healthcare system

The integration of IP over BSNs in healthcare will improve quality and efficiency of the treatment in various ways. We assume that IP over BSNs integrated system will be used in general hospital area and home area during patients moves inside these facilities. There are various potential applications for patient monitoring. The various benefits will overcome using Internet based small embedded devices.

4.1 Treatment quality improvement

The patient's conditions are carefully monitored, while doctor and patient visit inside an operating room or a hospital but not while they are in outside hospital, for instance home or abroad visit. The same can be true when they are outside hospital. However, it is possible that patients' condition gets worse while they are in unmonitored field, and it's vital. With the availability of IP over BSNs integrated systems, it is possible to monitor patients' conditions in such scenarios and to notify doctors when patient's conditions degenerate suddenly. To make this kind of integrated global connectivity can allocate current position of the patients, and their health conditions monitored by doctor using internet based equipments. Various types of BSNs, depends on the patient, we need to provide a flexible technologies to deal biomedical data in a plug-and-play mode. Global health monitoring systems have monitored patient's biomedical data and position identification inside a smart hospital/ home. In other words, the systems need to maintained a global connectivity to discover the available BSNs and examined biomedical data while the doctor not in to the hospital.

4.2 Medication error reduction

The present an important problem in healthcare is to reduce biomedical errors include nurse's treatment mistakes, their check and order mistakes and so on. If any case, the technical system identifies the patient condition and verifies treatment orders then some of biomedical error will be solve. An important dispute in global health care monitoring system to reduced the biomedical errors. But if the global monitoring system supports doctors during patient monitoring applications, some of the biomedical errors will be kept. These kinds of error require real-time transactions for quality improvement applications. Therefore, IP integration with BSNs makes real time patient identification during dynamically movement and vital biomedical data information.

4.3 Accurate medical record

In hospital, nurses are keeping accurate biomedical records of the patient is a foundation of medical treatment. If biomedical records are not kept accurately, it wills accidents but patient die. In addition, BSNs devices can store accurate records condition of patient in to the server. The IP integrated BSNs system will enable the identification of biomedical data to them. In the case, patient condition history data is inquired to doctor from global systems then also he can monitor for server data base.

4.4 Accurate location tracking

The present monitoring system has their basic limitations is that they offer coarse and often unreliable location information. On the other hand, location tracking technologies such as GPS can accurately locate a patient but not identify it. The global monitoring system using more IP-based BSNs in smart hospital/home are will enable more accurate and reliable patient's location tracking. There are several ways to integrate these pieces of information.

4.5 Cost reduction

The management of both cost reduction and quality of treatment is an important challenge. In a potential area is to reduce biomedical administration. IP over BSNs is used to identify the biomedical data and make global connectivity. The patient monitoring and change of biomedical data is an important, semantics.

4.6 Security reduction

Security is always a big issue in Information Technology field and there are several cases as attackers have been crash system. Thus, we have also considers security protocols to prevent global IP based healthcare system. We have used Time stamp and nonce into fragmentation packets to prevent healthcare data.

5. Conclusion

This chapter has presented the combination of IT over embedded devises for global healthcare monitoring applications. The chapter had presented two schemes, which are SHA (Smart Hospital Area) networks and SH (Smart Home) networks, parallel it is presenting internet connectivity over biomedical devices to collect globally biomedical date and the benefits of global communication system for healthcare monitoring applications. It is a unique news-style approach to implementation at hospitals and other smart home across the country. These installations are profiled because they significantly improve clinical outcomes, reduce costs or raise the efficiency of a healthcare provider or doctor. Recent research has also focused on the development of ubiquitous sensor networks (USN) and pervasive monitoring systems for cardiac patients.

6. Acknowledgment

This work was supported by NAP of Korea Research Council of Fundamental Science & Technology

7. References

Otto, C.; Jovanov, E. (2006). *An Implementation of the WBAN Health Monitoring Protocol for ZigBee Compliant TinyOS Messaging,* Electrical and Computer Engineering Dept.,University of Alabama in Huntsville, Alabama.

Elder Population to Dramatically Incérasse in Developing Nations Avalable from http://www.californiaelderlawattorneyblog.com/2009/07/elder-population-to-dramatical.html.

Guang-Zhong Yang,(2006). *Body Sensor Networks,* springer-verlog London, 2006.

Kushalnagar, N., Montenegro, G., and C. Schumacher (2007). *IPv6 over Low-Power Wireless Personal Area Networks (6LoWPANs): Overview, Assumptions, Problem Statement, and Goals,* RFC 4919.

Montenegro, G., Kushalnagar, N., Hui, J., and D. Culler, (2007). *Transmission of IPv6 Packets over IEEE 802.15.4 Networks,* RFC 4944.

Hui, J.; Culler, D.; Chakrabarti, S. (2009). *6LoWPAN: Incorporating IEEE 802.15.4 into the IP architecture,* IPSO White Paper No. 3. IP for Smart Objects (IPSO) Alliance, USA.

Singh D. ; Lee H-J., Chung W-Y. (2009). *An energy consumption technique for global healthcare monitoring applications,* ACM- International Conference on Interaction Sciences: Information Technology, Culture and Human, pp. 539-542,.Seoul, Korea.

Singh D. ; Lee H-J. (2009). *Database Design for Global Patient Monitoring Applications using WAP"* Proceding in 4th ACM International Conference on Computer Sciences and Convergence Information Technology, pp.25-32, Seoul, Korea.

Singh D. ; Lee H-J., Chung W-Y. (2009). *Secure IP-Ubiquitous Sensor Network for Healthcare Applications Monitoring In-Home Area,* The Second International Conference on the Applications of Digital Information and Web Technologies, pp. 335-337, London.

Singh D. ; Ping Q-S., Tiwary U. S., Lee H-J., Chung W-Y. (2009). *Global Patient Monitoring system using IP-enable Ubiquitous Sensor Network.* World Congress on Computer Science and Information Engineering, pp. 524-528. Los Angeles, USA.

Singh D. ; Singh M., Singh. S., Q-S., Tiwary U. S., Lee H-J. (2009). *IP-based Ubiquitous Sensor Network for In-Home Healthcare Monitoring.* IEEE-International Conference on Multimedia, Signal Processing and Communication Technologies, pp. 201-204, Aligarh, India.

Singh D. ; Tiwary U. S., Lee H-J., Chung W-Y. (2009). *Global Healthcare Monitoring System using 6lowpan Networks.* IEEE-International Conference on Advanced Communication Technology, pp.113-117, Phoenix Park, Korea.

Singh D. ; Ping Q-S., Singh M., Tiwary U. S., Lee H-J., Chung W-Y. (2008*) IP-enabled Sensor Networks for Patient Monitoring, IEEE*-International Conference on Wireless Communication and Sensor Networks, pp.127-130, IIIT Allahabad, India.

9

Legislation, Standardization and Technological Solutions for Enhancing e-Accessibility in e-Health

Pilar Del Valle García, Ignacio Martínez Ruiz, Javier Escayola Calvo, Jesús Daniel Trigo Vilaseca and José García Moros
Aragon Institute for Engineering Research (I3A), University of Zaragoza (UZ), Zaragoza, Spain

1. Introduction

"It is usual to consider human dignity as the basis for human rights. In this sense, this term is used to refer to a number of features that characterize humans and that serve to express their uniqueness. [...] Thus, the idea of human dignity rests on a human being characterized by his or her capacity and performance in carrying out a particular social role. This has been translated into the conception of rights. Indeed, human rights theory has been founded on a model of the individual, characterized mainly by his or her "capacity" to reason, "capacity" to feel and "capacity" to communicate. It is this model that is (and which has traditionally been) the prototype of the moral agent, that is the prototype of a subject able to participate in moral discourse. [...] This is what we often refer to as moral "capacity", being also a trait of individuals as moral agents" [1].

In recent decades advances in Assistive Technology (AT) and in Information and Communication Technology (ICT) have influenced the lives of people with disabilities or special needs. Developments in the knowledge and understanding of disability, and changes in the social and legal framework —as a result of the "Rights of People with functional diversity " and the "Right to an Independent and Dignified Life"— have led to Electronic Accessibility (e-Accessibility) and Universal Design (design for all).

For years, the terminology used in the field of functional diversity resulted, more often than not, in undesirable results both at the legal level and in the sphere of political action. For this reason, since the mid 1970's people with functional diversity have voiced their objections to words such as "disability" and "handicap", words which were too closely confined to a medical and diagnostic approach and which barely reflected the shortcomings and imperfections of society itself in its response to the phenomenon of disability.

In 1980, the World Health Organization (WHO) [2] created the International Classification of Impairments, Disabilities, and Handicaps (ICIDH) to provide a unifying framework for classifying human functioning and disability as health components. After international revision efforts coordinated by the WHO, the World Health Assembly on May 22, 2001, approved the International Classification of Functioning, Disability and Health (ICF). Functioning and disability are viewed as a complex interaction between the health condition of the individual and the contextual factors of the environment as well as personal factors.

The picture produced by this combination of factors and dimensions is of "the person in his or her world." The classification treats these dimensions as interactive and dynamic rather than linear or static. It allows for an assessment of the degree of disability, although it is not a measurement instrument. It is applicable to all people, whatever their health condition. The language of the ICF is neutral as to etiology, placing the emphasis on function rather than condition or disease. It also is carefully designed to be relevant across cultures as well as age groups and genders, making it highly appropriate for heterogeneous populations. The ICF puts the notions of 'health' and 'disability' in a new light. It acknowledges that every human being can experience a decline in health and thereby experience some degree of disability. Disability is not something that only happens to a minority of humanity. Thus, the ICF 'mainstreams' the experience of disability and recognizes it as a universal human experience. By shifting the focus from cause to impact it places all health conditions on an equal footing allowing them to be compared using a common metric - the ruler of health and disability. Furthermore, the ICF takes into account the social aspects of disability and does not see disability only as a 'medical' or 'biological' dysfunction. By including contextual factors in which environmental factors are listed, the ICF allows the impact of the environment on a person's functioning to be recorded [3].

As the XXI century progresses, so too does the concept of design for all which involves contemplating the possible requirements of all patients including the elderly and people with disabilities. Design for all is "*the intervention in environments, products and services with the aim that everyone, including future generations, regardless of age, gender, capabilities or cultural background, can enjoy participating in the construction of our society, with equal opportunities participating in economic, social, cultural, recreational and entertainment activities while also being able to access, use and understand whatever part of the environment with as much independence as possible*" [4]. This new concept appears a suitable way to ensure equal opportunities for all citizens and their active participation in society. Design for all means overcoming the stigma of difference that has been traditionally associated with people with functional diversity and it assumes that their conditions regarding the environment are on the same level as other more common and shared conditions such as age, the ability to undertake activity or the temporary restriction of some function. This assumes that the human dimension is not defined by capabilities, or measures, but should be viewed more generally in such a way that diversity is the norm rather than the exception. Therefore, the values of this new paradigm lead to a new culture in which disability-related needs (even if they remain the guide and the motivation) are no longer the absolute centre and reason for action. Everyone is susceptible to limitations or conditioning factors at certain times. Therefore, the idea of design for all is to think of those with the greatest needs and thus benefit everyone. Thus, products such as phones with increasingly large keys, remote controls with large and simplified buttons, talking lifts, etc. have become increasingly popular in recent years.

Within the broad field of disability, e-Accessibility is one aspect that is becoming increasingly relevant at present. The problems involved in bringing technology to people with functional diversity makes it necessary to implement a user experience along with an interface specific to their needs, avoiding any kind of a problem with the hardware required to interact with medical devices in telemedicine cases. While the potential of AT and ICT is growing, e-Accessibility is more urgently necessary to enable people with disabilities to take part in almost any living environment. In 2006, the International Conference on Computers Helping People with Special Needs (ICCHP) [5] summarized this process with an equality equation (Equality = e-Quality) [6] symbolizing how much equal opportunities in society depend on e-Accessibility. Providing e-Accessibility should be seen as a global challenge in the global economy. Given these challenges, the ICCHP puts special emphasis on the problems of people with disabilities in countries with political, economic and social difficulties. It is in those countries where access to AT and ICT is most hindered.

The computer world is also a market in which people with disabilities are becoming very important potential customers (as demonstrated, for example, by Microsoft's international agreements [7] to adapt its operating system and carry out awareness campaigns about the importance of accessibility in new technologies). In this context, the ISO 9241 family of standards provides for accessibility in communication, directly or indirectly. These standards cover the design of equipment and services for people with a wide range of sensory capabilities, physical and cognitive, including those who are temporarily disabled and elderly people. The technological requirements to be met by services and applications in order to be e-accessible are described in this family of standards.

With this background, a scheme of ideas is proposed below in Figure 1, divided into six sectors, which details the relationship between the different fields that a person with

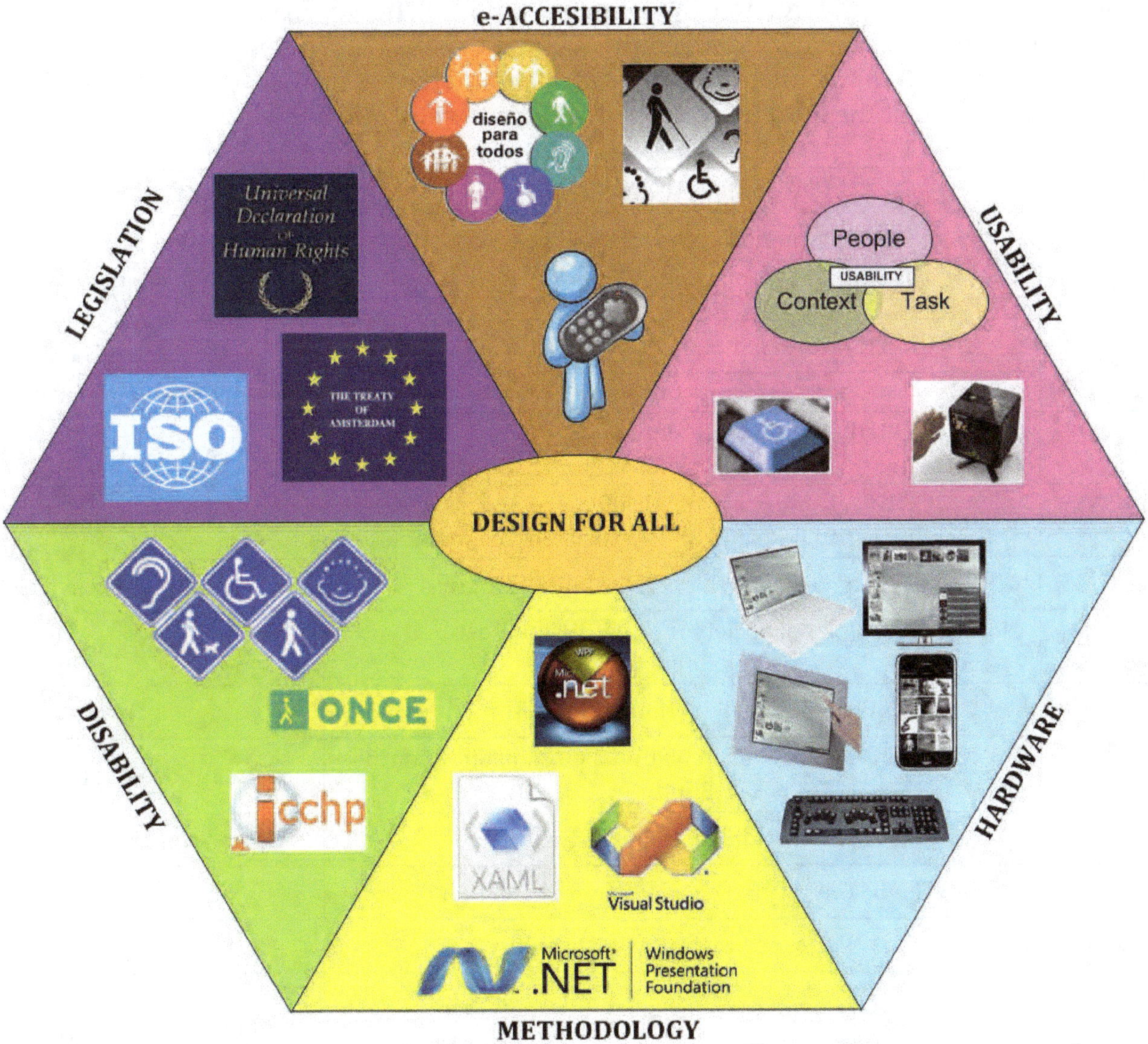

Fig. 1. Outline of ideas for e-Health solutions design based on the paradigm of design for all

functional diversity finds around him. This outline of ideas follows the paradigm of design for all, taking people with special needs as the centre of the design, which will determine the developed software applications. In this broad context, the first sector in Figure 1 covers types of disabilities, the barriers faced and their foundations. In the area of legislation, all the laws that protect the rights of people with disability are reviewed. In the section on e-accessibility, the concept of design for all allows new designs to be developed according to recommendations on how to bring new technologies closer to the specific requirements of people with disability. The area of usability defines the ease with which people can use a particular tool or other human-made object to achieve a particular goal. Thus, the design of new e-Health solutions has to comply with the specific characteristics of usability for people with disability. The hardware section covers the design of a graphical interface that applies to any platform and has the necessary adaptive hardware for people with disability. Finally, the methodology area covers technical guidelines to be followed with different systems, programming tools and communication standards.

To conclude this introduction, it should be noted that great efforts have been made in recent years by major international companies driving the development of AT, design for all and the adoption of open standards to enable people with functional diversity to improve their opportunities for independence and employability through technology. This tremendous boost has been led in recent years by various initiatives, institutions, companies and organisations, some of the most important of which are shown in Table I.

	Accessible Technology	http://accessibletech.org
	ADA. Americans with Disabilities Act	http://adaresources.org
	Disability.gov	www.disability.gov
	DPI. Disabled Peoples' International	www.dpi.org
	European Congress on Visual Disability	www.eurovisionrehab.com
	ICCHP. International Conference on Computers Helping People with Special Needs	www.icchp.org
	ICDVRAT. International Conference Series on Disability, Virtual Reality and Associated Technologies	www.icdvrat.reading.ac.uk
	International Women and Disability Congress	www.micongreso.gva.es
	ISLRR. International Society for Low Vision Research and Rehabilitation	www.islrr.org
	NFB. National Federation of the Blind	www.nfb.org
	ONCE Foundation. Spanish National Organization for the Blind	www.fundaciononce.es
	WFD. World Federation of the Deaf	www.wfdeaf.org
	WFDB. The World Federation of the Deafblind	www.wfdb.org
	WID. World Institute on Disability	www.wid.org
	World Congress of Inclusion International	www.inclusion-international.org

Table 1. International initiatives that promote e-Accessibility and usability

This chapter presents a comprehensive review of the most recent advances in legislation, standardization and technological solutions for enhancing e-Accessibility in e-Health. In Section 2, the current state of the legislation in this field is reviewed. Section 3 describes and analyzes the main characteristics of ISO 9241, the standard that regulates the legal implementation of the design requirements for e-Accessibility. Finally, the recommended technology requirements, as well as the specialized medical devices and products for each type of disability, are presented and discussed in Section 4.

2. State of the art. Legislation

This section analyzes and details the current state of the international law on e-Accessibility, usability and disability. Accessibility of ICT products and services has become a priority in Europe as a result of demographic change. Due to the fact that people are living longer, it is calculated that by the year 2025 there will be 113.5 million people over the age of 65 in the European Union [8]. It is estimated that there are approximately 100 million elderly people and 50 million people with disabilities in Europe, 15% of the total population (800 million approx.). To this percentage must be added the population which is temporally disabled due to illness or injury, and people that have disabilities such as dyslexia or allergies. A recent study in the United States [9] revealed that 60% of working-age adults could benefit from using accessible technologies because they experience impairments or difficulties when using current technologies.

The concept of disability has undergone a profound transformation in recent years. Historically perceived from a health and social protection perspective, it is currently based on a bio-psycho-social vision. Society cannot and should not ignore the contributions, expertise and creativity of each and every one of its members. Thus, and according to the recent United Nations Convention, people with functional diversity are "those people with long-term physical, mental, intellectual or sensory impairments which, in interaction with various attitudinal and environmental barriers, hinders their full and effective participation in society on an equal basis with others"

The directives of the European Union (EU) state that the equal treatment principle requires the absence of any direct or indirect discrimination based on religion or belief, racial or ethnic origin, disability, age or sexual orientation. The principle of non-discrimination is a general principle of EU law included in several legal texts. Disability as a human problem that affects all of us equally, regardless of the factors surrounding us, is a principle encoded in Human Rights documents that protect all of us. The principles of non-discrimination and human rights have been enshrined in several fundamental texts.

The Universal Declaration of Human Rights of 1948 established that: *"everyone is entitled to all the rights and freedoms set forth in this Declaration, without distinction of any kind, such as race, colour, sex, language, religion, political or other opinion, national or social origin, property, birth or other status. Furthermore, no distinction shall be made on the basis of the political, jurisdictional or international status of the country or territory to which a person belongs, whether it be independent, trust, non-self-governing or under any other limitation of sovereignty" [Article 2] and that "all are equal before the law and are entitled without any discrimination to equal protection of the law. All are entitled to equal protection against any discrimination in violation of this Declaration and against any incitement to such discrimination"* [Article 7] [10].

The juridical basis of non-discrimination for disability is detailed in the Treaty of Amsterdam [October 2nd, 1997]. The Intergovernmental Conference that drew up the Treaty of Amsterdam offered an even stronger guarantee by including a declaration in the Final Act stating that Community institutions must take account of the needs of people with a disability when adopting measures to be incorporated into Member States' legislation: "*without prejudice to the other provisions of this Treaty and within the limits of the powers conferred by it upon the Community, the Council, acting unanimously on a proposal from the Commission and after consulting the European Parliament, may take appropriate action to combat discrimination based on sex, racial or ethnic origin, religion or belief, disability, age, or sexual orientation*" [Article 13] [11].

Furthermore, the Charter of Fundamental Rights of the EU -proclaimed during the Nice Summit of December 7th, 2000- states the principle of non-discrimination for people with disability: "*any discrimination based on any ground such as sex, race, colour, ethnic or social origin, genetic features, language, religion or belief, political or any other opinion, membership of a national minority, property, birth, disability, age or sexual orientation shall be prohibited*" [Article 21] [12].

Subsequently, the Commission of the European Communities presented the *e*Europe 2002 Action Plan [13] to the Council, the European Parliament, the Economic and Social Committee and the Committee of the Regions. This Action Plan was focused on exploiting the advantages offered by the Internet and therefore on increasing connectivity. Three years later the *e*Europe 2005 Action Plan [14] was adopted with the main objective of stimulating the development of services, applications and contents, while accelerating the deployment of secure access to broadband Internet. The ongoing *i*2010 [15] deals with the growth and deployment of the Information Society and audiovisual policies in the EU. Its purpose is to coordinate the actions of the member states to facilitate digital convergence and to face the challenges linked to the Information Society. For developing this strategic framework, the Commission has carried out extensive consultations about previous initiatives and instruments such as the aforementioned *e*Europe projects and the "*Communication on the future of European regulatory audiovisual policy*".

Figure 2 shows a timeline providing a graphic summary of the legislation discussed in this section.

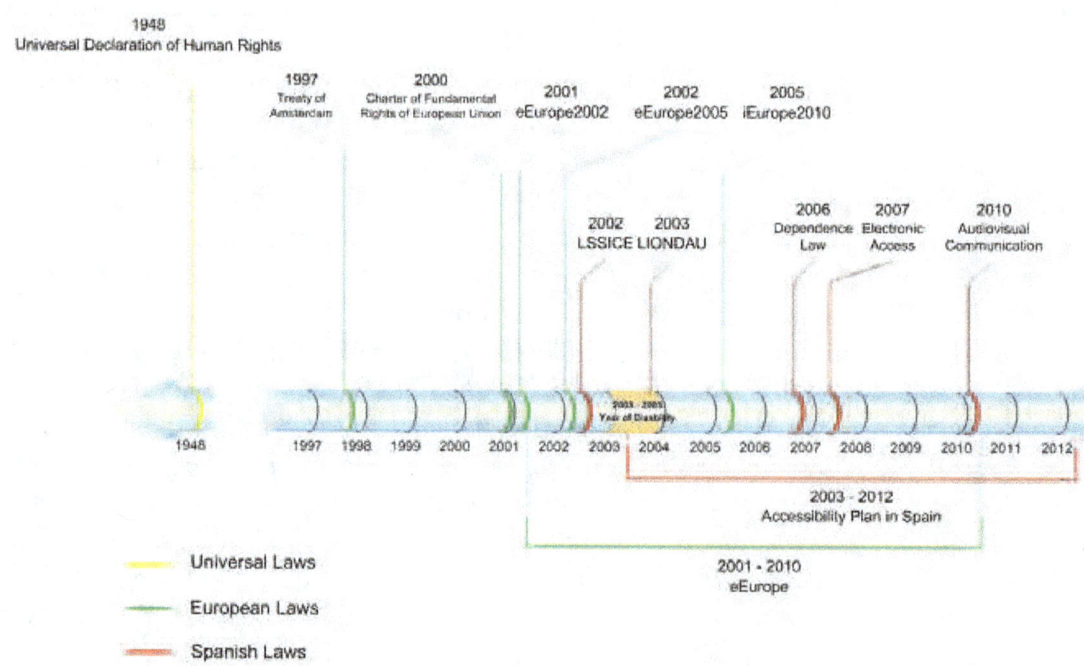

Fig. 2. Timeline summary of the legislation

3. Standardization on e-Accessibility for e-Health. ISO 9241

The standard that regulates the legal implementation of the design requirements in the area of e-Health is ISO 9241 [16]. ISO 9241, among other specifications, provides design guidelines for human-centred web-based user interfaces with the aim of increasing e-Accessibility and usability. ISO 9241-151:2008 [17] provides guidance on the human-centred design of software Web user interfaces with the aim of increasing usability. Web user interfaces address either all Internet users or closed user groups such as the members of an organization, customers and/or suppliers of a company or other specific communities of users. ISO 9241-171:2008 [18] provides ergonomics guidance and specifications for the design of accessible software for use at work, in the home, in education and in public places. It covers issues associated with designing accessible software for people with the widest range of physical, sensory and cognitive abilities, including those who are temporarily disabled, and the elderly. It addresses software considerations for accessibility that complement general design for usability as addressed by ISO 9241-110 [19], ISO 9241-11 [20] to ISO 9241-17 [21], ISO 14915 [22] and ISO 13407 [23].

Finally, ISO 9241-20:2008 [24] is intended for use by those responsible for planning, designing, developing, acquiring, and evaluating information/communication technology (ICT) equipment and services. It provides guidelines for improving the accessibility of ICT equipment and services such that they will have wider accessibility for use at work, in the home, and in mobile and public environments. It covers issues associated with the design of equipment and services for people with a wide range of sensory, physical and cognitive abilities, including those who are temporarily disabled, and the elderly.

Thus, depending on the type of disability involved, the ISO 9241 standard-based design will require other technologies (in addition of assistive products and equipment) to be consistent for the user. Figure 3 shows a relationship diagram for different types of visual, hearing, physical and speech disabilities.

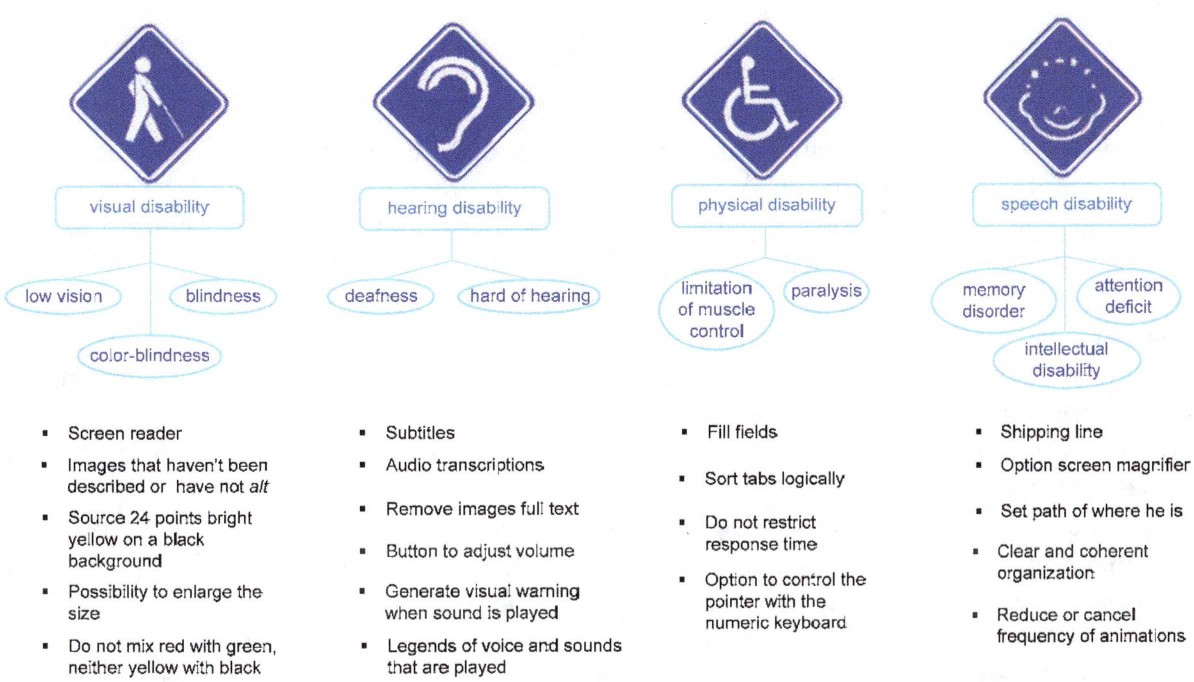

Fig. 3. Relationship diagram "technology - type of disability"

Independently of the type of functional diversity, there are a number of technological requirements that apply equally to all categories because they affect the overall philosophy of communication between man and computer: ergonomic design, customizable settings, multiple channels, etc. Here are the main general requirements to be considered in the design for all established by ISO 9241:

- **Messages**: an interface must be concise, coherent and consistent in order to reduce the effort required by the user to work with his or her computer. Short, simple messages are recommended. It is also desirable that the same message always has the same text, appears in the same area of the screen and has the same compositional elements. The reaction time to events is highly variable from one user to another. Therefore, it is counterproductive to display messages that automatically disappear over time. The speed with which the message is generated is also very important and this particularly affects voice messages. There should be consistency between what we hear and what actually occurs.
- **Channel redundancy:** this solves many of the problems of accessibility. It is commonly used as an indicator that a task is finished or as a warning of some kind of error. Hearing-impaired users lose this information so it should be accompanied by a visual signal of the event. Not only must there be a redundant output channel, but also in the input. It should be possible to operate with the mouse only, with the keyboard only, only with push button only and with speech recognition systems only.
- **Data entry:** this is done similarly in text mode or graphics mode user interfaces, although in the latter case an "edit box" item must be created. In both cases, the written text must be able to be scrolled by the cursor so that the screen reader can synthesize it to voice mode or convert it into Braille. For data entry fields, the accompanying identification labels must be aligned horizontally with the first line of the field so that they can be readily associated by screen reader users.
- **Customising the keyboard:** the keyboard is an essential peripheral so that all aspects of accessibility must be considered carefully. Users must have access to any element of the interface from the keyboard. Also, the use of simultaneous actions should be avoided or else an alternative sequential method should be provided to achieve the same result. To speed up keyboard operations, menus should be circular.
- **Icons:** for people with visual impairments it is uncomfortable to perceive icons and other small objects in the workspace, so the operating system should be enabled to change their sizes and positions, either independently or in groups. Icons must also have an associated label, facilitating the identification and understanding of their role.
- **Windows**: the management tasks of the windows (refresh, move, resize, etc.) are usually operated with the mouse but for users with low accuracy skills or who are blind, the use of the mouse is a disadvantage. Therefore, the standard requires that all these operations should also be able to be done with the keyboard. In the specific case of toolbars, which cannot be accessed by keyboard, it requires that all operations be accessible through the menu option.
- **User support services**: operating systems provide support services used by many applications. This assistance is usually in text format, but must also include the possibility of incorporating pictures or sign language.
- **System services:** in general, the standard requires that the operating system should provide the user with access to any input device that it uses and recommends that it also provide a voice recognition system. Similarly, output data should be handled by

both video and audio so that blind users can access the same information. All options should be activated on an optional basis so that the same software platform can be used interchangeably by a wide range of users with different needs. In addition, the services of the operating environment should be designed so as to be able to ensure that applications built upon it can be accessible.

- **Keyboard controller:** this is responsible for communications between computer and keyboard, and is a point at which many features that facilitate accessibility can be incorporated. People with accuracy problems in the use of their arms, fingers or hands have greatest difficulty in the use of the keyboard, followed by people with mental and visual functional diversity. These different issues need to be considered.
- **Mouse driver**: this must be able to modify the movement direction of the pointer so that the user can operate it in the most ergonomically comfortable manner. Likewise, it should be possible to modify the speed and acceleration of the pointer, differentiating between horizontal and vertical speed, click acceptance time and the time between two clicks.
- **Applications:** it should be borne in mind that, despite recent advances, users with accessibility issues sometimes need to use special devices or programs, so the standard requires applications to cooperate with these access tools. To avoid problems of consistency and coordination between applications, every application should have a choice of finish. Moreover, to achieve a completely accessible interface, all the services and requirements set forth so far are not enough. In addition, applications should be designed so that the number of steps required to access any option is minimized and do not require the simultaneous use of more than one input device, with particular emphasis on the most frequently used options. Thus, any user will achieve greater efficiency.

The principal requirements established by ISO 9241 for each type of functional diversity are as follows:

- **Visual disability.** The main barrier for people with visual impairment in accessing information is that such information is presented visually. Many users use screen readers to communicate with computers. Screen readers provide a description in either speech or Braille of windows, controls, menus, images, texts and other information that may appear on the screen. Some of the barriers for blind people in accessing content on the web are:
  - Images without alternative texts to describe their content.
  - Complex images, such as bar charts or statistics, without detailed descriptions.
  - Multimedia (videos, animations, etc.) without text or audio descriptions.
  - Tables whose content is incomprehensible when read sequentially (cell to cell in the order they appear in the code language or complete lines as presented on the screen).
  - Lack of independence of devices that cannot properly use the application with input devices other than the mouse (e.g., keyboard). The mouse is a pointing device impossible to use for people who cannot see where the cursor is.
  - Non-standard formats of documents that can be problematic for screen readers.
  - Font size with absolute measures that cannot be altered.
  - Design of pages when changing the font size leads to layout problems and difficult navigation.
  - Low-contrast images or text that cannot easily be changed using a user style sheet.

    - Text added by images rather than directly which makes it difficult to increase the size for easy reading.
    - Using colour to highlight text without using other additional formatting elements (such as italic, bold or underlining).
- **Hearing disability**. People with hearing difficulties but who are not deaf have problems with changes and certain frequency ranges, and in identifying and distinguishing certain sounds. They typically use the "Show Sounds" option already provided by some operating systems that offers visual information related to the sounds generated in the use of the computer. Besides having problems detecting auditory information, deaf users are often unable to speak in ways that are recognized by computer speech recognition systems. The barriers are:
    - Lack of subtitles or transcripts of audio content.
    - Lack of pictures to help understand the content of pages. Pages with too much text and no pictures can hinder understanding for people whose primary language is sign language rather than spoken or written language.
    - Need for voice input on some websites.
- **Physical disability**: physical disabilities are those that affect the proper mobility of people. Chronic degenerative diseases are characterized by the following symptoms: tremors (hands, arms, legs, jaw and face), rigidity in the limbs and trunk, slowness of movement and postural instability. Some of the barriers affecting people with functional motor disabilities are:
    - Icons, buttons, links and other elements of interaction are too small, making them difficult to use for people with limited dexterity in their movements.
    - Lack of independence of devices that cannot properly handle web pages with the keyboard instead of the mouse.
- **Ageing disability**: ageing is associated with a gradual loss of skills that can turn into a decrease in vision, hearing, memory, coordination and physical skills. The limitations derived from the environment cannot be considered as disabilities, but rather as environmental conditions that restrict opportunities of access to new technologies. Some limitations derived from the environment are:
    - Small screens, making visualization of applications designed for higher resolutions difficult.
    - Monochrome or black and white monitors that mask information based on colour alone.
    - Working environments that do not allow the perception of sound content of the application (high level of background noise, etc). To overcome this limitation, it is necessary to provide transcripts or subtitles.
    - Environments with poor lighting or limited visibility conditions that require increasing the font size, zoom, and contrast or changing the style of web pages.
    - Absence of a mouse to use the computer so that the keyboard must be used. Applications should be designed to enable device independence.

4. Technological solutions for disability in relation to e-Health

ICTs have improved our quality of life and recent progress in e-Health issues is already evident. However, people with visual, hearing, physical and speech disabilities do not completely enjoy all the potential benefits of e-Health, since these e-Health designs or developments do not consider their specific needs.

The aids provided by specific technological requirements for people with disabilities are classified according to the logic of the operation: alternatives (to allow replacement of a methodology or tool method, or tool "alternatives" that can be used by the subject), enhancement (to supplement the shortage of functional resources in subjects to perform an action or to "enhance" the low productivity of these) and substitutes (to allow the replacement of an absent or damaged functionality in the subject by another which the subject does have) [25].

This section will present and discuss the recommended technology requirements for each type of disability:

- **Psycho-cognitive diversity and ageing people**: providing solutions to the difficulties people have in learning and understanding abstract or complex concepts, the establishment of relationships between concepts, carrying out tasks with complex structures, the use of short term memory, interpretation and memorization of long sequences of operations, the ability of understanding of language, etc. These include many resources of the ICT environment: environment control, safety control, telemedicine, telecommuting, distance education and training, adapted jobs, etc.
- **Physical diversity:** incorporating solutions to issues related to mobility and manipulation including mobility and transportation, hygiene and personal care, household tasks, computer access, support for autonomy, etc.
- **Sensory diversity:** very different solutions that target visual diversity (including mobility aids, reading aids, writing aids) and hearing diversity (personal communication, telephony, communication in general, etc...)

There is great awareness in companies about new developments conforming to the standards that establish guidelines to implement the idea of design for all [26]. The general objective is to develop technologies for building channels of communication and interaction between people with some kind of special need and their environment. Different products and assistive devices [27] include many technological resources that are explicitly designed, manufactured in standard mode, or adapted from those already manufactured. These products can help people with functional diversity to overcome or mitigate their disabilities, providing access to greater autonomy and improved quality of life. An analysis of the most significant specialized medical devices and products is given below grouped by type of functional diversity [28]-[30].

4.1 Psycho-cognitive disability and ageing people

Some of the recent advances in this context of e-Health include special types of mouse with devices that allow moving the digital cursor over the screen through foot movements, or context keyboards (see Figure 4). These context keyboards are designed with pictograms instead of letters on every key in order to develop the augmentative communication of the patient through images that help to represent her/his needs [31].

Another milestone is the photo-sharing model, used by many parents with autistic children, which allows children to construct sentences through a book containing photographs of real objects collected through their own experiences. Grace [32] is an iPhone application based on a system of communication through images with which it is expected to help autistic people improve their social skills. It has more than 300 symbols and pictures stored on the iPhone terminal reflecting current day-to-day vocabulary of society. It also allows new pictures to be added at any time as the vocabulary grows.

Among applications for elderly people, the Cogknow project [33] aims to help minimize the overall risk of exclusion of older people with dementia, focusing the action on several aspects of their lives: memory, continuity of social contact, ability to perform daily activities, and increased safety. A mobile device (Smartphone or Pocket PC) has been developed which allows the elderly to remember their daily activities (using images), and to easily contact their families by simply clicking on the picture of the person they want to communicate with. Furthermore, the same device will act as a Global Positioning System (GPS) locator so that the carer or relative can monitor the movements of the user.
The large touch screens that allow applications to be opened and managed with a simple hand gesture are only a foretaste of what our relationship with technology will be in the coming years. Some other highlights of the technology applied to user interface design are shown in [34], and an example of these advances is the Gesture Cube [35], see Figure 5. While touchpads are now handled by dragging the fingers over the screen according to certain paths and geometries, the interface of the future will be handled by gestures alone. As its name suggests, the Gesture Cube senses and interprets hand movements and it can operate with various devices. The user moves the hand towards or away from the cube or waves the hand in front of it, while a series of sensors instantly detect the hand position and transmit the coordinates to the electronics installed in the interior. Thus, certain preset movements can be programmed to perform certain actions such as opening a program.

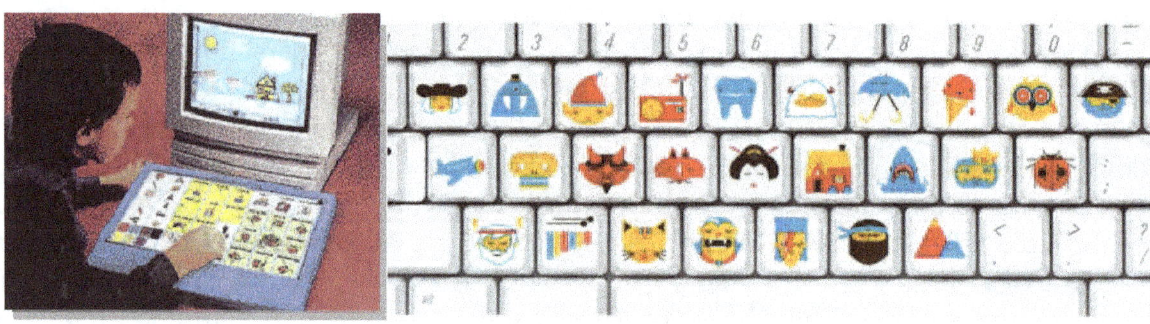

Fig. 4. Context keyboards (figures extracted from their respective websites, see references)

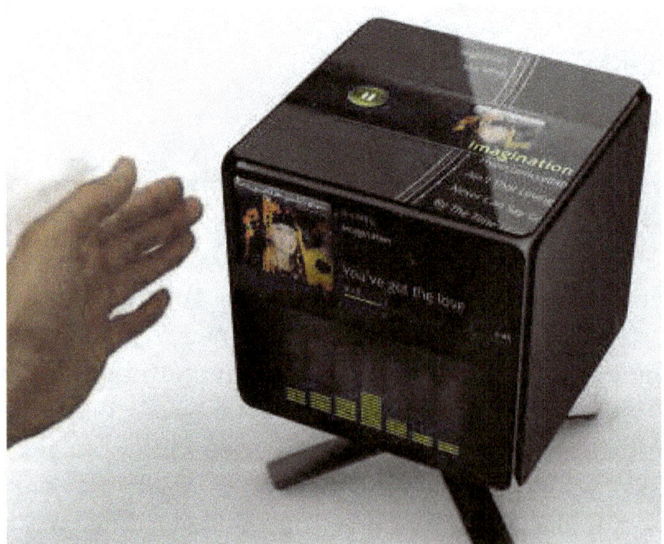

Fig. 5. Gesture Cube (figure extracted from website, see references)

4.2 Physical disability

There have been many medical advances in this field. Some highlights are glucose analyzers/meters (with strips including a capillary action that automatically acquire the blood and a beep to warn that the application is completed, the test result appearing on the display and also spoken through a synthetic voice), digital talking body thermometers (suitable for armpit, oral and rectal use with memory of the last measurement), or Head Pointer systems (suitable for people who have good head control and are able to use the computer keyboard with the head). The most significant advances are listed below:

- **Licorn**. This is a helmet with a built-in metal rod holding a small stylus or pencil. This is for operating the computer keyboard for people with good head control.
- **Ergonomic mice and push-buttons**. Special ergonomic mice operated by ball, tablet or plaque, keys, even the floor, wireless, head, joystick, push buttons, touch screen, voice, eyes, etc. With head mice, the user's head movements are processed by the system that moves the cursor on the computer screen. In mouse control by the iris, the system allows the user to place the mouse pointer anywhere on the computer screen simply by looking at that point. There are also virtual mice whose movement and click options appear on the screen operated by a push-button.

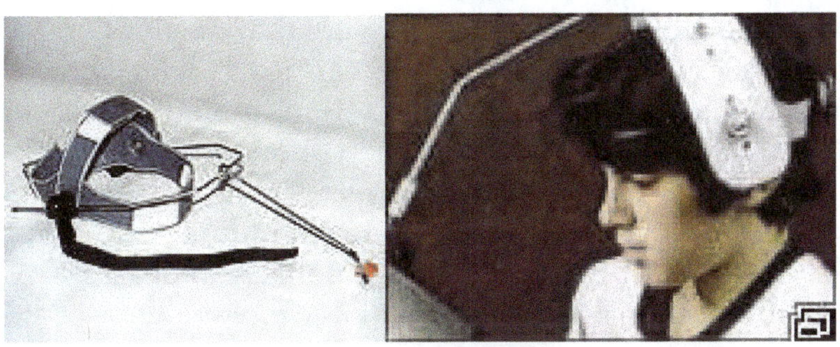

(a) Licorn

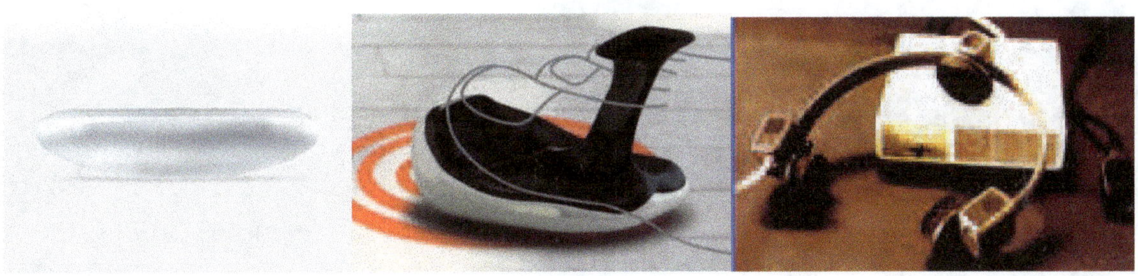

(b) Ergonomic mice

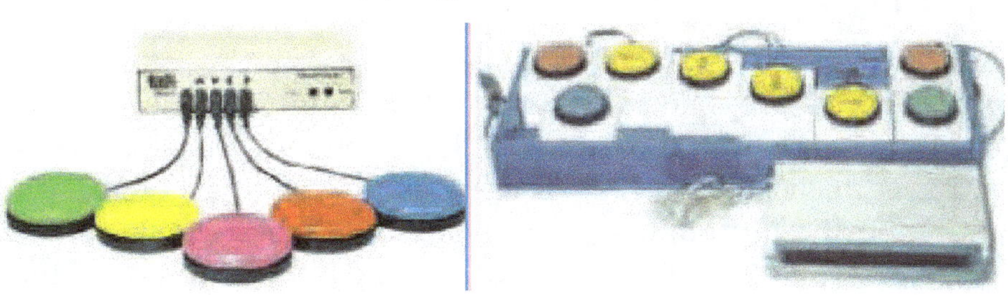

(c) Push-buttons

Fig. 6. Hardware devices for physical disability (figures extracted from their respective websites, see references)

4.3 Sensory (visual, hearing and speech) disability

Typhlotechnology is the adaptation and accessibility of ICTs for their use and implementation by people with blindness and visual impairment. A very detailed review of technological advances in typhlotechnology developed for people with visual functional diversity was given in [36]. Some other highlights of the technology applied to visual impairment were reviewed for this work and are collected in [37]-[46]. The most significant are listed below:

- **USB Braille keyboard** [47], for people with visual disability. As shown in Figure 7(a), this allows Braille letters to be entered, either completely replacing the conventional keyboard or working simultaneously with it. Braille input keys are arranged in a central ergonomic manner in two groups of 4 keys. The extra keys around the Braille keys correspond to a standard MF2 keyboard regard in terms of their function and form. The keyboard allows the combination of cells of six and eight points to generate characters following the American National Standards Institute (ANSI) Braille table.
- **CdBraille** [48], see Figure 7(b), is a relief printing system for Compact Disc (CD) and Digital Video Disc (DVD). This technology allows printing the surface of CDs and DVDs in Braille language.
- **Nokia Braille reader** [49], see Figure 7(c), is an application for touch screen phones that allows people with blindness or reduced vision to be able to write, read and send text messages. This system operates through software that displays on the screen a series of black and white circles on which the fingers can rest. Light vibrations can be felt that allow users to decipher the message. This is a Braille reader that translates text messages and reproduces them on touch screen phones with haptic feedback.
- **Loadstone GPS** [50] is a program to help blind people; it combines GPS and voice recognition systems, developed by two blind programmers. It is free and open source with the aim of "helping the blind to get from point A to point B". Another option also based on GPS is Mobile Geo [51], which is still in development.

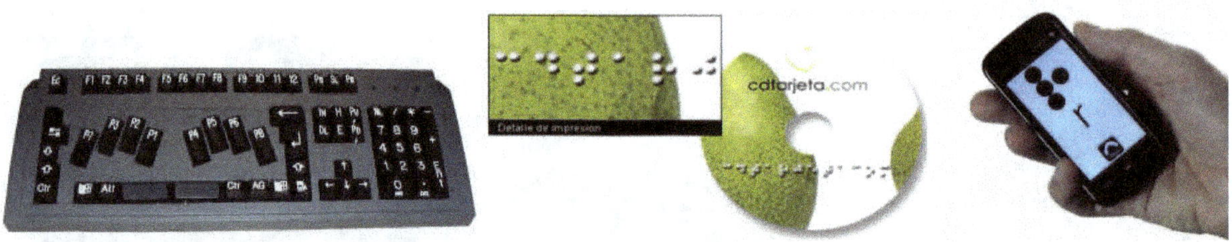

(a) USB Braille Keyboard (b) CdBraille (c) Nokia Braille

Fig. 7. Advances for physical disability (figures extracted from their respective websites, see references)

Some other highlights of the technology applicable in cases of hearing disability have been reviewed for this work and are collected in [52]-[53]. The most significant are listed below:

- A recent example, made in Spain, is the Barakaldo phone 010, which serves people with hearing and speech disabilities [54]. These groups can communicate with their local councils or authorities through a new system. Through their mobile phones and Personal Digital Assistants (PDAs), they can chat with the operators of the service.
- The Telesor system [55], allows public and private organizations to provide telephone services to people with hearing or speech disabilities, in a manner equivalent to that offered to a hearing person through voice phone. This ensures that all inhabitants with hearing or speech disabilities can communicate through their mobile devices (cell

phones and PDAs) with public and private telephone services. This communication is always made in real time via text and character to character communication mode. It is necessary to install a free widget on the mobile phone that will provide the functionality and user interface required.

- The cochlear implant is a device designed to reproduce the function of the cochlea through implanted electrodes. It uses a few external components (microphone, processor and transmitter) whose function is to collect, process and transmit sound to the electrodes. Cochlear implants, therefore, are designed to help people with profound deafness who are unable to benefit from hearing aids.

Finally, specific medical devices adapted for sensory disabilities and their associated hardware are described below (see Figure 8):

- Glucose analyzer (see Figure 8(a)). The strips are equipped with a capillary action that automatically places the blood in the alveoli of reaction. Very little blood is required. A beep alerts the user that the application of the blood has been completed. After 30 seconds the test result appears on the display in large print and is spoken by a synthetic voice.
- Talking thermometer (see Figure 8(b)). The talking digital body thermometer has an audible alert and memorises the last measurement.
- Talking blood pressure monitor (see Figure 8(c)). This uses a digital Liquid Crystal Display (LCD) and an oscillometric measurement method. The measurement process is accompanied by the addition of brief pre-recorded messages. There are also sound signals to indicate the end of the measurement. There are other models with facilities for language selection or disabling playback voice messages. The monitor announces the results shown on screen, whether they are valid as if there is an error. The date and time of measurements stored in the memory are recorded.
- Braille blood pressure monitor (see Figure 8(d)). Shenzhen ND Industrial Design has developed this blood pressure monitor made of a soft, flexible material which can be placed around the wrist. The results are shown in Braille by means of dots corresponding to the data being generated on the surface. Designed for people who have impaired vision, blindness, difficulty in hearing or who are completely deaf [56].
- Medicine dispenser (see Figure 8(e)). Adapted to the thread on a medicine bottle, this dispenses 5 ml doses of the liquid. The fluid passes through a small chamber with 5 ml capacity to facilitate accurate measurement.
- Pill organizer (see Figure 8(f)). On the upper side are the initials of the days of the week in Braille. Each day has four boxes with the Braille letters "a", "b ", "c" or "d", corresponding to 4 different times of day (morning, noon, afternoon and evening) when the medication is taken.
- Braille keyboard (see Figure 8(g)). Tecnalia has developed for ONCE a small wireless Bluetooth technology Braille keyboard. This application may be used by people with visual disabilities in both desktops and laptops as well as on PDAs and mobile phones [57].
- Screen magnifier (see Figure 8(i)). This type of adaptation is probably the first that appeared on the market and involves enlarging the characters and other content on the screen by up to six or seven times their normal size. This application requires screen magnifier software and manual handling equipment.
- Image magnifier. This equipment has an expansion chamber which projects the image of the object captured on a screen. Depending on their visual ability, the image magnifier allows users to adjust contrast, colour, sharpness, brightness and focus,

according to their own needs. For older people, the use of the magnifier means recovering their eyesight for many tasks that allow them to be independent.

- Screen magnification software. This software extends by up to twenty-five times the original size of the objects visible on the screen in all Windows applications. The screen magnifier ZoomText is character magnification software that allows the user to see text and drawings through a virtual magnifying glass at the size required.
- Voice reader (see Figure 8(h)). The Korean Sungwoo Park has developed an audible reader for the blind and called it Voice Stick. The device is a handheld scanner that combines Optical Character Recognition (OCR) and text-to-speech technology. It can read literally any text and convert it into audio which the user receives through headphones [58].
- Screen readers. These are a form of AT potentially useful for people who are blind or have vision problems, or learning difficulties. They are often combined with other AT applications such as screen magnifiers. The choice of screen reader is determined by several factors, including the platform or the cost. There are so many that we summarize the most important in a descriptive table (see Table 2).

Name	Author	S.O.	Notes
95Reader	SSCT	Windows	Japanese.
Blindows	Audiodata	Windows	Supports *Microsoft* Active Accessibility and Java Access Bridge.
HT Reader	HT Visual	Windows	Include support for MSAA and PDF.
iZoom	Issist	Windows	Screen Magnifier. Includes support for Mozilla Firefox.
Linux Screen Reader	GNOME	GNOME	Supports AT-SPI.
LookOUT	Choice Technology	Windows	Also available integrated with screen magnifier.
Magic	Freedom Scientific	Windows	Magnifier that can be used with JAWS.
Mobile Speak	Code Factory	Symbian, Windows Mobile	Supervisor by cells.
PC-Talker	Kochi System Development	Windows	Japanese Reader. Supports MSAA and Flash.
PCVoz	EzHermatic	Windows	Supports MSAA.
Simply Talker	EcoNet International	Windows	Trial version available.
Virgo	BAUM Retec AG	Windows	Supports MSAA and Java Access Bridge.
Virtual Vision	MicroPower	Windows	Supports MSAA.
VoiceOver	Apple	Mac OS X	Distributed with Mac OS X, uses the Apple Accessibility API.
Window-Eyes	GW Micro	Windows	Supports MSAA.
ZoomText	Ai Squared	Windows	Magnifier that includes support for voice synthesizer.

Table 2. Medical devices for physical disability

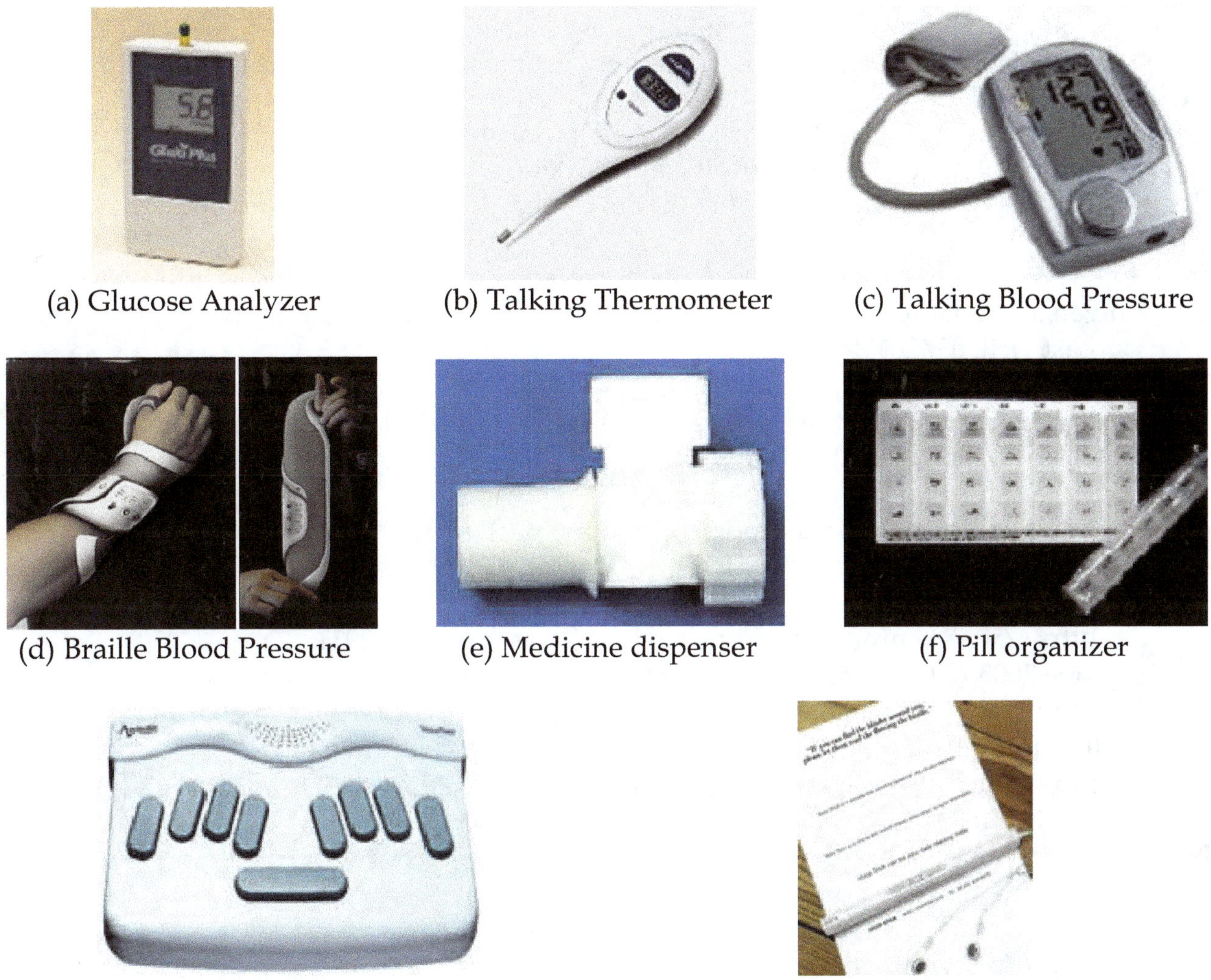

(a) Glucose Analyzer (b) Talking Thermometer (c) Talking Blood Pressure

(d) Braille Blood Pressure (e) Medicine dispenser (f) Pill organizer

(g) Braille Keyboard (h) Voice Reader

Fig. 8. Medical devices for physical disability (figures extracted from their respective websites, see references)

5. Acknowledgements

This work was partially supported by projects TIN2008-00933/TSI of the Innovation and Science Ministry (MICINN) and European Funds for Regional Development (EFRD), TSI-020100-2010-277 and TSI-020302-2009-7/Plan Avanza I+D of Ministry of Industry, Tourism and Trade.

6. References

Romañach Cabreo J., Palacios A. El modelo de la diversidad. La Bioética y los Derechos Humanos como herramientas para alcanzar la plena dignidad en la diversidad funcional. Ediciones Diversitas - AIES, 84-964-7440-2, 2008.

World Health Organization (WHO). http://www.who.int/en/. Last visit: 03/2011.

International Classification of Functioning, Disability and Health (ICF). http://www.who.int/ classifications/icf/en/. Last visit: 03/2011.

Design for all. http://www.designforall.org. Last visit: 03/2011.

International Conference on Computers Helping People with Special Needs (ICCHP). "e-Accessibility: Equality = e-Quality". ICCHP. www.icchp.org/2006/. Last visit: 03/2011.

Windows® API Code Pack for Microsoft® .NET Framework http://archive.msdn.microsoft.com/WindowsAPICodePack. Last visit: 03/2011.

Design for all. www.designforall.org/en/downloads/dossier-DfA-Fd-ang.pdf. Last visit: 03/2011.

Villarino, P. & Cayo, L. Discapacidad: Nuevas realidades, nuevos términos. CERMI, 2004.

The Universal Declaration of Human Rights. http://www.un.org/en/documents/udhr/. Last visit: 03/2011.

Treaty of Amsterdam. http://europa.eu/legislation_summaries/institutional_affairs/treaties/amsterdam_treaty/index_en.htm. Last visit: 03/2011.

Charter of Fundamental Rights of the EU. 2000. http://www.europarl.europa.eu/charter/pdf/ text_es.pdf. Last visit: 03/2011.

Commission of the European Communities. "eEurope 2002 Action Plan: accessibility of public websites and their content (2002/C 86/02)". http://www.europarl.europa.eu/sides/. Last visit: 03/2011.

—. "eEurope 2005 Action Plan: An Information Society for all". http://www.csae.map.es/csi/pdf/eeurope2005_es.pdf. Last visit: 03/2011.

—. "i2010: A European Information Society for growth and employment". http://europa.eu/legislation_summaries/information_society/c11328_es.htm. Last visit: 03/2011.

ISO9241. Ergonomics of human-system interaction. www.iso.org/iso/catalogue_detail.htm?csnumber=37031. Last visit: 03/2011.

—. Part 151: Guidance on World Wide Web user interfaces. http://www.iso.org/iso/iso_catalogue/catalogue_tc/catalogue_detail.htm?csnumber=37031. Last visit: 03/2011.

—. Part 171: Guidance on software accessibility http://www.iso.org/iso/iso_catalogue/catalogue_tc/catalogue_detail.htm?csnumber=39080. Last visit: 03/2011.

—. Part 110: Dialogue principles http://www.iso.org/iso/iso_catalogue/catalogue_tc/catalogue_detail.htm?csnumber=38009. Last visit: 03/2011.

—. Part 11: Guidance on usability http://www.iso.org/iso/iso_catalogue/catalogue_tc/catalogue_detail.htm?csnumber=16883. Last visit: 03/2011.

—. Part 17: Form filling dialogues http://www.iso.org/iso/iso_catalogue/catalogue_tc/catalogue_detail.htm?csnumber=16889. Last visit: 03/2011.

ISO 14915 Software ergonomics for multimedia user interfaces http://www.iso.org/iso/iso_catalogue/catalogue_tc/catalogue_detail.htm?csnumber=25578. Last visit: 03/2011.

ISO 13407 - Human-centred design processes for interactive systems http://www.iso.org/iso/catalogue_detail.htm?csnumber=21197. Last visit: 03/2011.

ISO 9241. Part 20: Accessibility guidelines for information/communication technology (ICT) equipment and services. http://www.iso.org/iso/iso_catalogue/catalogue_tc/catalogue_detail.htm?csnumber=40727. Last visit: 03/2011.

Soto Pérez F.J., Hurtado Montesinos M.D. Tecnologías de ayuda y atención a la diversidad: oportunidades y retos.

INREDIS. http://www.inredis.es/Default.aspx. Last visit: 03/2011.

Roca Dorda J., Roca González J., Del Campo Adrián M.E. De las ayudas técnicas a la tecnología asistiva.

Enderle J., Blanchard S., Bronzino J. Introduction to biomedical engineering. Singapore Academic Press, 2000. 0-12-238660-4.

Marazzi, A. "Presentan una tecnología que leerá órdenes enviadas por el cerebro de personas con discapacidades" 6 de Abril de 2010. http://gizmologia.com. Last visit: 03/2011.

Marquez, X. "Concepto de mouse para usar con tu pie" 4 de Abril de 2010. http://gizmologia.com. Last visit: 03/2011.

Tecnalia. Corporación tecnológica. http://www.tecnalia.info/. Last visit: 03/2011.

Widgetbox. http://www.widgetbox.com/. Last visit: 03/2011.

Ferrer-Roca O., Vilarchao-Cavia J., Troyano-Luque J.M., Clavijo M. "Virtual Sonography Through the Internet: Volume Compression Issues". (J Med Internet Res 2001;3(2):e21) www.jmir.org/2001/2/e21/. Last visit: 03/2011.

Emedmobile. http://www.emedmobile.com/. Last visit: 03/2011.

BL Healthcare. TCx Interactive System. http://www.blhealthcare.com/TCx-I_dedicated%20system_solution.html. Last visit: 03/2011.

Arregui Noguer B., Grau Sabaté X. , Pérez Bueno L. Tecnología y discapacidad visual : necesidades tecnológicas y aplicaciones en la vida diaria de las personas con ceguera y discapacidad visual. Madrid : Organización Nacional de Ciegos Españoles, Consejo General 2004, 2004. 84-484-0125-5.

Redaccion. San Sebastián, escaparate de lo último en tecnología social. Diario Vasco. 03 de Diciembre de 2009. http://www.hoytecnologia.com/noticias/Sebastian-escaparate-ultimo-tecnologia/143753. Last visit: 03/2011.

Sánchez J., Aravena G., Flores H. AUDIOMEMORICE: Desarrollo de la memoria de niños con discapacidad Visual a través de audio. Santigo-Chile : Sánchez, Jaime, 2003.

Higueras, E. Desarrollan un sistema de visualización braille a pantalla completa. s.l. : Tendencias Informáticas. Facultad de Informática de la UPM, 2010. http://www.tendencias21.net/Desarrollan-un-sistema-de-visualizacion-braille-a-pantalla-comp leta_a4268.html. Last visit: 03/2011.

Stack Overflow. How can you program if you're blind? Stack Overflow. 2010. http://stackoverflow.com/questions/118984/how-can-you-program-if-youre-blind. Last visit: 03/2011.

Shipman M., Yang P. Electroactive Polymer Design Opens Door To 'Full Screen' Displays For The Blind. North Carolina State University News. 29 de Marzo de 2010. http://news.ncsu.edu/ releases/wmsdispignabraille/. Last visit: 03/2011.

Ghosh T., Chakraborti P. , Di Spigna N., Winick D. , Yang P., Franzon P. The Integration of novel EAP-based Braille cells for use in a refreshable tactile display. San Diego: 12th International Conference on Electroactive Polymer Actuators And Devices, 2010.

Diseño para Todos. Grafica para ciegos. Junio de 2010. http://www.disenoparatodos.com/proyectosz/grafica_para_ciegos.htm. Last visit: 03/2011.

Pardo, L. Aerozoom mejora la lupa de Windows 7. s.l. : NeoTeo, 2010. http://www.neoteo.com/aero zoom-mejora-la-lupa-de-windows-7.neo. Last visit: 03/2011.

Toshiba. Internet Journal of emerging Medical Technologies. Coming Soon: Touchscreen Phones for The Blind. 21 de Mayo de 2010. http://www.medgadget.com/archives/2010/05/coming_soon_ touchscreen_phones_for_the_ blind.html. Last visit: 03/2011.

Toto, S. Japanese researchers develop mini brain wave measuring device. NODE. 6 de Abril de 2010. http://www.crunchgear.com/2010/04/06/japanese-researchers-develop-mini-brain-wave-measuring-device/. Last visit: 03/2011.

Antarq Tecnosoluciones. Antarq Tecnosoluciones. La alternativa a la discapacidad. Junio de 2010. http://www.antarq.com.mx/. Last visit: 03/2011.

Web Cdbraille. http://www.cdbraille.com. Last visit: 03/2011.

Finnish Federation of the Visually Impaired. http://www.nkl. fi/yleista/english.htm. Last visit: 03/2011.

Portaltic/EP. Una mujer crea una aplicación del iPhone para sus dos hijos autistas.

Loadstone - GPS. http://www.loadstone-gps.com/. Last visit: 03/2011.

Proyecto TELPES. Soluciones de Teleasistencia para Personas Sordas. Ciudadanía Digital del Plan Avanza. 2008-2010.

Sign SmithTM products featuring SigningAvatar® characters. Vcom3D, Inc. http://www.vcom3d.com /signsmith.php. Last visit: 03/2011.

El teléfono 010 de Barakaldo. http://deia.com. Last visit: 03/2011.

Telesor. http://www.telesor.es/. Last visit: 03/2011.

Shenzhen ND Industrial Design Co. http://www.sz-nd.com/ecompany.htm. Last visit: 03/2011.

Tecnalia - Corporación tecnológica. http://www.tecnalia.info. Last visit: 03/2011.

Sungwoo Park http://www.coroflot.com/public/individual_details.asp?individual_id=188883&sort_by=1&. Last visit: 03/2011.

10

Semiconductor II-VI Quantum Dots with Interface States and their Biomedical Applications

Tetyana Torchynska[1] and Yuri Vorobiev[2]
[1]*ESFM – National Polytechnic Institute, México D. F.*
[2]*CINVESTAV-IPN, Unidad Querétaro, Querétaro, QRO., México*

1. Introduction

Nanocrystals of group II-VI semiconductors, known as quantum dots (QDs), in which electrons and holes are three dimensionally confined within the exciton Bohr radius of the material, are characterized by the exceptional optical properties, such as broad absorption and sharp emission bands as well as size-tunable photoluminescence in the visible spectral range.

The most popular are CdSe/ZnS QDs due to their bright and unique emission with the wide excitation spectra and narrow emission bandwidths (Bailey et al., 2004; Dybiec et al., 2007; Jamieson et al., 2007; Kune et al., 2001; Norris et al., 1996; Tessler et al., 2002). The II-VI QDs have been investigated in versatile photonic applications including solar cells (Choi et al., 2006; Kongkanand et al., 2008; Lopez-Luke et al., 2008), optical fibre amplifiers (Liu et al., 2007), color displays using light-emitting diode arrays (Huang et al., 2008: Klude et al., 2002; Zhao et al., 2006), optical temperature probes (Liang et al., 2006; Walker et al., 2003), as well as in biology and medicine (Alivisatos et al., 2005; Grodzinski et al., 2006; Hoshino et al., 2007; Murcia et al., 2008; Portney & Ozkan, 2006; Wang et al., 2007).

Note that metal, semiconductor, polymer and ceramic nanoparticles in general have gained essential interest for biological and medical applications (Brigger, et al., 2002). Polymer and ceramic nanoparticles have been widely used as drug carriers, whereas metal nanoclusters and semiconductor QDs have been applied mainly for imaging and therapy. Among various nanoparticles, semiconductor QDs attracted much attention due their exceptional optical properties. In comparison with organic dyes and fluorescent proteins, the semiconductor quantum-confined core/shell nanostructures, such as CdSe/ZnS QDs, are brighter, more stable against photo bleaching, have multicolor emission in dependence on core sizes and can be excited for this emission with a single light source. The size-tunable properties allow one to choose an emission wavelength that is well suited to experimental conditions and to synthesize the QD-based probe by using an appropriate semiconductor materials and nanocrystal sizes.

In biology and medicine the semiconductor QDs have been used: for the fluorescence resonance energy transfer (FRET) analysis (Bailey et al., 2004; Jamieson et al., 2007; Zhang et al., 2005), in gene technology (Gerion et al., 2002; Han et al., 2001; Pathak et al., 2001), fluorescent labeling of cellular proteins (Dubertret et al., 2002; Dubertret et al., 2003; Hanaki et al., 2003), cell tracking (Bailey et al., 2004; Jamieson et al., 2007), pathogen and toxin detections (Lee et al., 1994; Yang et al., 2006), the bioconjugation to different antibodies and the targeted imaging and the delivery of anticancer drugs (Ebenstein et al., 2004; Ferrari et al., 2005; Torchynska 2009a; Torchynska et al., 2009b; Torchynska et al., 2010; Vega Macotela et al., 2010), the tissue, arterial and venous imaging (Larson et al., 2003; Wu et al., 2002), as well as in vivo animal imaging (Gao et al., 2004; Parungo et al., 2005).

The capping by wide band gap semiconductor (ZnS) of CdSe alone is not sufficient to stabilize the core, particularly in biological solutions, but the additional covering of ZnS shell with polymers or ZnS shell silanization provide increasing in QD stability and a reduction in non-specific adsorption. As a result the core/shell CdSe/ZnS QDs covered with polymers or silanized have improved essentially the efficiency of using of fluorescent markers in biological applications (Ebenstein et al., 2004; Larson et al., 2003; Torchynska, 2009a; Torchynska et al.,, 2010).

The conjugation of biomolecules with QDs has been achieved, as a rule, through covalent bonds using functional groups (linkers) on the QD surface (Gerion et al., 2001; Parak et al., 2002; Wolcott et al., 2006) or with the help of electrostatic interaction between QDs and biomolecules in self-essembled cases (Clapp et al., 2004; Ji et al., 2005; Torchynska 2009a). The essential set of publications related to the study of QD bioconjugation using PL spectroscopy revealed that the PL intensity of QDs decreased (Guo et al., 2003; Ji et al., 2005; Torchynska et al., 2009a; Vega Macotela et al., 2010) or increased (Torchynska et al., 2009a; Torchynska et al., 2009b) owing, as supposed, to the energy exchange between QDs and biomolecules. The shape of PL spectra of these bioconjugated QDs was not changed (Guo et al., 2003; Ji et al., 2005; Torchynska et al., 2009a; Torchynska et al., 2010). However up to now the full impact of bioconjugation processes on optical properties of CdSe/ZnS QDs is not understood completely.

The chapter presents the results of theoretical and experimental investigations of the authors related to the effect of QD dimensions and structure upon their photoluminescence spectra, as well as the influence of bioconjugation on QD emission and Raman scattering spectra, with an emphasis on the role of interface states in recombination processes in QDs. Besides, it contains a brief review of the data published by QDs inventors, producers and investigators necessary for the presentation and discussion of original results.

2. Synthesis of II-VI semiconductor core/shell QDs and encapsulation

A set of methods of growing CdSe, CdTe.... QDs have been reported (Crouch et al., 2003; Heine et al., 1998; Lou et al., 2004; Murray et al., 1993; Murray et al., 2000; Murray et al., 2001; Nordell et al., 2005; Park et al., 2004; Rosenthal et al., 2007; Yoon et al., 2005; Yu et al., 2005). The essential elements of these methods involve appropriate metallic or organometallic precursors (zinc, cadmium or mercury) with corresponding chalcogen precursors (sulfur, selenium or tellurium) in a coordinating solvent at high temperatures (Danek et al., 1994; Heine et al., 1998; Lou et al., 2004; Malik et al., 2005; Murray et al., 1993; Murray et al., 2000; Murray et al., 2001; Nann et al., 2002; Peng et al., 2001). The pyrolysis of organometallic precursors of cadmium and Se (or Te) introduced in (Murray et al., 1993; Murray et al., 2000) continues to be a wide used method for synthesizing CdSe or CdTe QDs. Typically CdSe (or CdTe) QDs were synthesized at 230–300 °C by the reaction between dimethyl cadmium (CdMe2) dissolved in trioctylphosphine (TOP) and TOPSe (or TOPTe) dissolved in TOP or in trioctylphosphine oxide (TOPO). The nucleation process is realized after the thermal decomposition of precursor reagents and the supersaturation of formed "monomers" that is relieved by nuclei generation. Monomer concentrations then are below the critical value for the nucleation, as result, the existing particles only grow without the formation of new nucleus (Murray et al., 2001). Time is a key parameter: longer reaction times result to a larger average particle size. Finally the formation of QDs takes place in these reactions, from which individual sizes of QDs were isolated by size-selective precipitation. The most successful system for the preparation of QDs with the high emission efficiency and mono dispersed particles includes a complex mixture of surfactants: stearic acid, TOPO, hexadecylamine, tributylphosphine (TBP), and dioctylamine (Qu & Peng, 2002). CdSe QDs having relatively small size (2-5 nm) absorb and emit light in the visible region (Fig.1), as well as CdSe QDs having a core-diameter 5 -8 nm and CdTe QDs absorb and emit light in the deep-red to IR regions, making them potential candidates for in vivo imaging and photodynamic therapy of cancer.

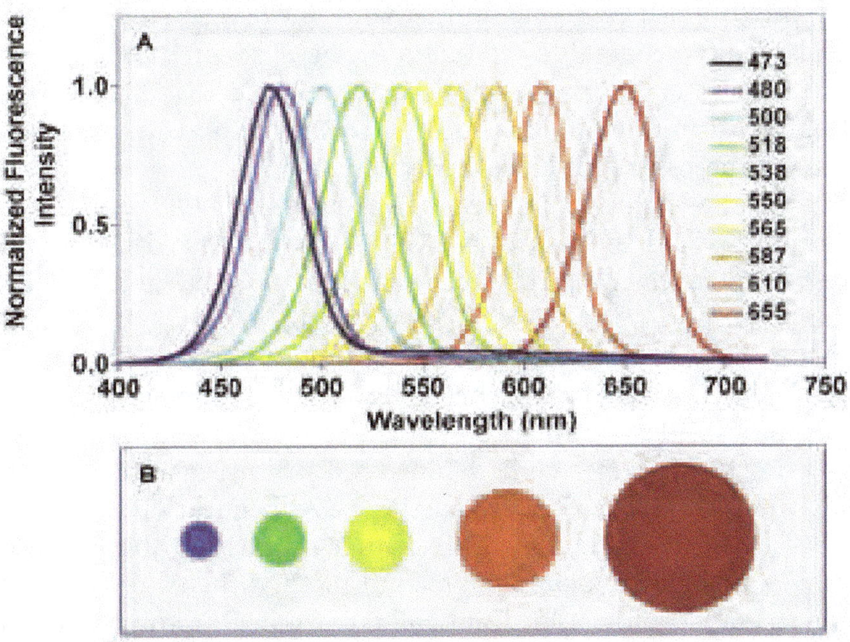

Fig. 1. Size-tunable fluorescence spectra of CdSe quantum dots (A), and illustration of the relative particle sizes (B). From left to right, the particle diameters are 2.1 nm, 2.5 nm, 2.9 nm, 4.7 nm, and 7.5 nm. (Smith & Nie, 2004)

Dimethyl cadmium is extremely toxic, expensive, unstable, explosive and pyrophoric, making the mentioned reactions difficult to control. Alternative cadmium precursors such as cadmium oxide, cadmium acetate, have been proposed as safer and greener cadmium precursors (Bilu et al., 2005a; Bilu et al., 2005b; Hai et al., 2009; Park et al., 2008; Peng et al., 2001; Qu et al., 2001). Recently (Peng et al., 2001) the synthesis of CdSe nanocrystals from CdO and elemental Se was realized, as an example of green chemistry with relatively safe materials, but the hazards associated with the CdO and Se have not been avoided.

The state of the surface impacts very strongly on optical and electrical properties of semiconductors that require embedding semiconductor clusters in a passivating medium (Alivisatos et al., 1996).

It is well known that the emission intensity of CdSe QDs increases essentially when the CdSe (or CdTe) cores are capped inside a shell of high bandgap material, such as ZnS, to form a CdSe/ZnS core-shell QDs. There are some more advantages for core/shell QDs in comparison with core-only QDs. The chemical and physical stabilities of core QDs increase when conjugated or shelled by higher band-gap semiconductors and polymers (Dabbousi et al., 1997; Kim et al., 2003; Peng et al., 1997).

Many types of core/shell QDs were developed such as CdSe/ZnS, CdSe/$Zn_{0.2}Cd_{0.8}S$, CdSe/CdS and CdTe/CdSe etc. Let us discuss the preparation of ZnS shells on CdSe cores as the best example presented in (Dabbousi et al., 1997). A solvent mixture (10:1) composed of TOPO and TOP was prepared by heating TOPO at 190 °C under vacuum, cooling to 60 °C and adding TOP. The CdSe QD suspension was prepared in hexane, transferred into the solvent mixture, and hexane was distilled out. A solution of diethyl zinc and hexamethyldisilathiane in TOP were added into the CdSe QD suspension kept at 140–220 °C, and ZnS shells were grown at this temperature. When required thickness of ZnS shells was obtained, controlled by absorption spectrum, the reaction was stopped by adding 1-butanol. The reaction mixture was cooled to room temperature, and the core/shell CdSe/ZnS QDs were separated by precipitation from a mixture of 1-butanol and methanol (Dabbousi et al., 1997). Shelling CdSe QDs with CdS resulted in considerable red-shifts in the absorption and photoluminescence bands of CdSe/CdS QDs in comparison with CdSe/ZnS QDs (Kim et al., 2003; Peng et al., 1997). Due to hydrophobic capping of QDs prepared by the methods mentioned above, further surface modification was necessary for biocompatibility.

Encapsulation has typically included incorporating core/shell QDs into organic polymers (Chin 2004; Fogg et al., 1997; Greenham et al., 1997; Huynh et al., 1999; Huynh et al., 2002; Mattoussi et al., 1999; Zenkevich et al., 2007) or inorganic glasses (Darbandi et al., 2005; Eisler et al., 2002) for the protection from environmental degradation or for added functionality and/or device applications. For biological and medical applications the main attempt related to performing hydrophilic capping of core/shell QDs and to prevent their precipitation.

Typically, the QDs synthesized in organic solvents have hydrophobic surface ligands such as trioctylphosphine oxide (TOPO), trioctylphosphine (TOP), tetradecylphosphonic acid (TDPA), or oleic acid (William et al., 2006). Two strategies have been applied to disperse QDs in aqueous buffers. The first method includes the exchange of the hydrophobic monolayer on the QD surface on the hydrophilic ligands. At the second method the native hydrophobic ligands can be retained on the QD surface. Additionally on the QD surface the adsorption of amphiphilic polymers, which includes hydrophilic segments such as polyethylene glycol (PEG) or multiple carboxylate groups, has been performed. A set of polymers have been reported, such as octylamine-modified polyacrylic acid (Yu et al., 2003), PEG-derivatized phospholipids (Dubertret et al., 2002), block copolymers (Gao et al., 2004), and amphiphilic polyanhydrides (Kirchner et al., 2005). The core/shell QDs are negatively charged if dihydrolipoic acid (DHLA) or octylamine-modified polyacrylic acid have been used as a surface-capping agent (Jaiswal et al., 2003; Wu et al., 2003). All these polymers provide relatively simple surface-modification of QDs for approaching biological compatibility.

Recently, the interest appears to the coating of emitting QDs with a layer of transparent silica (Chin 2004; Fogg et al., 1997; Greenham et al., 1997; Huynh et al., 1999; Huynh et al., 2002; Mattoussi et al., 1999; William et al., 2006; Zenkevich et al., 2007). Silica coating is expected to bring many advantages due to the thin silica layer (Fig. 2). A protective capping material on the QD surface increases the mechanical stability, enables a transfer into various organic and aqueous solvents, and protects QDs against oxidation and agglomeration; as well it improves the QD biocompatibility. Actually the surface of silica can be easily modified to link bioconjugators.

3. Optical properties of II-VI semiconductor core/shell QDs

The high quality nanoscale CdSe crystals has allowed at the middle of 90th of last century to resolve and study the QD size dependence of up to eight excited states in QD absorption spectra. This study was carried out for the strong confinement regime when the QDs are small compared to the exciton Bohr radius and absorption transitions are between discrete quantum size levels of electrons and holes in QDs (Efros et al., 1996; Norris et al., 1996). Let us consider absorption and photoluminescence spectra of CdSe QDs of different sizes presented in (Efros et al., 1996; Norris et al., 1996). The samples were prepared using the technique described in (Mural et al., 1993) and presented in n.2 of this chapter. Using this method nearly monodispersed wurtzite crystallites of CdSe (σ «5%) were prepared with the surface passivated by an organic tri-*n*-octylphosphine/tri-*n*-octylphosphine oxide ligands. The effective radii of studied QDs were determined in the range from 12 to 56 Å using small angle X-ray scattering and TEM measurements (Efros et al., 1996). The samples were isolated and redispersed into a mixture of *o*-terphenyl in tri*n*butylphosphine ~200 mg/ml to form an optically clear glass located between sapphire separated by a 0.5 mm thick Teflon.
Fig. 3 and Fig. 4 present the normalized absorption and full luminescence spectra for the set of CdSe QD's with radius between 12 and 56 Å, excited by a 300 W Xe arc lamp with broad beam (~50nm FWHM) to prevent the size selection of QDs (Efros et al., 1996; Norris et al., 1996).

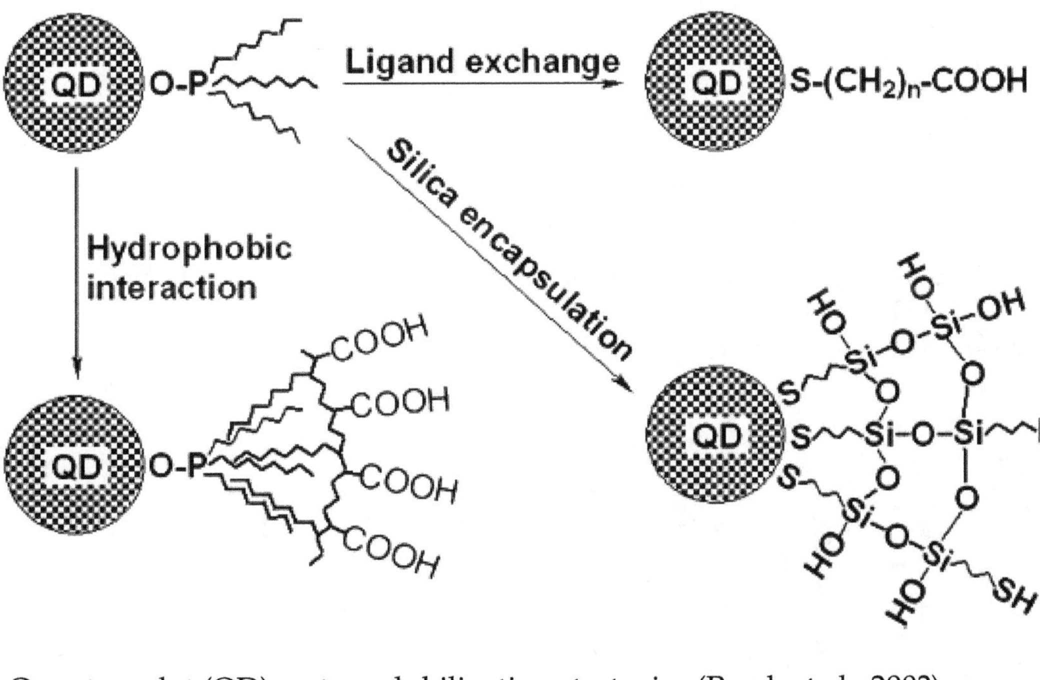

Fig. 2. Quantum dot (QD) water solubilization strategies (Parak et al., 2002).

It is clearly seen from figure 3 the shift of absorption and emission spectra into low energy side with the QD size increasing. The resulting full luminescence, excited at above QD band-edge absorption, contains contributions from all crystallites in the QD ensemble and is inhomogeneously broadened without distinct phonon structure. The full luminescence and absorption spectra show a strong size dependence of the Stokes shift, which varied from 100 meV for small QD sizes to 25 meV for large QD sizes (Efros et al., 1996). The high energy excited states are clearly seen in QD absorption spectra as well. The comparison of theoretically predicted and experimentally detected results has shown that energy and transition dynamics of band-edge emission can be quantitatively understood in terms of the intrinsic band-edge exciton (Efros et al., 1996; Norris et al., 1996). The long lifetimes of the band-edge luminescence (~1μs at 10K) was attributed to the exciton thermalization to a dipole forbidden +/- 2 dark exciton states.

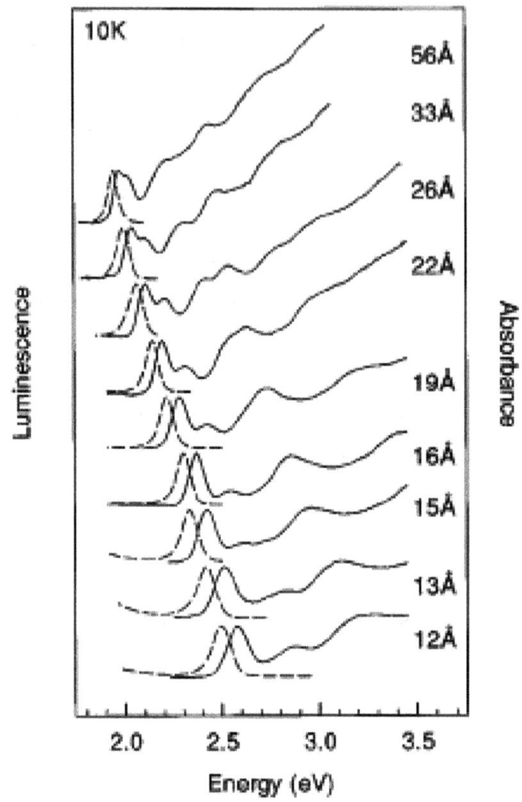

Fig. 3. Normalized absorption and full luminescence spectra for CdSe QD's between 12 and 56 Å in radius. The absorption spectra are indicated by solid lines; the corresponding luminescence spectra by dotted lines. (Efros et al., 1996).

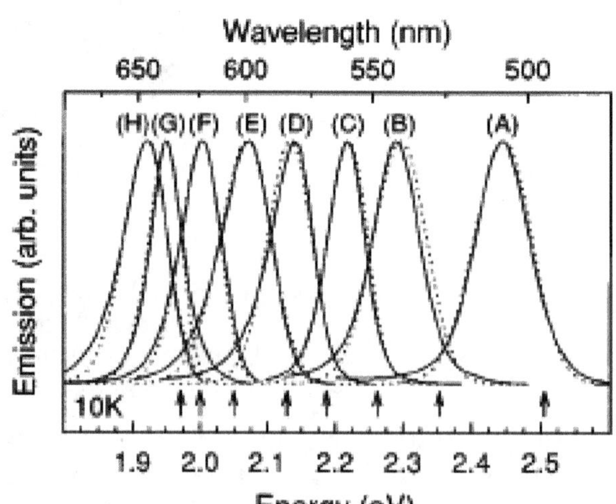

Fig. 4. Full luminescence spectra for QD size series from 15 Å(A) to 50 Å (H) (solid lines). Arrows indicate the PL excitation positions and dotted lines show the best fit obtained by the global fitting procedure (Norris et al., 1996).

With the size control that can now be achieved for CdSe QDs, the capping of lower band-gap (CdSe, CdTe....) core nanocrystals with a higher band-gap (CdS, ZnSe, ZnS...) shells is an attractive possibility that leads to the core/shell QDs with improved luminescence, higher stability (protected from the surrounding environment), and perfect electrically connection (Korton et al., 1990, Hoener et al., 1992, Hines & Guyot-Sionnest, 1996). In early 90th the CdSe nanocrystals have been successfully capped with ZnS (Kortan et al., 1990; Hines et al., 1996) and ZnSe (Hoener et al., 1992) for modification the surface passivation conditions. An advantage of ZnS shell in comparison with CdS shell is that ZnS forms at lower temperatures than CdS and ZnS and CdSe do not alloy well. The last aspect leads to the large lattice mismatch (12%) between two materials CdSe/ZnS (Madelung, 1992). The ZnS-capped CdSe exhibited enhanced band-edge luminescence, and an order of magnitude increased the quantum yield (Kortan et al., 1990), as well as decreased the surface trap concentration detected for the CdSe-TOPO QDs in the 700-800 nm spectral range and a much reduced tendency to permanent bleaching (Hines et al., 1996; Gong et al., 2007).

With the growth of ZnS shell on the surface of CdSe core absorption and emission spectra changed ((Hines et al., 1996; Gong et al., 2007; Rakovich et al., 2003). Fig. 5 shows the variation of absorption and emission spectra of CdSe QDs with the core size of 4.0 nm as the thickness of ZnS shell increased from roughly 0.3 to 1.7 nm (Rakovich et al., 2003). It is clear that emission and first absorption peaks monotonically shift into low energy spectral range together with broadening of absorption peaks when the ZnS shell thickness enlarges (Rakovich et al., 2003). A red-shift of absorption and emission spectra upon passivation at the shell formation is explained by a weakening of the carrier confinement in CdSe QDs due to its partial tunneling into the ZnS shell (Dabbousi et al., 1997; Dzhagan et al., 2008). The red-shift is larger when the shell becomes thicker (Dzhagan et al., 2008). Comparable shifts in the optical spectra of CdSe/ZnS and CdSe/CdS are obtained because of a weaker tunneling of the core-confined carriers into the shell made of a wider bandgap material (Dzhagan et al., 2008).

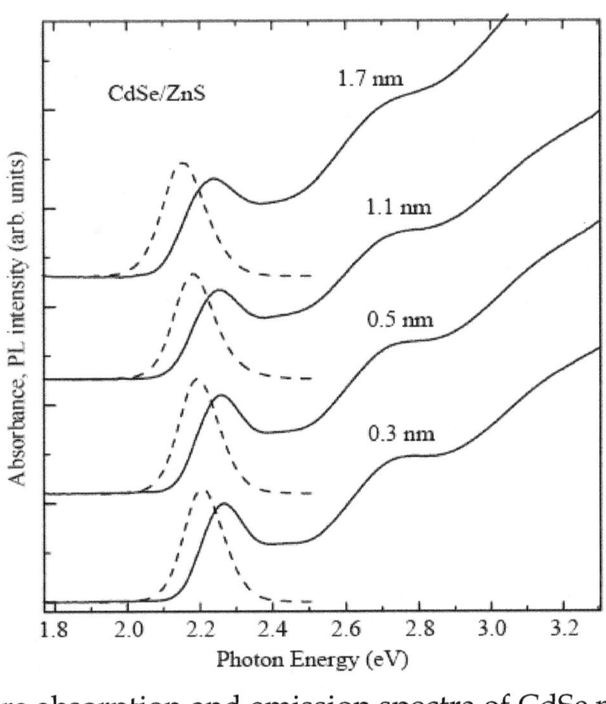

Fig. 5. Room-temperature absorption and emission spectra of CdSe nanocrystals with different thicknesses of ZnS shell (in nanometers. Rakovich et al., 2003).

The Raman scattering in CdSe QDs has been studied efficiently during last two decades (Alivisatos et al., 1989; Baranov et al., 2003; Dzhagan et al., 2007; Dzhagan et al., 2008; Hwang et al., 1999; Meulenberg et al., 2004; Torchynska et al., 2007; Torchynska et al., 2008). The original CdSe QDs passivated by organic molecules reveal a Raman peak related to scattering by the longitudinal optical (LO) phonon at about 206-210 cm^{-1} (Meulenberg et al., 2004), which is red-shifted from its bulk value of 213 cm^{-1} due to phonon confinement (Meulenberg et al., 2004; Tanaka et al., 1992), as well as a weaker mode arising from the second order (2LO) appeared at 415 cm^{-1}(Meulenberg et al., 2004). The shift of a LO phonon Raman peak from 210 cm^{-1} down to 205 cm^{-1} and LO Raman peak softening with decreasing QD sizes from 3.0 nm to 1.6 nm was theoretically predicted in (Meulenberg et al., 2004). But the different sample passivation produces a different magnitude of LO phonon shift suggesting a variance in the nature of the phonon confinement with passivant type and/or the strain effects due to effective compressive or tensile surface stresses in QDs (Meulenberg et al., 2004).
The effect of ZnS shell thickness in the range 1.0-3.5 ML on the phonon spectra in CdSe QDs was studied in (Baranov et al., 2003). The Raman lines of LO and 2LO phonons of the CdSe core and the line of LO phonons of the ZnS shell at about 350 cm^{-1} with intensity comparable to that of 2LO CdSe peak are clearly seen in the Raman spectrum (Fig. 6). It is shown that the line of ZnS LO phonons at 350 cm^{-1} partly overlaps the second order Raman lines of the CdSe core, but it can be distinguished even at the ZnS shell thickness of 0.5 ML.

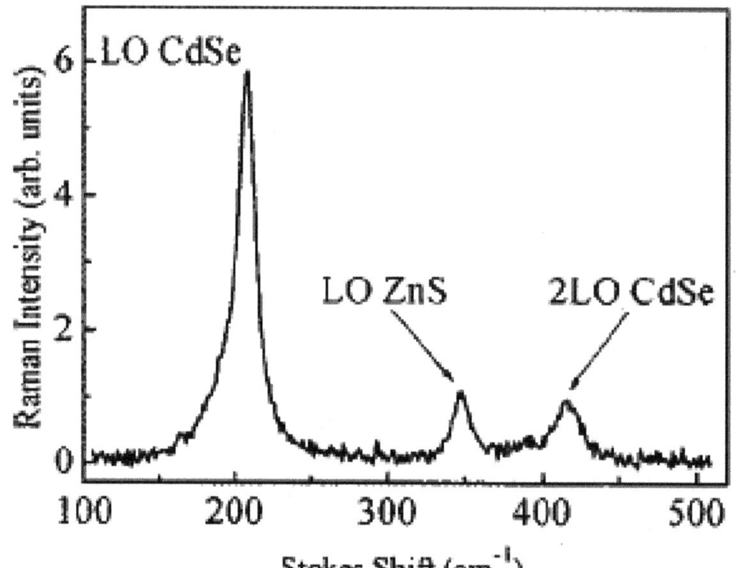

Fig. 6. Raman spectrum of CdSe/ZnS QD's with a shell thickness 3.4 ML excited by a 476.5-nm line of an Ar laser (Baranov et al., 2003).

The Raman spectrum transformation in dependence on the shell types (CdS, ZnS) and the order of shell atom deposition: CdSe/ZnS1 (Zn then S), CdSe/ZnS2 (S then Zn) or CdSe/CdS2 (S then Cd) were studied in (Baranov et al., 2003; Dzhagan et al., 2007). After passivation with CdS the LO phonon Raman peak at 206 cm^{-1} and an additional Raman peak around 270 cm^{-1} have been revealed (Fig. 7). The Raman peak at 270 cm^{-1} was assigned to Cd–S vibrations in the shell (Dzhagan et al., 2008). The phonon confinement and lattice mismatch-induced strain can induce the shift of LO phonon Raman lines in thin-layer superlattices and in core/shell QDs by more than 20 cm^{-1} (Dinger et al., 1999). The authors supposed that the Cd-S vibration related Raman peak appeared at 270 cm^{-1}, which downward shifted on 30 cm^{-1} from the bulk value of the CdS LO phonon, 305 cm^{-1}, due to the formation of an alloyed layer at the interface between CdSe core and CdS shell.

The interdiffusion during the ZnS shell growth was also assumed for CdSe/ZnS QDs, which revealed a similar Cd–S mode (Dzhagan et al., 2008). The role of sulfur as an initiator of the interdiffusion was supported by the fact that the CdS-like peak was observed to be stronger (Fig.7) for the samples where sulfur atoms were deposited first (CdSe/ZnS2). The larger lattice mismatch for the CdSe/ZnS interface can further stimulate interdiffusion. The red shift of the CdSe LO phonon peak after passivation (Fig. 7) was explained by the formation of an intermixed core/shell interface as well. The late effect is accompanied by the quenching of QD emission intensity.

4. Theoretical analysis of the emission spectra of QDs using mirror boundary conditions in the quantum mechanical description

To explain the emission spectra of QDs observed, the corresponding system of electronic energy levels for them should be known. Theoretical analysis of the energy spectra and optical properties of nanosized semicoinductor sphere was published first in 1982 (Efros & Efros, 1982), and the discussed core-shell II-VI semiconductor QDs present ideal material for comparison of theory with experiment.

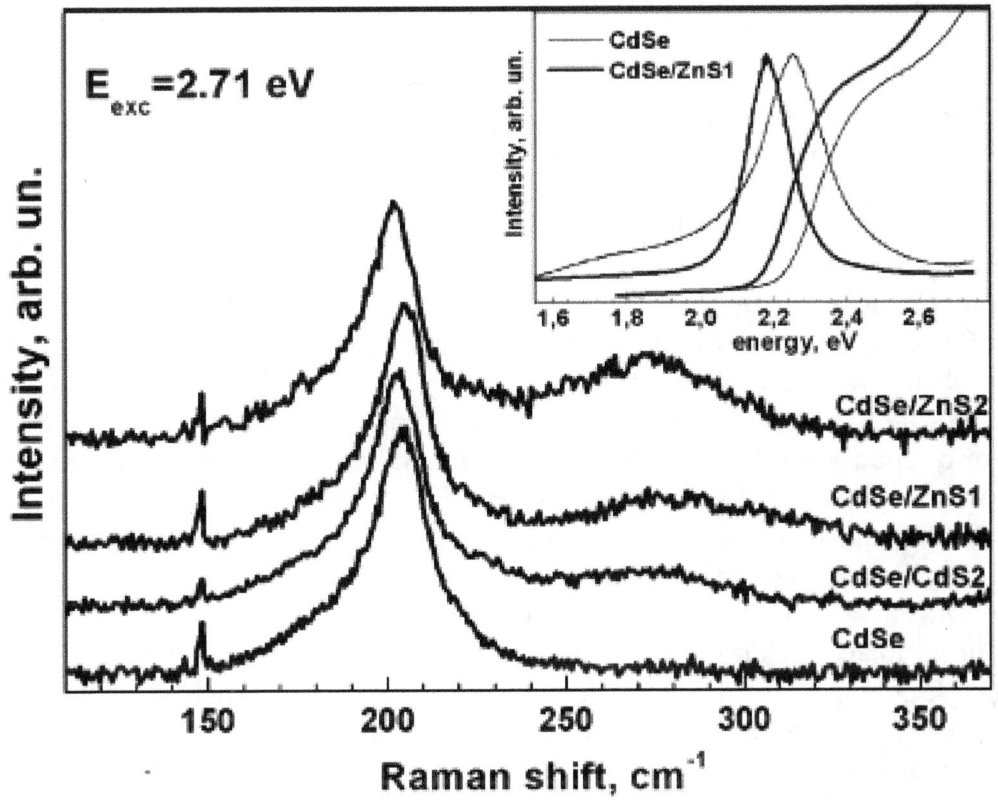

Fig. 7. Normalized Raman spectra of CdSe and core-shell QDs. Inset: Absorption and PL of CdSe and CdSe/ZnS QDs (Dzhagan et al., 2008).

However, during almost two decades of investigation of these objects, no one publication appeared related to such a comparison. As we shall see, the reason for that is simple: the calculations performed in (Efros & Efros, 1982; Gaponenko, 1998) predict much larger energy levels separations than those observed experimentally. We attribute this discrepancy to the boundary conditions used for description of a spherical QDs in all previous publications: namely, the traditional "impenetrable walls" boundary conditions. Another point is that the effective mass approximation normally used in these calculations, could be questioned in case of nanosized semiconductor particles. We have shown that both the agreement of theory with experiment and the applicability of the effective mass approximation could be greatly improved using another type of boundary conditions, as we call them, **even mirror boundary conditions**. We assume that a particle (electron) confined in a QD is specularly reflected by its walls; the assumption is based on the data of STM (Schmid et al., 2000) showing a clear interference pattern near the surface of a solid created by incident and reflected de-Broglie waves for an electron; an attempt to treat walls of a quantum system as mirrors was made previously (Liboff and Greenberd, 2001; Liboff, 1994) in so-called "quantum billiard" problem; however, the analytical form of the conditions employed in these papers was different from ours and much more complicated.
In our **treatment of QD boundary as a mirror**, the boundary condition will equalize values of particle's Ψ-function in an arbitrary point inside the QD and the corresponding image point in respect of mirror-reflective wall. In a general case, one can allow Ψ-functions to coincide by their absolute value, since the physical meaning of the wave function is connected to $\Psi^*\Psi$. Thus, depending on the sign of the equated values of Ψ, one will obtain **even** and **odd** mirror boundary conditions. For the case of odd boundary condition incident and reflected waves cancel each other at the boundary, so that one will obtain the case equivalent to that of impenetrable walls with zero Ψ-function at the boundary, representing "strong" confinement case. However, experimental data (Dabbousi et al., 1997) show that it is not always so – there is a possibility that a particle may penetrate the barrier, and then return again into the confined volume. Thus, the wave function will not vanish at the boundary, and the system will be considered as a "weak" confinement as long as particle flux through the boundary is absent (Liboff, 1994).
Application of the new boundary conditions for such weak confinement case will yield solution different from those for QD with impenetrable boundaries. Supposedly, the resulting energy spectrum would be also different, which may offer better explanation of some experimental data. Therefore, here the treatment is focused on weak confinement case with even mirror boundary conditions, which is a timely and very important task that, to our point of view, will be important for bringing theory and experiment together. In the considered quantum dot with mirror-reflective boundaries, as a particle (electron, hole) is approaching the wall from inside, its image will also do so from the outside, meeting with the particle at the boundary. Due to the specular reflection, the actual particle continues to move along the trajectory of its image inside the QD whereas the image keeps on moving outside, virtually expanding a QD into a lattice of reflected cells. Formation of such virtual periodic structure extension greatly favours the effective mass approximation. Thus, to investigate the specific features of the problem, we consider only the **even** form of mirror boundary conditions here.
Assuming the potential inside the quantum box (QD) equal to zero and using the common variable separation method, we look for a solution of the stationary Schrödinger equation $\Delta\Psi + k^2\Psi = 0$ (with $k^2 = 2mE/\hbar^2$ and particle mass m) in the form

$$\Psi = \prod_j \Psi_j(x_j) = \prod_j (A_j \exp(ik_j x_j) + B_j \exp(-ik_j x_j)) \cdot \quad (1)$$

Here x_j describe the coordinates x, y, z and k_j – the components of wave vector **k**. For our case of a **spherical QD**, following the treatment made in (Efros & Efros, 1982; Gaponenko, 1998) we apply the common methodology of a particle confined in a three-dimensional square well potential (for example, Schiff, 1968). The wave function in polar coordinates has a form

$$\Psi(r,\theta,\varphi) = R(r)\ Y_{l,m}(\theta,\varphi) \quad (2)$$

The angular part $Y_{l,m}$ is similar to that of hydrogen atom. The energy spectrum is determined by solution of the radial part of equation R(r), which is expressed in spherical Bessel functions of half-odd-integer order for the new variable $\rho = \alpha r$; for our purposes it will be sufficient to analyze the first of them

$$j_0(\rho) = \sin\rho/\rho \quad (3)$$

with $\rho/r = \alpha = \hbar^{-1} (2mE)^{1/2}$.
For the case of the impenetrable walls of a QD, the boundary condition is $\sin \alpha r = 0$ (for sphere radius $r = a/2$ and diameter a). Thus, one will have $\alpha a/2 = \pi n$ yielding the energy spectrum (in agreement with (Efros & Efros, 1982; Gaponenko, 1998))

$$E = \frac{h^2}{2ma^2} n^2 = \frac{h^2}{8ma^2}(2n)^2, n = 1,2,3,... \quad (4)$$

Here m is the effective mass of a particle confined in a QD. As one can see, the parameter α has the meaning of a wave vector, i.e. if we introduce de-Broglie wavelength λ, then $\alpha = 2\pi/\lambda$. The condition obtained $a = n\lambda$ requires an integer number of wavelengths fit along the diameter of the sphere.
To introduce the mirror boundary condition, we employ the spherical reflection laws to find the position "x" of the reflected image of the point characterized with a radius vector "r" nearby the wall, so that x = 0 and r = 0 will correspond to the centre of a sphere. For the standard expression for spherical mirror

$$(r - a/2)^{-1} + (x - a/2)^{-1} = -4/a.$$

so that

$$x = a\, r/(4r - a).$$

If the particle given by r-value locates in direct vicinity of quantum dot wall, one should set $r = a/2 - \delta$ having $\delta << a/2$. In this case $x \approx a/2 + \delta$, meaning that at negligibly small distances between the mirror and the object, a spherical mirror behaves similarly to the planar one. Under these assumptions, the mirror boundary condition will have the form

$$\Psi(a/2 - \delta, \theta, \varphi) = \Psi(a/2 + \delta, \theta, \varphi) \quad (5)$$

Using spherical Bessel functions for the radial eigen-function, we obtain from (5) the condition $\cos \alpha\, a/2 = 0$, which gives $\alpha\, a/2 = \pi(2n + 1)/2$, and the energy spectrum

$$E = \frac{h^2}{8ma^2}(2n+1)^2, n = 0,1,2,... \quad (6)$$

As one can see, now the diameter of the sphere can include only **odd** number of half-wavelengths. This expression is different from the previous one: in (4) we have the coefficient $h^2/8ma^2$ multiplied by squares of even integers, whereas (6) feature the squares of odd integers only. For large quantum numbers this difference is not essential, but for small "n" it is pronounced, reaching 400% for the lowest energy state.

Since the form of the energy spectra obtained with mirror boundary conditions does not differ from that obtained with traditional methodology, we will use the classification of quantum confinement types for a spherical QDs employed in (Efros & Efros, 1982; Gaponenko, 1998) and discuss only the strong confinement case with $a/2 << a_B$, where a_B is the Bohr radius for an exciton:

$$a_B = \frac{\hbar^2 \varepsilon}{\mu e^2}$$

with reduced mass $\mu = (m_e m_h)/(m_e + m_h)$, electron and hole masses $m_{e,h}$ and dielectric constant of the material ε. Following the argumentation of (Efros & Efros, 1982; Gaponenko, 1998), the current case can be considered as a simplification when one can use the expressions for energy spectra obtained (4, 6) with the corresponding effective mass m. The reason for that is that the separation between the quantum levels is of the order $\hbar^2/ma^2$, which is large compared to the Coulomb interaction energy between an electron and a hole that is proportional to $e^2/\varepsilon a$. Therefore, we can ignore the Coulomb interaction, taking only the aforementioned energy spectra expressions for the case of quantum confinement effect.

According to (Efros & Efros, 1982; Gaponenko, 1998), the optical absorption threshold for the spherical semiconductor QD is given by the expression

$$\hbar \omega_{01} = E_g + \frac{h^2}{2\mu a^2} \tag{7}$$

which corresponds to the spectrum (4) with n = 1 for the case of impenetrable walls. For the spherical quantum well with mirror-reflecting walls we use the expression (6), which for the optical absorption threshold (n = 0) will yield:

$$\hbar \omega_{01} = E_g + \frac{h^2}{8\mu a^2} \tag{8}$$

Among the great amount of papers devoted to various QDs, not many present the experimental values of energy levels together with the exact well dimensions. Luckily, such data can be found for CdSe/ZnS core-shell quantum dots. They are pronouncedly spherical, with exactly known dimensions and positions of the lower energy levels.

We assume that in these core-shell QDs the carrier reflections conditions are fulfilled at the CdSe/ZnS boundary, as discontinuity of electrical potential causes reflection of the particle flux. Thus, one can safely hypothesize the walls of CdSe quantum well could be considered as effective mirror surface confining the particles.

To compare the experimental data with the theory, we use the following parameters of CdSe (Gaponenko, 1998; Haus et al., 1993): $m_e/m_o = 0.13$, $m_h/m_o = 0.45$ (m_o - the free electron mass), material dielectric constant around 10. For the band gap, we take recently found value of E_g = 1.88 eV (Esparsa-Ponce et al., 2009) (while the previous value of 1.84 eV (Gaponenko,

1998; Haus et al., 1993) is also not much different). The reduced mass corresponding to the effective masses cited is $\mu = 0.1\ m_o$, resulting in the Bohr radius for the exciton to be about 5.3 nm. The spherical nanocrystals of CdSe described above featured radii between 1.15 and 2.75 nm, keeping the strong confinement condition valid for all the cases considered.

The Table 1 below summarizes the experimental data on spherical QDs of CdSe together with the calculated data. The absorption threshold wavelength λ_{01} for nanocrystals with diameter a = 2.85 nm was taken from (Hines & Guyot-Sionnest, 1996), the rest of the experimental data proceed from (Dabbousi, 1997). The photon energy $\hbar\omega_{01}$ corresponds to the absorption threshold, which differs by the energy difference ΔE from the band gap (i.e., supplying the degree of an actual quantum confinement effect). The values of $\Delta E_{calc} = \hbar\omega_{01} - E_g$ were calculated after expression (8) for QD with mirror-reflecting walls.

a, nm	2.3	2.85	4.2	4.8	5.5
λ_{01}, nm	470	515	555	582	612
$\hbar\omega_{01}$, eV	2.64	2.41	2.24	2.13	2.1
ΔE, eV	**0.76**	**0.53**	**0.36**	**0.25**	**0.22**
ΔE_{calc}, eV (8)	**0.72**	**0.47**	**0.22**	**0.17**	**0.13**

Table 1. Comparison of theoretical and experimental data on light absorption in CdSe nanocrystals

As one can see, the energy values calculated using the expression (8) obtained for mirror-reflecting walls of a quantum well yields very good correlation with the experimental data, while the expression (7) obtained for the case of traditional impenetrable wall case gives the values about 4 times larger.

In Fig. 8 we present a data set for CdSe nanocrystals taken from (Invitrogen, 2010), showing the dependence of emitted photon energy upon well diameter a (curve 1). Curve 2 corresponds to the energy (8), displaying a good agreement with the experimental data.

In our previous publications we have shown that the mirror boundary conditions could be successfully applied to other geometries of QDs, such as hexagonal, triangular and pyramidal (Vorobiev et al., 2009; Vorobiev et al., 2010; Vorobiev et al., 2011).

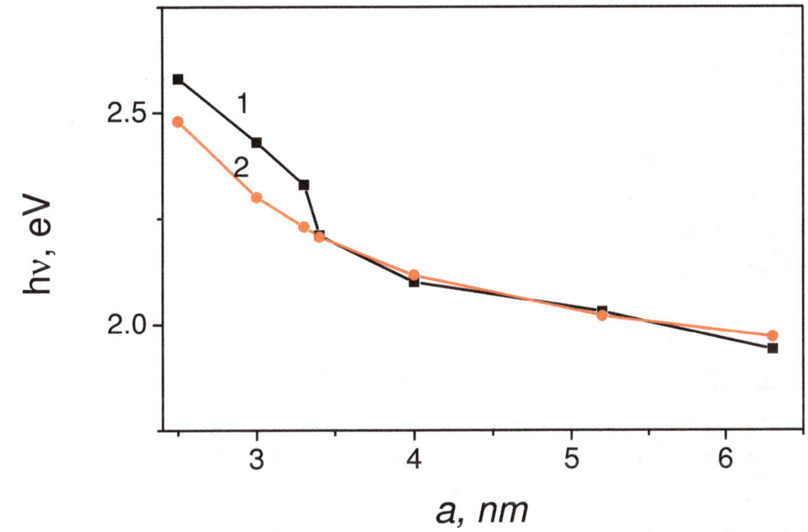

Fig. 8. Experimental (1) and calculated (2) exciton energy in CdSe QDs.

Thus we can conclude that the method used can be considered as a simple and reliable approach for solution of the Schrödinger equation describing the particles confined in the semiconductor quantum dots, in particular, for the framework of effective mass approximation. Our theoretical predictions feature very good agreement with the experimental data for the spherical CdSe nanocrystals, while the traditional impenetrable wall approximation yields much overestimated results. The mirror boundary conditions are easy to implement, which allows simplifying consideration of a large variety of QD geometries and obtaining analytical expressions for the energy spectra for the different types of nanosystems.

5. The process of QD bioconjugation for imaging, labelling and sensing

As we mentioned above in n.2, the preparation of water-soluble II-VI core/shell QDs is an important step for many biological applications. QDs, as a rule, can be grown easily in hydrophobic inorganic solvents (see n.2). Then the methods of solubilisation are applied based mainly on exchange of the technological hydrophobic surfactant layer with a hydrophilic one (Bruchez et al., 1998; Gerion et al., 2001; Kim et al., 2003), or the preparation of a second surface QD layer by the adsorption of bifunctional linker molecules, which provide both hydrophilic character and functional groups for bioconjugation. In second method the layers are used, such as: the amphiphilic molecule cyclodextrin (Pellegrino et al., 2004), chitosan, a natural polymer with one amino group and two hydroxyl groups (Calvo et al., 1997; Miyzaki et al., 1990), PEG-derivatized phospholipids, encapsulation in phospholipid micelles (Dubertret et al., 2002), addition of dithiothreitol (Pathak et al., 2001), organic dendron (Guo et al., 2003; Wang et al., 2002), oligomeric ligands (Kim et al., 2003), or poly (maleicanhydride alt-1-tetradecene), as well as silica and mercaptopropionic acid (MPA) (Bruchez et al., 1998; Gerion et al., 2001). MPA achieves the conjugation through carboxyl groups, and silica through thiol groups on its surface. It is essential that, for example, phospholipid and block copolymer coatings tend to increase the diameter of CdSe–ZnS QDs from ~4–8 nm before encapsulation to ~20–30 nm (Chan et al., 1998; Medintz et al., 2005). Fig. 9 presents the schemes widely used for conjugation of proteins to QDs (Medintz et al., 2005).
The numbers of steps were used for preparing QDs to bioconjugation: the mixture of QDs during some time with the bifunctional linker in solution, the extraction from the organic solvent by centrifugation and re-dissolving QDs in an appropriate conjugation buffer (Chan et al., 1998). This algorithm was used initially for such linker molecules as: mercaptoacetic acid, glutathione and histidine, mercaptosuccinic acid, dithiothreitol, and for bifunctional compounds containing sulfhydryl groups (Aldana et al., 2001; Pathak et al., 2001). The disadvantage of this procedure is the slow desorption of linker molecules that causes the QD precipitation and long-term storage problems (Jamieson et al., 2007; Mattoussi et al., 2000). To improve the long-term stability of biocompatible QDs a set of methods has been proposed, such as (Jamieson et al., 2007): (a) the use of engineered recombinant proteins joint electrostatically to a QD surface which were modified with dihydrolipoic acid, (b) the use of hydrophilic organic dendron ligands to create a hydrophilic shell of QDs, (c) the application of a micellar encapsulation procedure in which phospholipid molecules surround the TOPO coated QD surface, and (d) the conjugation of QDs to streptavidin via an amphiphilic polymer coating. The steady improvement in producing of biocompatible II-VI QDs made over the past 10 years has contributed essentially to the successful implementation of these new luminescent markers in biology and medicine.

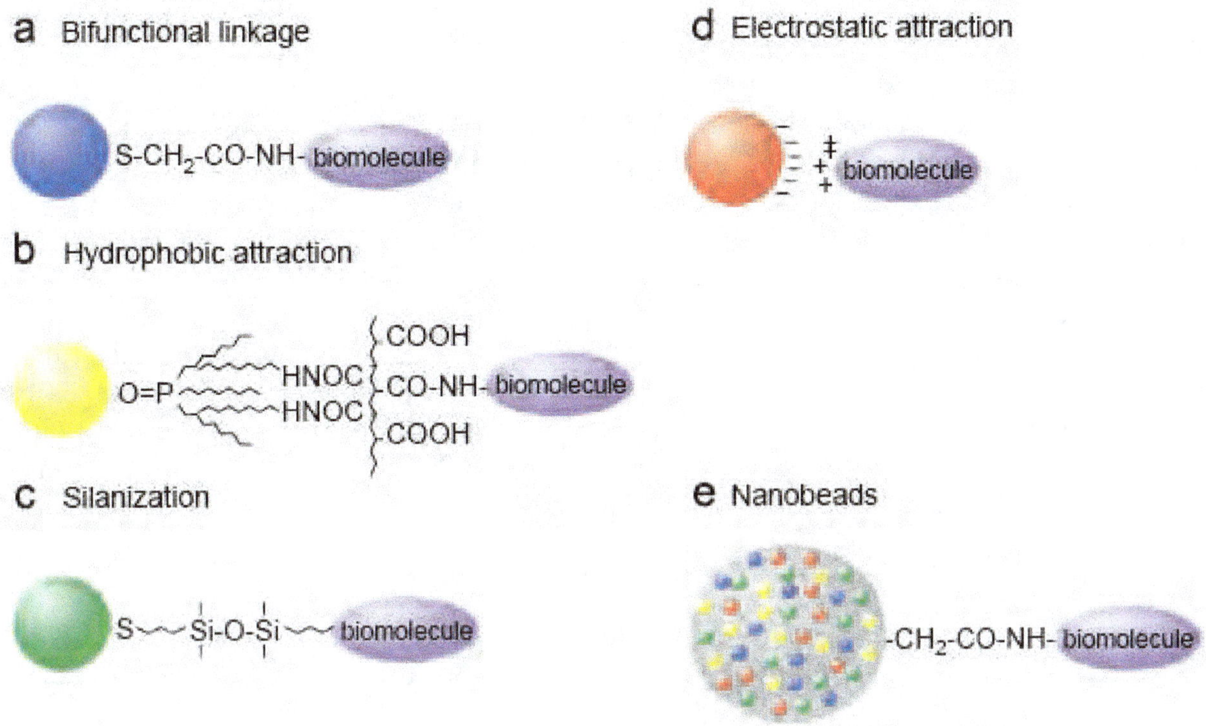

Fig. 9. A schematic presentation of different approaches of QD conjugation to biomolecules (Jamieson et al., 2007; Medintz et al., 2005): (a) Use of a bifunctional ligand such as mercaptoacetic acid for linking QDs to biomolecules. (b) TOPO-capped QDs bound to a modified acrylic acid polymer by hydrophobic forces. (c) QD solubilisation and bioconjugation using a mercaptosilane compound. (d) Positively charged biomolecules linked to negatively charged QDs by electrostatic attraction. (e) Incorporation of QDs into microbeads and nanobeads.

6. PL spectra of nonconjugated core/shell CdSe/ZnS QDs with interface states

The ability to cover core/shell II-VI QDs with polymers and biomolecules is a critical step, as we mentioned above, in producing efficient bio-luminescent markers. We have shown early (Torchynska et al., 2009 a, b and c) that core/shell CdSe/ZnS QDs with radiative interface state are very promising for the spectroscopic confirmation of the bioconjugation process. These systems permit to detect both the variation of PL intensity at the bioconjugation, that ordinary has been monitored, and the transformation of emission spectra related to the change of a full width at half maximum (FWHM) (Torchynska b and c; Vega Macotela et al., 2010a) and PL peak positions, as well as the transformation of Raman scattering spectra (Torchynska et al., 2007; Torchynska et al., 2008; Vega Macotela, 2010b; Diaz-Cano et al., 2010).

The nature of radiative interface states in the core /shell CdSe/ZnS QDs has to be investigated. To study the origin of interface states, the PL spectra of CdSe/ZnS QDs covered by the amine-derivatized PEG polymer with core emission at 525, 565, 605 and 640 nm have been investigated in dependence on the size of CdSe cores. Then PL spectra of 565 and 605 nm QDs have been studied in dependence on a set of factors, such as: i) the size of CdSe cores, ii) the temperature of PL measurements (10 and 300K), iii) the state of bioconjugation and iv) the time of aging in ambient air.

Commercially available core-shell CdSe/ZnS QDs, covered with amine-derivatized polyethylene glycol (PEG) polymer, are used in a form of colloidal particles diluted in a phosphate buffer (PBS) with a 1:200 volumetric ratio. Studied QDs are characterized by the sizes: i) 3.2-3.3 nm with color emission at 525-530 nm (2.34-2.36 eV), ii) 3.6-4.0 nm with color emission at 560-565 nm (2.19-2.25 eV), ii) 5.2-5.3 nm with emission at 605-610 nm (2.03-2.08 eV) and iv) 6.3-6.4 nm with color emission at 640-645 nm (1.92-1.94 eV). Some parts of CdSe/ZnS QDs (named 565P and 605P) were bioconjugated that we will discuss in next section. Other parts of CdSe/ZnS QDs (named 525N, 565N, 605N and 640N) have been left nonconjugated and serve as a reference object. Nonconjugated CdSe/ZnS QDs in the form of a 5 mm size spot were dried on a polished surface of crystalline Si substrates as described earlier in (Torchynska et al., 2009 a, b and c; Vega Macotela et al., 2010a). PL spectra were measured at 300 K and some of them at 10 K at the excitation by a He-Cd laser with a wavelength of 325 nm and a beam power of 20 mW using a PL setup described in (Torchynska et al., 2009 a, b and c; Vega Macotela et al., 2010a).

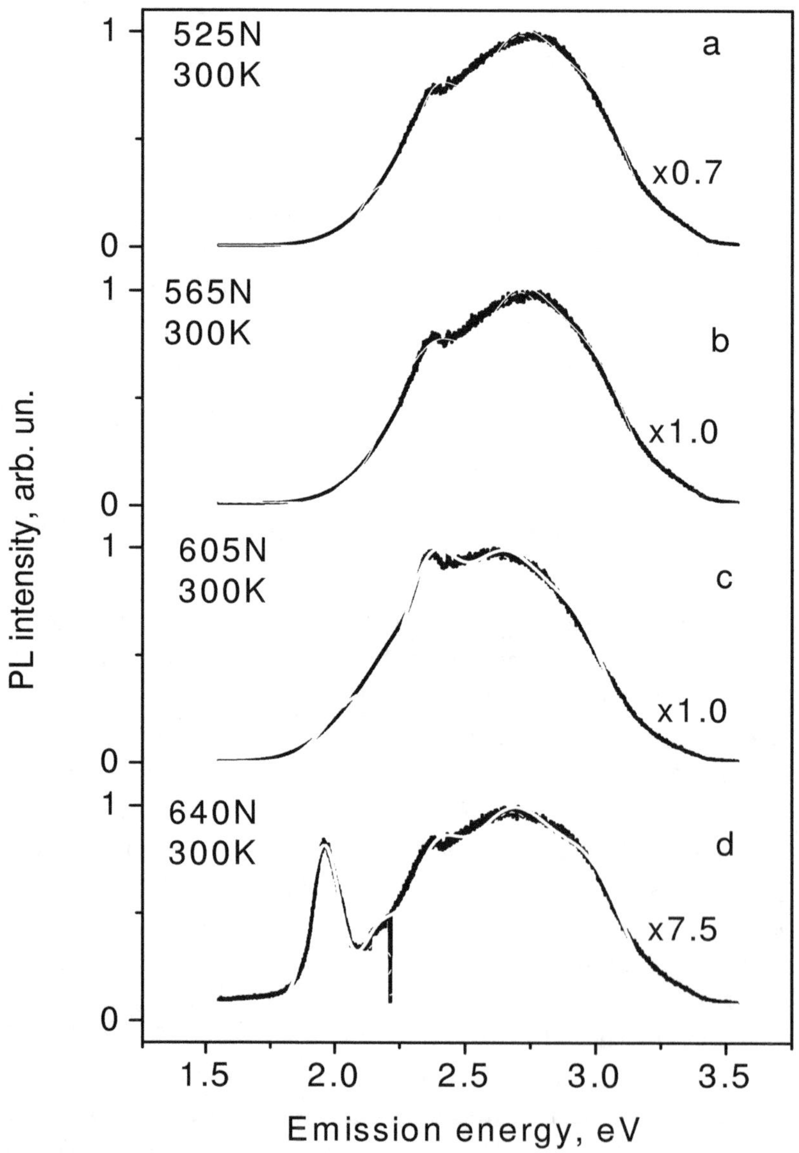

Fig. 10. CdSe/ZnS QDs of different sizes with interface states

Normalized PL spectra of nonconjugated CdSe/ZnS QDs measured at 300 K demonstrate the broad PL band in the spectral range of 1.80-3.20 eV with a main maximum at 2.37 eV and with shoulders (or small peaks) (Fig. 10). This broad PL band does not depend on the size of CdSe QD cores (Fig. 10). It is clear that the broad PL bands are a superposition of elementary PL bands. The deconvolution procedure has been applied to PL spectra permitting to represent them as a superposition of five elementary PL bands (Fig. 11a,b). The peaks of elementary PL bands are at 2.02, 2.17, 2.33, 2.64 and 3.03 eV (Fig. 11a) for 605N QDs and at 1.99, 2.19, 2.35, 2.64 and 3.03 eV (Fig. 11b) for 565N QDs. PL bands with the peaks at 2.02 eV (605N) and 2.19 eV(565N) relate to emission of ground state excitons in the CdSe cores of corresponding QDs. The nature of other PL bands needs to be studied.

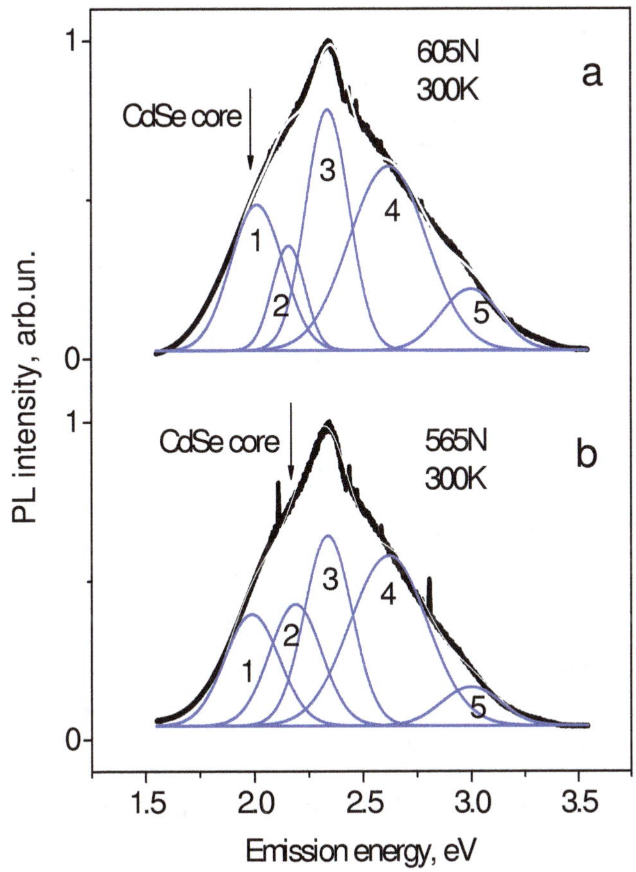

Fig. 11. The deconvolution results for 605N QDs (a) and 565N QDs (b)

The high energy PL bands can be assigned to the electron-hole recombination via: i) excited states in the CdSe core ii) defects in the CdSe core or ZnS shell and/or iii) interface states at the ZnS/polymer interface. The PL spectrum of nonconjugated (605N) CdSe/ZnS QDs has been studied at a low temperature (10 K) with the aim to clarify the nature of high energy PL bands (Fig. 12). As one can see in Fig. 12 the PL spectrum does not change essentially at temperature decreasing. The result of deconvolution has shown that only the PL band related to a CdSe core shifts from 2.02 eV (300 K) up to 2.12 eV (10 K) due to increasing the optical band gap in a CdSe core at 10 K. The temperature variation of CdSe core peak energy was found to be 2.2 10^{-4} eV/K that is less than the value obtained earlier (3.3 10^{-4} eV/K) for the CdSe/ZnS QDs (Rusakov et al., 2003) with the thickness of ZnS shell from the range of 0.3-1.7 nm. The last fact is related, apparently, to the higher thickness of ZnS shell (2 nm) in studied CdSe/ZnS QDs

(Invitrogen, 2010). Simultaneously the high energy PL bands do not change their spectral positions that testify that high energy PL bands are not connected with the defect-related states or excited states in semiconductors (CdSe or ZnS). Thus high energy PL bands can be assigned to the currier recombination via the interface states at the ZnS/polymer interface.

The permanent position of high energy PL bands in QDs with different CdSe core sizes (Fig. 10, Fig. 11), the independence of their PL peaks versus temperatures (10 K or 300 K) (Fig. 12) permit to assign the high energy PL bands to the radiative recombination of photogenerated carriers via interface states related to the ZnS/polymer interface.

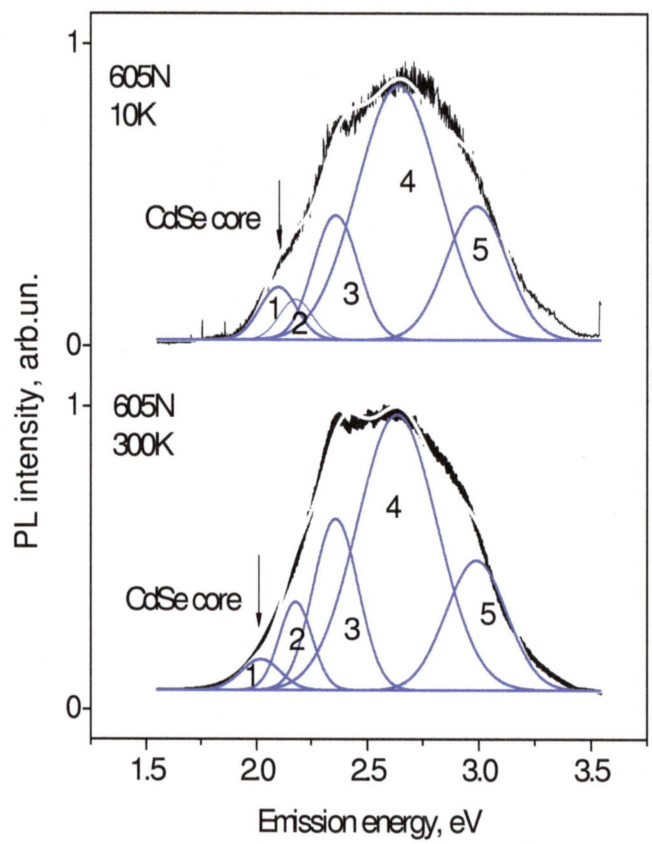

Fig. 12. PL spectra of 605N QDs measured at the temperature of 10 K (a) and 300 K (b).

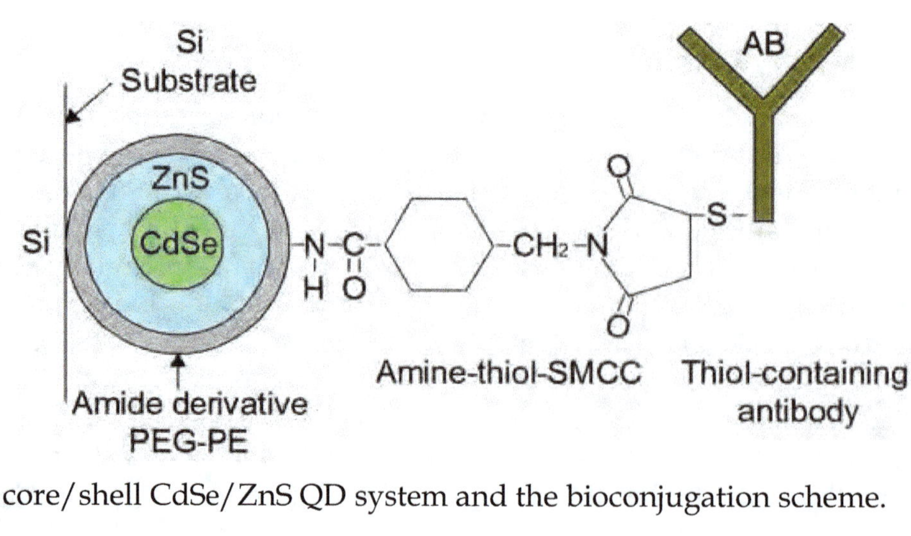

Fig. 13. The core/shell CdSe/ZnS QD system and the bioconjugation scheme.

7. The PL spectra of bioconjugated core/shell CdSe/ZnS QDs with interface states

The part of 565 nm CdSe/ZnS QDs has been bioconjugated (named 565P) to the mouse anti PSA (Prostate-Specific Antigen) antibodies, mAb Z009, Ms IgG2a. The part of 605 nm QDs has been bioconjugated (605P) to the anti IL10 (Interleukin 10) antibodies, rat IgG2a, clone JES3-12G8, code MCA2250. At the bioconjugation the commercially available 565 nm and 605 nm QD conjugation kits have been used (Invitrogen, 2010). This kit contains amine-derivatized PEG polymer coated QDs and the amine-thiol crosslinker SMCC. The conjugation reaction is based on the efficient coupling of thiols that present in reduced antibodies, to reactive maleimide groups which exist on the QD surface after the SMCC activation (Fig. 13). Bioconjugated CdSe/ZnS QDs in the form of a 5 mm size spot were dried on a polished surface of crystalline Si substrates (Fig. 13).

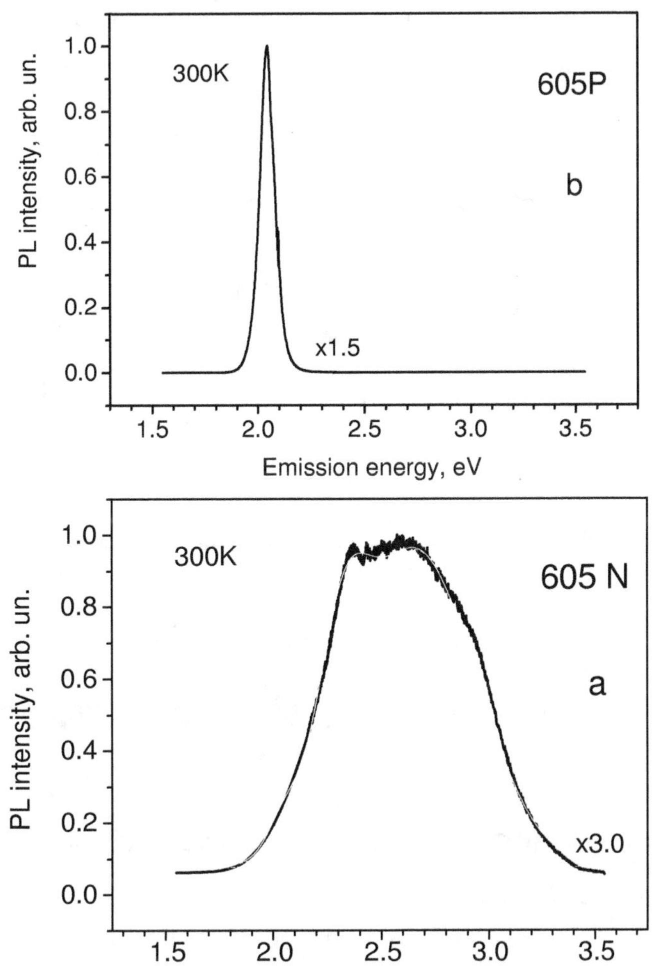

Fig. 14. Nonconjugated (a) and bioconjugated (b) 605 nm CdSe/ZnS QDs (Torchynska et al., 2009b).

Figures 14 and 15 present the PL spectra measured for bioconjugated and nonconjugated QDs. In fresh bioconjugated 605P (Fig. 14.b) and 565P (Fig. 15.b) samples we can see only the PL band 2.04 and 2.20 eV, respectively, related to the exciton recombination at ground states in the correspondent CdSe cores. The PL intensity of core PL band in 605P QDs increases at bioconjugation that manifests the change of multiplication coefficients from x3.0 in 605N QDs to x1.5 in 605P QDs for normalized PL spectra (Fig. 14). In contrary the PL intensity of core PL band in 565P QDs decreases at bioconjugation that manifests the change of multiplication coefficients from x2.0 in 565N QDs to x3.0 in 565P QDs for normalized PL spectra (Fig. 15). The FWHM of QD emission bands decreases at the bioconjugation in both types of QDs due to disappearing of the high energy PL bands related to the interface states. This effect was explained in (Torchynska et al., 2009a) on the base of re-charging of interface states at the QD bioconjugation with anti IL-10 antibodies.

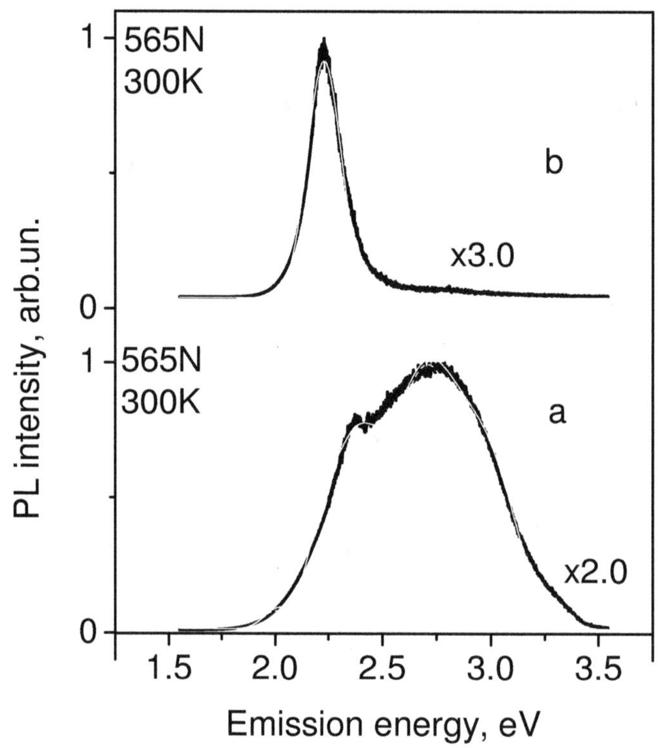

Fig. 15. Nonconjugated (a) and bioconjugated (b) 565 nm CdSe/ZnS QDs (Vega Macotela et al., 2010a).

8. The model of bioconjugation process for CdSe/ZnS QDs with interface states

The recombination process in CdSe/ZnS QDs can be considered as the competition of exciton recombination inside the CdSe core and the hot electron-hole recombination via radiative interface states (Fig. 16) at the CdSe/ZnS or ZnS/polymer interfaces (Torchynska et al., 2009a). The interface states (IS), responsible for the hole trapping in non-conjugated QDs, are negatively charged acceptor-like defects (IS^-) (Korsunskaya et al., 1980 a, b; Korsunskaya et al., 1982). Simultaneously, the interface states, responsible for the electron trapping in non-conjugated QDs, are positively charged donor-like defects (IS^+). The negative charge of acceptor-like interface states is due to their compensation by electrons from donor-like interface states in non-conjugated CdSe/ZnS QDs (Torchynska et al., 2009a).

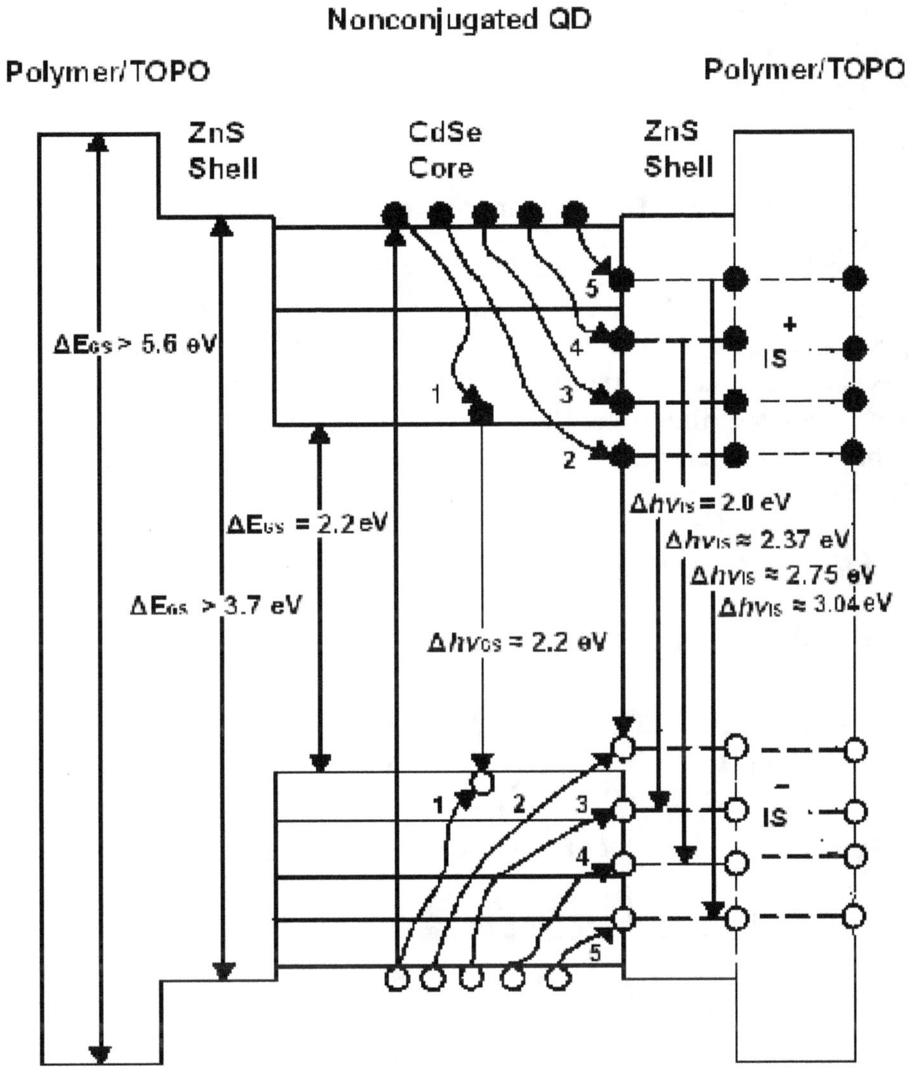

Fig. 16. The energy diagram of CdSe/ZnS core/shell QDs covered by PEG polymer in the nonconjugated state. Symbols IS^+ and IS^- present the charge of donor-like and acceptor-like interface states, respectively. Dashed lines show the ways of carrier tunneling from the CdSe/ZnS interface toward the ZnS/polymer interface.

The bioconjugation of proteins with QDs has been achieved through covalent bonds using functional groups (Fig. 13) on the QD surface (Parak et al., 2002) and/or with the help of electrostatic interaction (Ji et al., 2005). Actually the distribution of H^+ ions along the chain axis in antibody molecules is asymmetric (Antibodies, 2009) that is a reason for the appearance in biomolecules of dipole moments detected at the Raman scattering study (see n.10). It was supposed in (Torchynska et al., 2009a) that in bioconjugated CdSe/ZnS QDs the electrons from donor-like interface states accumulate at the QD surface (or in polymer) where they interact electrostatically with the positively charged antibodies. In this case the electrons from donor-like states do not compensate the acceptor-like interface states of QDs (Fig. 17). Simultaneously, the hot electron-hole recombination flow via neutral acceptor-like interface states decreases dramatically and the PL intensity of exciton emission inside CdSe core increases. Thus, this model assumes that the QD bio-conjugation process is accompanied by the re-charging of acceptor-like interface states in QDs (Fig. 17).

Actually this effect we have seen in Fig. 14 and Fig. 15 presented in this chapter. The PL intensity of high energy PL bands (2.37, 2.75 and 3.06 eV) related to interface states decreases tremendous in bioconjugated QDs that can be explained by recharging of interface states.

9. The aging of CdSe/ZnS QDs with interface states

Normalized PL spectra of nonconjugated CdSe/ZnS QDs measured at 300 K when the QD kits were obtained (1 day) and after the aging during 30-110 days demonstrate the broad PL band in the spectral range of 1.80-3.20 eV related to the exciton recombination in the CdSe core and the electron-hole recombination via the interface states (Fig. 18). The concentration of interface states increases due to the PEG polymer modification at the aging in ambient air that leads to the transformation of PL spectra of nonconjugated 605 nm QDs as it is presented in Fig. 18.

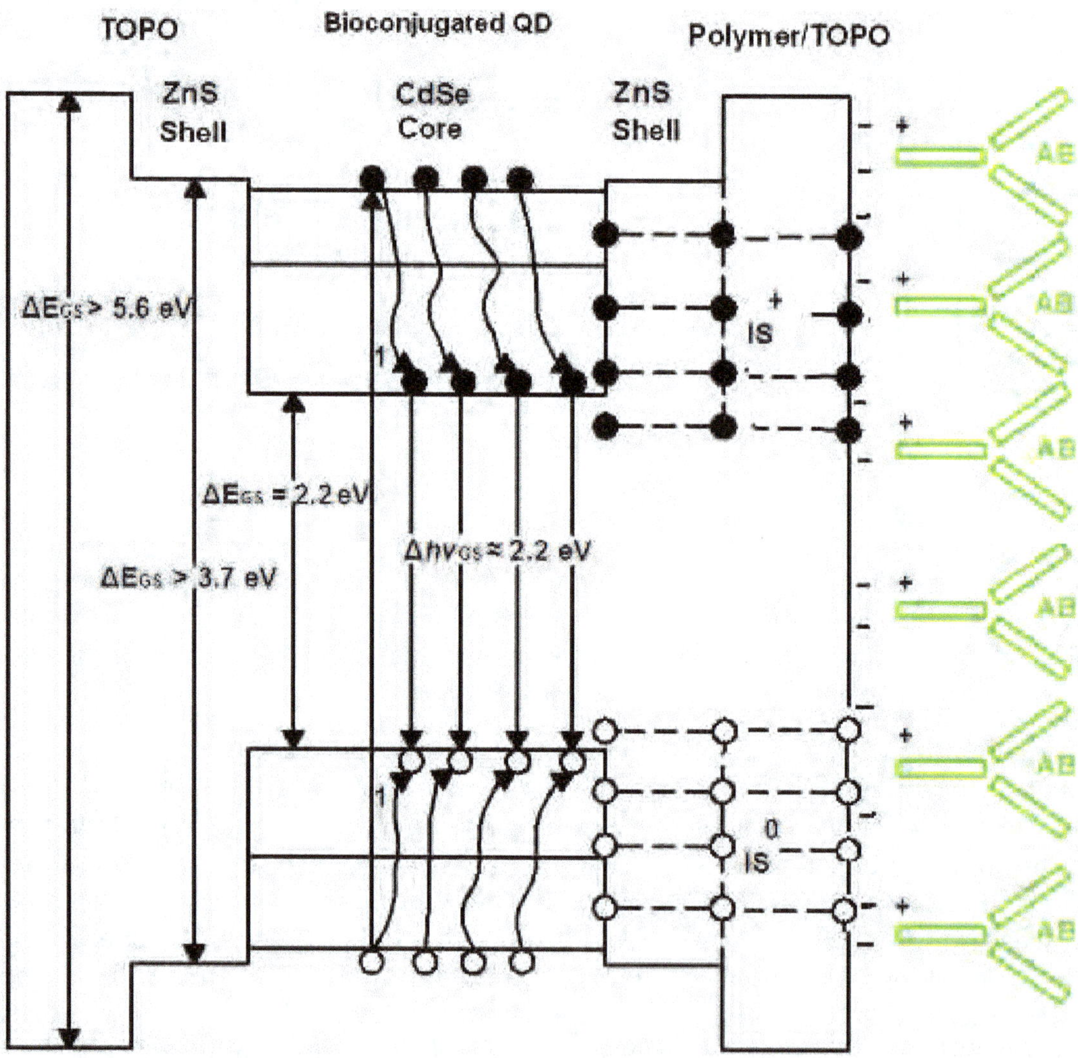

Fig. 17. The energy diagram of CdSe/ZnS QDs covered by polymer in the bioconjugated state. Symbols IS^+ and IS^0 present the charge of donor-like and acceptor-like interface states, respectively. Dashed lines show the ways of carrier tunnelling from the CdSe/ZnS interface toward the ZnS/polymer interface.

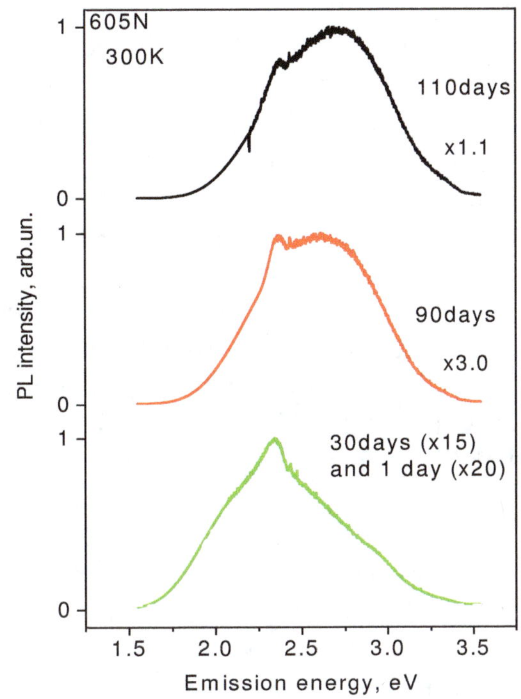

Fig. 18. PL spectra of 605N QDs measured in 1 day and after the 30, 90 and 110 days of aging in ambient air. Normalized PL spectra measured at 1 and 30 days coincide, but the multiplication coefficients are different (x20 for 1 day and x15 for 30 days).

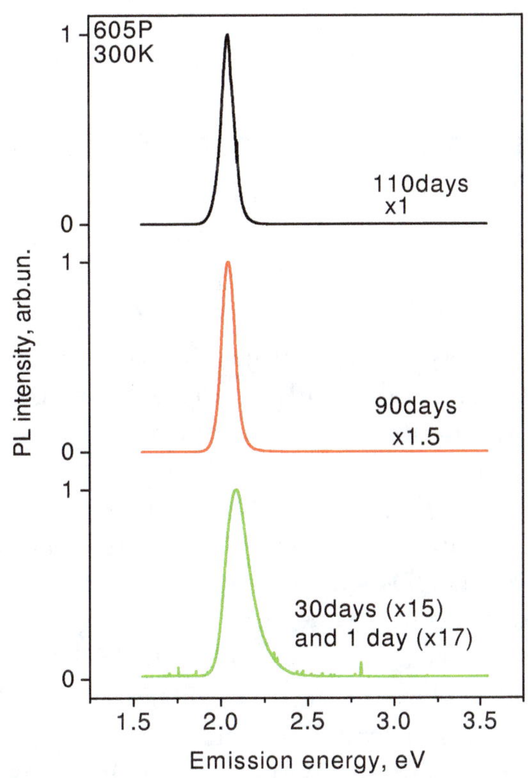

Fig. 19. PL spectra of 605P QDs measured in 1 day and after the 30, 90 and 110 days of aging in ambient air. Normalized PL spectra measured at 1 and 30 days coincide, but the multiplication coefficients are different (x17 for 1 day and x15 for 30 days).

Fig. 19 presents the PL spectra measured in different aging moments (1, 30, 90 and 110 days) for bioconjugated 605P QDs. In fresh bioconjugated 605P samples (1 day) we can see only the PL band 2.08 eV related to the exciton recombination at ground states in the CdSe core (Fig. 19). The PL intensity of this PL band increases essentially at bioconjugation that manifests the change of multiplication coefficients from x20 in 605N QDs to x17 in 605P QDs for normalized PL spectra measured in the 1 day (Fig. 18 and Fig. 19). At the aging the intensity of CdSe core PL band increases (30-110 days Fig. 19) and its peak position shifts to low energy (red shift) from 2.08 to 2.04 eV. The same coefficients (x15) of PL intensity enlargement in the nonconjugated 605N (Fig. 18) and bioconjugated 605P (Fig. 19) QDs with aging during 30-110 days in ambient air testifies that the reason of PL rise on this stage related to transparency increasing of PEG polymer for visible light (605 nm) at the aging.

Let us discuss the "red" shift of CdSe core emission (Fig. 19) for bioconjugated 605P QDs at the aging. It is well known that PL spectra of QDs can be influenced by the environment atmosphere, by thermal annealing or by optical excitation (Nassal et al., 2004). The PL shift can be a result of optically induced adsorption by polar molecules (Oda et al., 2006), or the chemical transformation of species on the QD surface (Cordero et al., 2000; Roberti et al., 1998). This shift can be stimulated by increasing the compressive strain in core/shell QDs at annealing or drying processes as well (Borkovska et al., 2009). We have seen that in non-conjugated QDs the polymer modification during aging in ambient air has induced: i) the enlargement of the concentration of interface states at the ZnS/polymer interface and ii) the rise of PEG polymer transparency for visible light. The physical aging of polymer is accompanied by the change of polymer density (Rowe et al., 2009; Shelby et al., 1998) and, due to this, by the variation of strain level at the ZnS/polymer interface. The last factor may be the reason of increasing of the concentration of interface states and the appearance of a red shift of QD emission with aging that has been detected in bioconjugated 605P QDs.

10. Raman scattering spectra of bioconjugated CdSe/ZnS QDs

Additionally to the emission study, other optical methods could give inportant information concerning the bioconjugated CdSe/ZnS QDs. Earlier we have shown that the study of Raman scattering of QDs bioconjugated to antibodies can be the powerful technique for the proof of actual bio-conjugation (Torchynska et al., 2007; Torchynska et al., 2008; Vega Macotela et al., 2010b; Diaz-Cano et al., 2010). Moreover in n.8 we supposed for the bioconjugation model of CdSe/ZnS QDs with interface states that antibody molecules are characterized by the dipole moments. This assumption is possible to confirm using the Raman scattering method as well.

Commercially available core-shell CdSe/ZnS QDs with emission at 565 nm and 605 nm were bioconjugated to anti PSA and anti IL-10 antibodies, respectively, as it described in n.7. Bioconjugated and nonconjugated QDs samples in a shape of small drops were dried on a surface of crystalline Si substrates (Fig. 14). Raman scattering spectra were measured at 300 K and the excitation by a He-Ne laser with a wavelength of 632.8 nm and a beam power of 20 mW using a setup described in (Torchynska et al., 2007 and 2008).

Fig. 20 and Fig. 21 present the Raman scattering spectra of CdSe/ZnS QDs bioconjugated to anti IL-10 (605P) and to anti PSA (565P) antibodies, respectively, as well as Raman spectra of nonconjugated (605N) and (565N) samples, for highest intensity Raman peak at 522 cm^{-1}. This peak related to the optical phonon line in a silicon substrate used for studied QD samples. The intensity of these Raman peaks in the nonconjugated 605N and 565 N QD samples is tenfold and threefold smaller than in the bio-conjugated 605P and 565P samples, respectively.

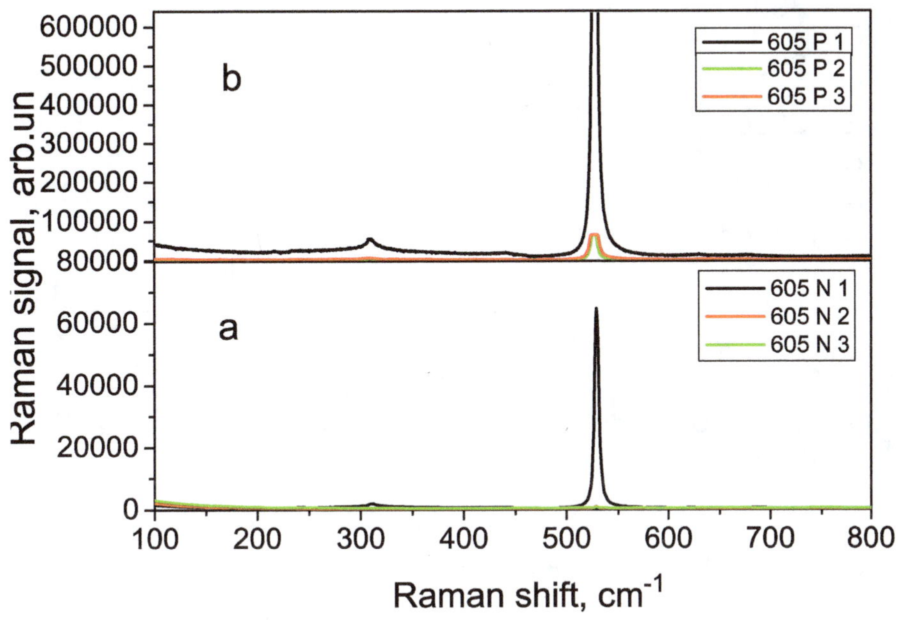

Fig. 20. The main Raman peak of Si substrate in nonconjugated (a) and bioconjugated (b) 605 nm CdSe/ZnS QD samples (Diaz-Cano et al., 2010).

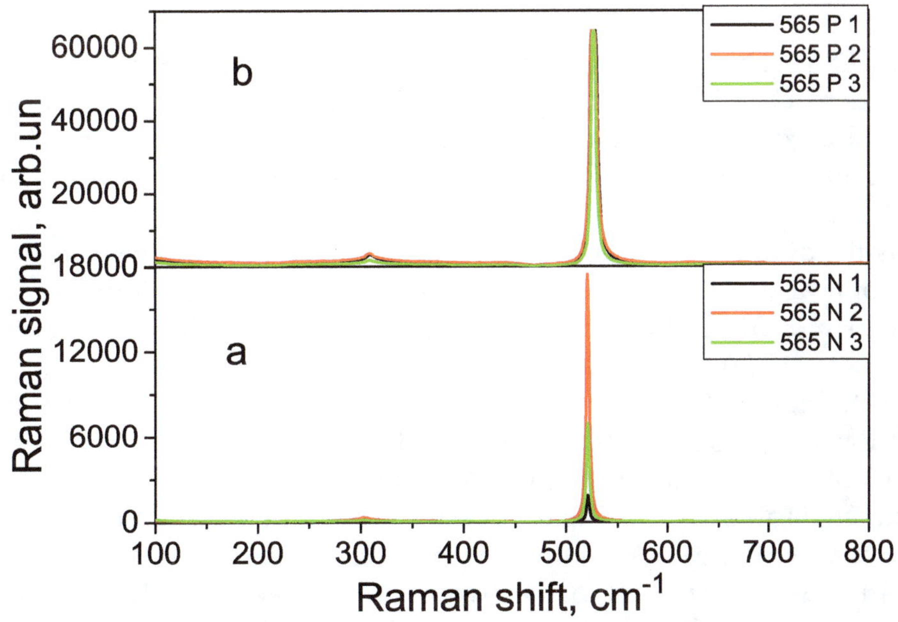

Fig. 21. The main Raman peak of Si substrate in nonconjugated (a) and bioconjugated (b) 565 nm CdSe/ZnS QD samples (Vega Macotela et al., 2010b).

In some 605 nm CdSe/ZnS QD samples it is possible to see the enlargement in bioconjugated states the intensity of Raman lines related to the CdSe core and ZnS shell of QDs in comparison with nonconjugated 605 nm QD samples (Fig. 22).

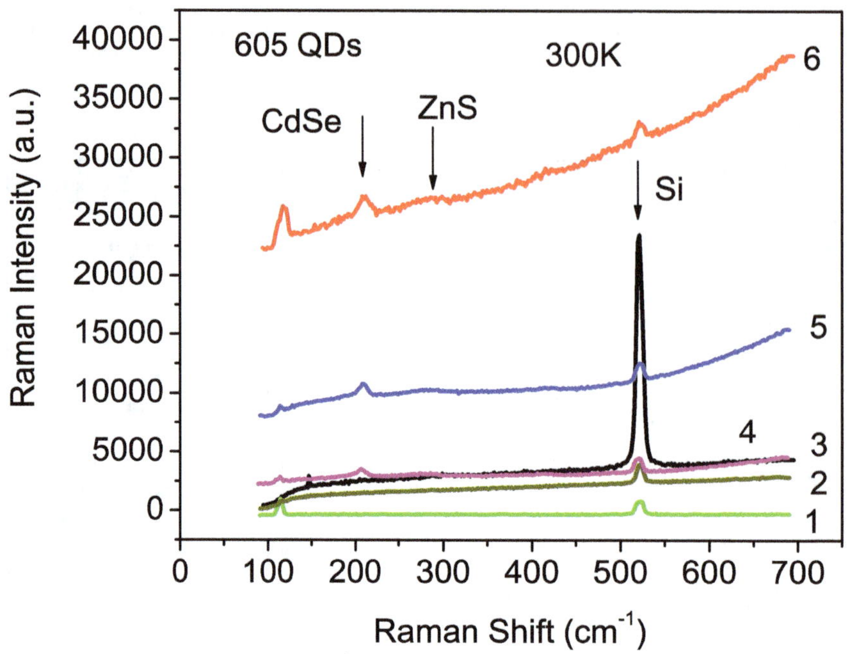

Fig. 22. Raman spectra of a set of nonconjugated (1,2,3) and bioconjugated to anti IL-10 mAb (4,5,6) 605 nm CdSe/ZnS QDs (Torchynska et al., 2008).

Fig. 23, Fig. 24, Fig. 25 and Fig. 26 present low intensity Raman peaks related to the Si substrate and obtained in spectral ranges 100-800 and 800-1050 cm^{-1} for nonconjugated (605N and 565N) and bioconjugated (605P and 565P) QD samples. All Raman peaks in the ranges 100-800 and 800-1050 cm^{-1} are characterized by the smaller intensities of Raman lines in nonconjugated QD samples (605N and 565N) than those in bioconjugated QD samples (605P and 565P).

Fig. 27 and Fig. 28 present low intensity Raman peaks related to the PEG polymer on the surface of CdSe/ZnS QDs. These Raman peaks, localized in the spectral range 1050-4000 cm^{-1}, are characterized by different tendencies for the CdSe/ZnS QDs bioconjugated to the anti IL-10 and to the anti PSA antibodies.To understand obtained Raman results the nature of all Raman peaks has to be discussed.

The silicon has the diamond crystal structure and, as a result, demonstrates one first-order Raman active optical phonon of symmetry Γ_{25}, located at the Brillouin-zone (BZ) center, with the frequency of 519-522 cm^{-1}, Fig. 20 and Fig. 21, Table 2 (Jonson & Loudon, 1964; Temple &Hathaway, 1973).

The Raman scattering in the region of 0-500 cm^{-1} in Si presents overtones of acoustic phonons. The Raman peaks at 230, 302, 435 and 469 cm^{-1} were assigned earlier (Temple &Hathaway, 1973) to the two TA phonon overtones scattered at L, X and near Σ critical points, respectively (Table 2). The Table 2 presents the frequencies of optical and acoustical phonons associated with the critical points of the silicon Brillouin zone. Raman peaks at 610 and 670 cm^{-1} in Si were assigned to the two-phonon peaks, which, as assumed, are the combinations of acoustic and optic phonons in the X and Σ directions (Table 2).

Raman peaks at 236, 308, 441, 620 and 677 cm^{-1} have been seen clearly in Raman spectra of non-conjugated and bio-conjugated QD samples in Fig. 23 and Fig. 24. Note that Raman peaks related to the CdSe cores (210-212 cm^{-1}) and to the ZnS shell (350 cm^{-1}) have been revealed only in some studied 605 nm QD samples (Fig. 22). The later may be the result of small quantity of 565 nm CdSe/ZnS QD materials.

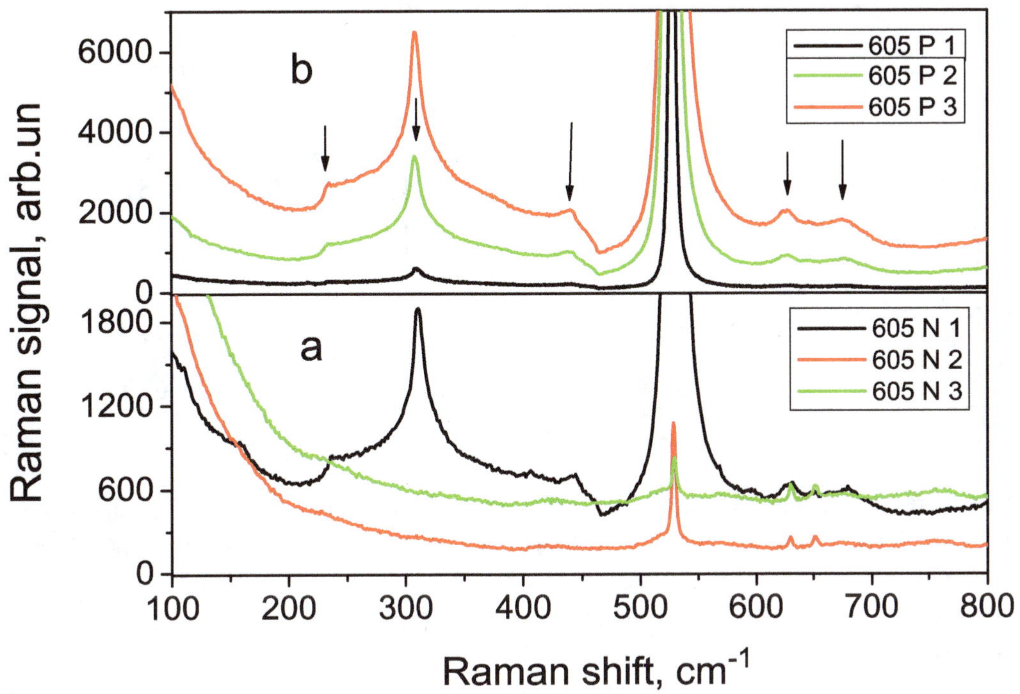

Fig. 23. Raman spectra of nonconjugated (a) and bioconjugated (b) 605 nm CdSe/ZnS QDs in the range related to the Si substrate (Diaz-Cano et al., 2010).

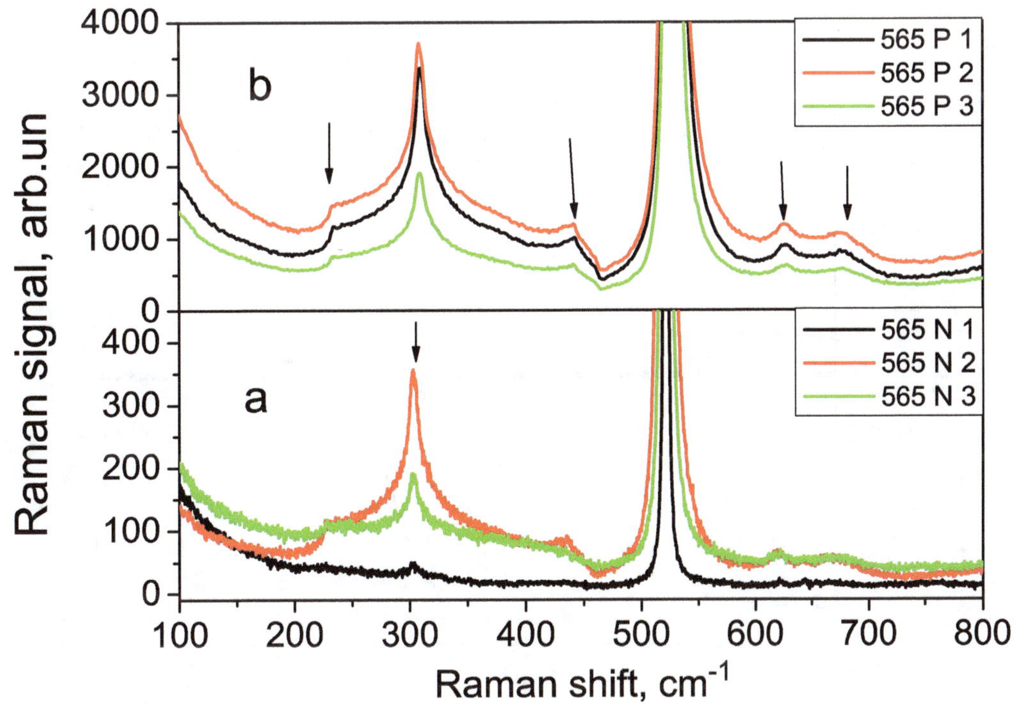

Fig. 24. Raman spectra of nonconjugated (a) and bioconjugated (b) 565 nm CdSe/ZnS QDs in the range related to the Si substrate (Vega Macotela et al., 2010b).

Critical points of Si BZ	Phonon frequencies from (Jonson & Loudon, 1964) (cm^{-1})	Phonon frequencies from (Temple &Hathaway, 1973) (cm^{-1})
Γ (0)	522	519
X (TO)	463	460
X(TA)	149	151
L(TO)	491	490
L(TA)	114	113
W(TO)		470
X(TA+TO)		610
Σ(TA+TO)		670

Table 2. Phonon frequencies at the critical BZ points of Si (Temple &Hathaway, 1973).

The Raman scattering in the 900-1050 cm^{-1} region in Si is attributed, as a rule, to overtones of optical phonons. The sharp increase in the Raman spectrum at 920 cm^{-1} or at 940 cm^{-1}, the shoulder at 975 cm^{-1} and sharp decrease at 1040 cm^{-1} were identified earlier (Temple &Hathaway, 1973) with the two TO phonon overtone scattering from the critical points at X, W, L and Γ, respectively (Table 2). In studied QD samples, as follows from Fig. 25 and Fig. 26, the Raman peak at 949 cm^{-1} and the shoulder at 980 cm^{-1} have been detected as well, which, apparently, related to two TO phonon overtones in Si from the critical points at W and L. Additionally, a set of small intensity Raman peaks at 837, 860, 1011 and 1039 cm^{-1} have been seen as well (Fig. 25 and Fig. 26). In bio-conjugated QD samples the intensity of Raman peak at 949 cm^{-1} and a shoulder at 990 cm^{-1} increase (Fig. 25 and Fig. 26). At the same time, the small intensity Raman peaks 837, 860, 1011 and 1039 cm^{-1} have disappeared (Fig. 25).

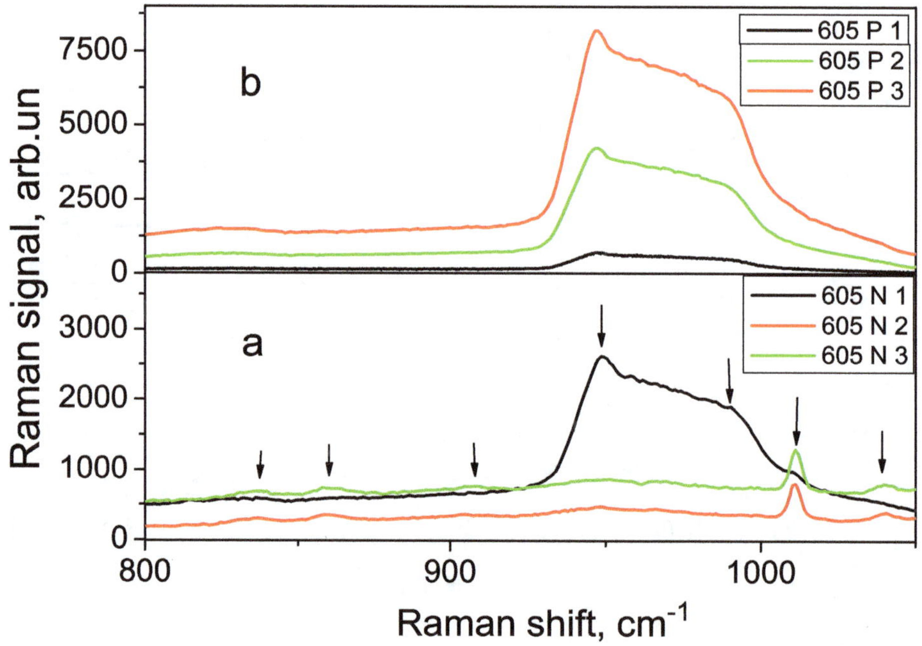

Fig. 25. Raman spectra of nonconjugated (a) and bioconjugated (b) 605 nm CdSe/ZnS QDs (Diaz-Cano et al., 2010).

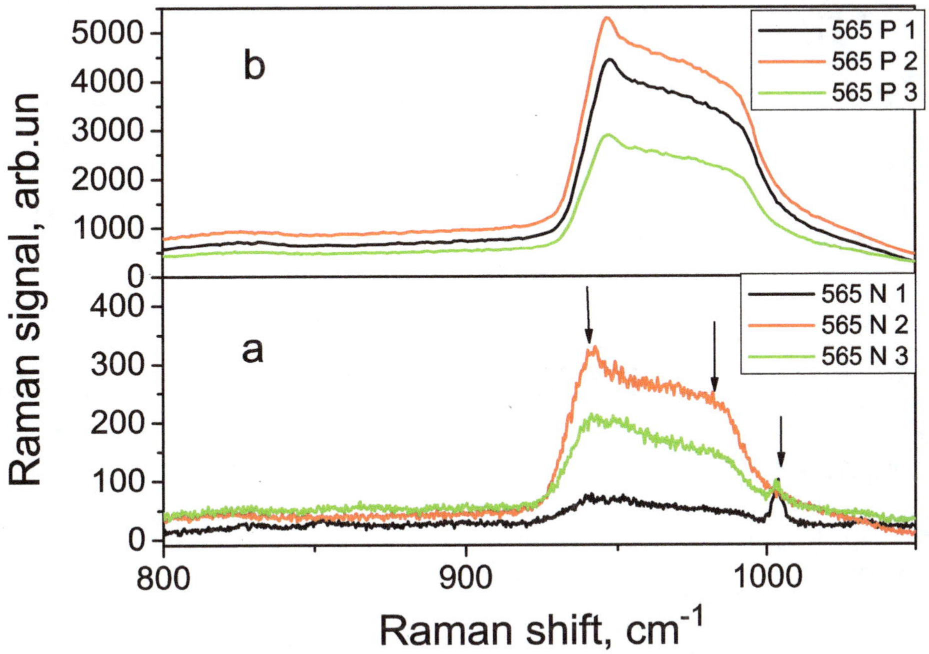

Fig. 26. Raman spectra of nonconjugated (a) and bioconjugated (b) 565 nm CdSe/ZnS QDs (Vega Macotela et al., 2010b).

In nonconjugated CdSe/ZnS QD samples (605N and 565N) in the range 1050-4000 cm^{-1} a set of Raman peaks at 1214, 1273, 1326, 1347, 1413, 1457, 1613, 1661 cm^{-1} and 2149-2430, 2752, 2880, 2939, 3061 and 3317-3380 cm^{-1} have been detected as well (Fig. 27 and Fig. 28). These Raman peaks and the small intensity Raman peaks revealed in Fig. 25a (837, 860, 1011 and 1039 cm-^{1}) can be assigned to the vibrations of different groups of atoms in the organic amine (NH_2)-derivatized PEG polymer [OH-(CH_2-CH_2-O)$_n$-H] covered the QD surface.

There are: 837, 860 and 1661 cm^{-1} - PEG skeleton vibrations (Kozielski et al., 2004), 1011 and 1039 cm^{-1} – stretching vibrations of COH groups, 1214, 1273, 1413 and 1457 cm^{-1} stretching vibrations of C-H bounds and deformation vibrations of C-H at 1326 and 1347 cm^{-1} (Kozielski et al., 2004; Nakamoto 1997), 1613 cm^{-1} - stretching vibrations of C=C bounds and 2149-2430 cm^{-1} - stretching vibrations of CO or C-N groups (Nakamoto, 1997), symmetric and anti-symmetric stretching vibrations of CH, CH_2 or CH_3 groups (2752, 2880, 2939 and 3061 cm^{-1}), as well as the stretching vibrations of (O-H) and (NH_2) groups at 3317-3380 cm^{-1}. To confirm that mentioned peaks related to PEG polymers, the QDs without PEG polymer have been studied as well, and, actually, these peaks have been not observed in Raman spectrum.

The intensity enhancement of Raman lines related to the Si acoustic and optical phonons in the bioconjugated QD samples can be attributed to the surface enhanced Raman scattering (SERS) effect (Aroca et al., 2004; Torchynska et al., 2007, 2008, 2009a). The surface electric field enhancement due to the realization of resonance conditions for the plasmon-, phonon- or exciton-polariton resonances is the known effect in nanocrystals of polar materials (Anderson, 2005). The stimulation of optical field near the interface of illuminated bioconjugated QDs and Si substrate leads to increasing dramatically the intensity of Si Raman lines and in some cases the CdSe core and ZnS shell Raman lines. This fact indicates that the anti IL10 and anti PSA antibodies are characterized by the **dipole moments** that permits them to interact with an electric field of excitation light at the Si surface and to participate in the SERS effect (Torchynska et al., 2007, 2008, 2009a).

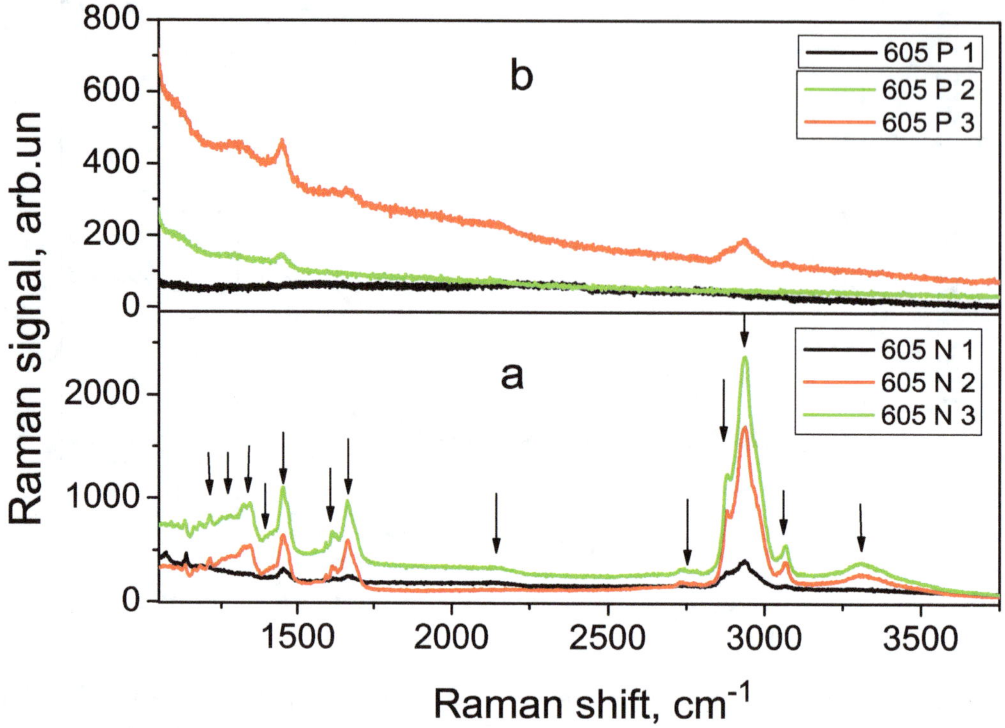

Fig. 27. Raman spectra of nonconjugated (a) and bioconjugated (b) 605 nm CdSe/ZnS QDs in the range of Raman shift related to the PEG polymer (Diaz Cano et al., 2010).

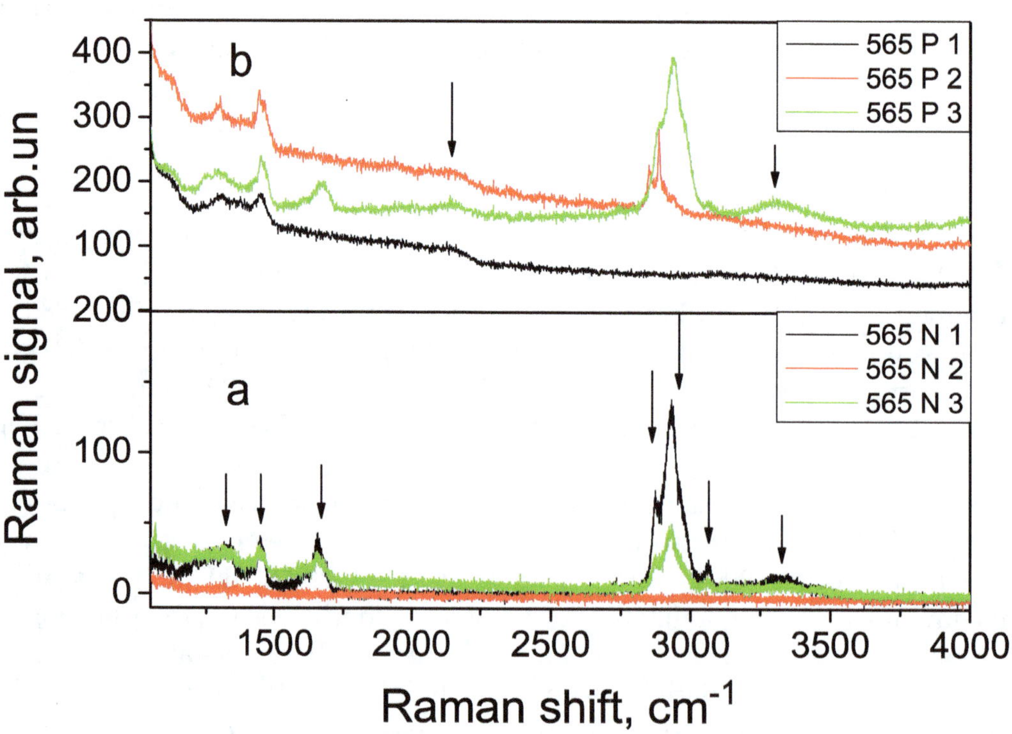

Fig. 28. Raman spectra of nonconjugated (a) and bioconjugated (b) 565 nm CdSe/ZnS QDs in the range related to the PEG polymer (Vega Macotela et al., 2010b).

The Raman line intensities of the peaks related to PEG polymer are smaller in nonconjugated 565 nm QD samples and a little bit increase in bioconjugated 565 nm QD samples (Fig. 28). In contrary the Raman line intensities of the peaks related to PEG polymer are high in nonconjugated 605 nm QD samples and decrease in bioconjugated 605 nm QD samples (Fig. 27). The last fact can indicate on scattering light re-absorption in anti IL-10 antibodies or on other resonance conditions for the vibrations of PEG atomic groups in these samples.

11. Conclusion

Thirteen years passed after the first demonstration of cell labelling experiments with colloidal quantum dots. Nowadays colloidal quantum dots are used to address a set of specific biological questions, as well as the numbers of medical applications, that plays an important role in basic life science. Although semiconductor QDs are unlikely to completely replace traditional organic fluorophores, QDs have secured their place as a viable technology in the biological and medical sciences. Their capability for single molecule and multiplexed detection, real-time imaging and biological compatibility, important for drug delivery and photo resonance therapy, makes II-VI material QDs a valuable technology in the scientific toolbox. Additionally II-VI QDs with interface states presented in this chapter permit to spread the experimental possibilities of the biological arsenal.

The work was partially supported by CONACYT Mexico (projects 000000000131184 and 00000000130387), as well as by the SIP-IPN, Mexico.

12. References

Aldana, J., Wang, Y.A., Peng, X.G. (2001). Photochemical Instability oof CdSe Nanocrystals Coated by Hydrophilic Thiols. *J. Am. Chem. Soc.*, Vol. 123, 8844-8850.

Alivisatos, A.P., Harris, D., Carroll, J., Steigerwald, M.L., Brus, L. (1989). Electrochemical Synthesis and Laser Induced Time Resolved Photoluminescence of CdSe/ZnS Quantum Dots. *Chem. Phys.*, Vol. 90, pp. 3463-3470.

Alivisatos, A.P. (1996). Semiconductor Clusters, Nanocrystals and Quantum Dots. *Science,* Vol. 271, pp. 933-937.

Anderson, M.S. (2005). Surface Enhanced Infrared Absorption by Coulping Phonon and Plasma Resonance. *Appl. Phys. Lett.*, Vol. 87, 144102.

Antibodies (2009). http://en.wikipedia.org/wiki/

Aroca, R.F., Ross, D.J., Domingo, C. (2004). Surface-Enhanced Infrared Spectroscopy. *Appl. Spectrosc.*, Vol. 58, pp. 324A-338A.

Bailey, R.E., Smith, A.M., Nie, Sh. (2004). Quantum Dots in Biology and Medicine. *Physica E,* Vol. 25, pp. 1-12.

Baranov, A.V., Rakovich, Yu.P., Donegan, J.F., Perova, T.S., Moore, R.A., Talapin D.V., Rogach, A.L., Masumoto, Y., Nabiev, I. (2003). Effect of ZnS Shell Thickness on the Phonon Spectra in CdSe Quantum Dots. *Phys.Rev. B*, Vol. 68, 165306.

Biju, V., Makita, Y., Nagase, T., Yamaoka ,Y., Yokoyama, H., Baba Y., Ishikawa, H. (2005a). Subsecond Luminescence Intensity Fluctuations of Single CdSe Quantum Dot. *J Phys Chem B*. Vol. 109, pp. 14350-14355.

Biju, V., Makita, Y., Sonoda, A., Yokoyama, H,. Baba, Y., Ishikawa, M. (2005b). Temperature-sensitive photoluminescence of CdSe quantum dot clusters. *J Phys Chem B,* Vol. 109, pp. 13899–13905.

Borkovska, L.V., Korsunska, N.E., Kryshtab, T.G., Germash, L.P., Pecherska, E.Yu.., Ostapenko, S., and Chornokur, G. (2009). *Semiconductors,* 43, 775 (2009).

Brigger, I., Dubernet, C., Couvreur, P. (2002). Nanoparticles in Cancer Therapy and Diagnosis. *Adv. Drug Deliv Rev.,* Vol. 54, pp.631-651.

Bruchez M, Moronne M, Gin P, Weiss S, Alivisatos AP. (1998). *Science,* Vol. 281, pp. 2013–2016.

Calvo P, RemunanLopez C, VilaJato JL, Alonso MJ. *J Appl Polym Sci* 1997;63:125–32.

Choi, S.-H., Song, H., Park, I.K., Yum, J.-H., Kim, S.-S., Lee, S. and Sung, Y.-E. (2006). Synthesis of Size-Controlled CdSe Quantum Dots and Characterization of CdSe-conjugated Polymer Blends for Hybrid Solar Cells.

Chin, I.L., Abraham, K.J., Chao Kang Chang, Yu Der Lee. (2004). Synthesis and Photoluminescence Study of Molecularly I mprinted Polymers Appended onto CdSe/ZnS Core-Shell. *Biosensors and Bioelectronics,* Vol. 20, pp. 127–131.

Chan, W.C.W., Nie, S. (1998). *Science,* Vol. 281, pp.2016-2018.

Clapp, A.R., Medintz, I.L., Mauro, J.M., Fisher, Br.R., Bawendi, M.G. and Mattoussi, H. (2004). Fluorescence Resonance Energy Transfer between Quantum Dot Donors and Dye-Labeled Protein Acceptors. *J. AM. Chem. Soc.* Vol. 126, pp. 301-310.

Cordero, S.R., Carson, P.J., Estabrook, R.A., Strouse, G.F., & Buratto, S.K. (2000). *J. Phys. Chem. B* 104, 12137 (2000).

Crouch, D., Norager, S., O'Brien, P., Park, J.H. and Pickett, N. (2003). New synthetic routes for quantum dots. *Phil. Trans. R. Soc. A,* Vol. 361, pp. 297-310.

Dabbousi, B.O., Rodriguez-Viejo, J., Mikulec, F.V., Heine, J.R., Mattoussi, H., Ober, R., Jensen, K.F., Bawendi, M.G. (1997). (CdSe)ZnS Core-Shell Quantum Dots: Synthesis and Characterization of a Size Series of Highly Luminescent Nanocrystallites. *J. Phys. Chem. B,* Vol.101 pp. 9463-9475.

Danek, M., Jensen, K.F., Murray, C.B. and Bawendi, M.G. (1994). Preparation of II–VI quantum dot composites by electrospray organometallic chemical vapor deposition. *J. Crys. Growth,* Vol. 145, pp. 714-720.

Darbandi, M., Thomann, R., Nann, T. (2005). Single Quantum Dots in Silica Spheres by Microemulsion Synthesis. *Chem. Mater.,* Vol. 17 pp. 5720-5725.

Diaz Cano, A., Jiménez Sandoval S., Vorobiev, Y., Rodriguez Melgarejo, F. and Torchynska, T.V. (2010). Peculiarities of Raman scattering in bioconjugated CdSe/ZnS quantum dots, *Nanotechnology,* Vol. 21, 134016.

Dinger, A., Hetterich, M., Goppert, M., Grun, M., Weise, B., Liang, J., Wagner, V., Geurts, J. (1999). *J. Cryst. Growth* Vol. 200, pp. 391-397.

Dubertret, B., Skourides, P., Norris, D.J., Noireaux, V., Brivanlou, A.H. (2002). In Vivo Imaging of Quantum Dots Encapsulated ij Phospholipid Micelles. *Science,* Vol. 298, pp. 1759-1762.

Dubertret, J.K., Mattoussi, H., Mauro, J.M., Simon, S.M. (2003). Long-term multiple color imaging of live cells using quantum dot bioconjugates. *Nat Biotechnol.,* Vol. 21, pp. 47-51.

Dybiec, M., Chomokur, G., Ostapenko, S., Wolcott, A., Zhang, J.Z., Zajac, A., Phelan, C., Sellers, T., Gerion, G. (2007). Photoluminescence Spectroscopy of Bioconjugated CdSe/ZnS Quantum Dots. *Appl. Phys. Lett.* Vol. 90, No. 26, 263112.

Dzhagan, V.M., Valakh, M.Ya., A E Raevskaya, A.E., Stroyuk, A.L., S Ya Kuchmiy, S.Ya. and D R T Zahn, D.R.T. (2007). *Nanotechnology* Vol. 18, 285701.

Dzhagan, V.M., Valakh, M.Ya., Raevskaya, A.E., .L. Stroyuk, A.L., Kuchmiy, S.Ya., D.R.T. Zahn, D.R.T. (2008). *Appl. Surf. Sci.*, Vol. 255, pp.725–727.

Ebenstein, Y., Mokari, T., Banin, U. (2004). Quantum-Dot-Functionalized Scanning Probes for Fluorescence-Energy-Transfer-Based Microscopy. *J. Phys. Chem. B.*, Vol. 108, pp. 93-99.

Eisler H.J.; Sundar V.C.; Bawendi M.G.; Walsh M.; Smith H.I.; Klimov V.I. (2002). Color-selective Semiconductor Nanocrystal Laser. *Appl. Phys. Lett.* Vol. 80, No. 24, pp. 4614-4616.

Efros, Al.L., Rosen, M., Kuno, M., Nirmal, M., Norris, D.J., and M. Bawendi, M. (1996). Band-edge Exciton in Quantum Dots of Semiconductors With a Degenerate Valence Band. *Phys. Rev. B*, Vol. 54, No. 7, 4843.

Éfros, Al.L., Éfros, A.L. (1982). Interband absorption of light in a semiconductor sphere. *Sov. Phys. Semicond.*, Vol.16(7), pp. 772-775.

Esparza-Ponce, H., Hernández-Borja, J., Reyes-Rojas, A., Cervantes-Sánchez, M., Vorobiev, Y.V., Ramirez-Bon, R., Pérez-Robles, J.F., González-Hernández, J. (2009). Growth technology, X-ray and optical properties of CdSe thin films. *Materials Chemistry and Physics*, Vol. 113, pp. 824-828

Gao, X.H., Cui, Y.Y., Levenson,R.M., Chung, L.W.K., Nie S.M. (2004). In Vivo Cancer Targeting with Semiconductor Quantum Dots. *Nat Biotechnol*, Vol. 22, pp. 969-976.

Gaponenko, S.V. (1998). *Optical Properties of Semiconductor Nanocrystals*, Cambridge University Press, ISBN 0-521-58241-5, Cambridge.

Gerion, D., Pinaud, F., Williams, Sh.C., Parak, W.J., Zanchet, D., Weiss, Sh. and Alivisatos, A.P. (2001). Synthesis and Properties of Biocompatible Water-Soluble Silica-Coated CdSe/ZnS Semiconductor Quantum Dots. *J. Phys. Chem. B*, Vol. 105, pp. 8861-8871 .

Gerion, D., Parak, W.J., Williams, S.C., Zanchet, D., Micheel, C.M., Alivisatos, A.P. (2002). Sorting Fluorescent Nanocrystals with DNA. *J Am Chem Soc.*, Vol. 124, pp. 7070-7074.

Grodzinski, P., Silver, M., Molnar, L.K. (2006). Nanotechnology for Cancer Diagnostics: Promises and Challenges. Expert Rev. Mol. Diagn., Vol. 6, No. 6, pp. 307-318.

Guo, W., Jack Li, J., Wang, J.A., Peng, X. (2003). Conjugation Chemistry and Bioapplications of Semiconductor Box Nanocrystals Prepared via Dendrimer Bridging. *Chem. Mater.*, Vol. 15, pp. 3125-3133.

Gao, X.H., Gui, Y.Y., Levenson, R.M., Chung, L.W.K., Nie, S.M. (2004). In Vivo Cancer Targeting and Imaging with Semiconductor Quantum Dots. *Nature Biotechnol.*, Vol. 22(8), pp. 969-976.

Greenham, N.C., Peng, X., Alivisatos, A.P. (1997). Charge Separation and transport in conjugated polymer/cadmium selenide nanocrystal composites studied by photoluminescence quenching and photoconductivity. *Synthetic Metals* 1997, Vol. 84, pp. 545-546.

Ferrari, M. (2005). Cancer Nanotechnology: Opportunities and Challenges. *Nature Reviews*, Vol. 5, pp. 161-171.

Fogg, D.E., Radzilowski, L.H., Dabbousi, B.O., Schrock, R.R.;, Thomas E.L., Bawendi, M.G. (1997). Fabrication of Quantum Dots/Polymer Composites. *Macromolecules* 1997, Vol. 30, pp. 8433-8439.

Hai, L.B., Nghia, N.X., Nga, P.T., Manh, D.H., Hanh, V.T.H. and Trang, N.T.T. (2009). Influence of Cd:Se Precursor Ratio on Optical Properties of Colloidal CdSe Tetrapods Prepared in Octadecene. *J. Phys: Conf. Ser.*, Vol. 187, 012027.

Han, M.Y., Gao, X.H., Su, J.Z., Nie, S. (2001). Quantum-Dot-Tagged Microbeads for Multiplexed Optical Coding of Biomolecules. *Nat. Biotechnol*, Vol. 19, pp. 631-635.

Hanaki, K., Momo, A., Oku, T., Komoto, A., Maenosono, S., Yamaguchi, Y., Yamamoto, K. (2003). Semiconductor quantum dot/albumin complex is a long-life and highly photostable endosome marker. *Biochem Biophys Res Commun*, Vol. 302, pp. 496-501.

Haus, J.W., Zhou, H.S., Honma, Komiyama, J.H. (1993). *Phys. Rev. B*, Vol. 47, pp. 1359-1365, 1993.

Heine, J.R., Rodriguez-Viejo, J., Bawendi, M.G. and Jensen, K.F. (1998). Synthesis of CdSe quantum dot ZnS matrix thin films via electrospray organometallic chemical vapor deposition. *J. Cryst. Growth,* Vol. 195, pp. 564-568.

Hines, M.A., Guyot-Sionnest, P. (1996). Synthesis and Characterization of Strongly Luminescing ZnS-Capped CdSe Nanocrystals *J. Phys. Chem.*, Vol. 100, pp. 468-471. Hwang, Y.N., Park, S.H., Kim, D. (1999). Size-dependent Surface Phonon Mode of CdSe Quantum Dots. *Phys. Rev.B*, Vol. 59, 7285.

Hwang, Y.N., Park, S.H., Kim, D. (1999). Size-dependent Surface Phonon Mode of CdSe Quantum Dots. *Phys. Rev.B*, Vol. 59, 7285.

Hong-Mei Gong & Zhang-Kai Zhou & Hao Song & Zhong-Hua Hao & Jun-Bo Han & Yue-Ying Zhai & Si Xiao & Qu-Quan Wang, *J Fluoresc* (2007) 17:715–720.

Hoener, C. F.; Allan, K. A.; Bard, A. J.; Campion, A.; Fox, M. A. Mallouk, T. E.; Webber, S. E.; White, J. M. *J. Phys. Chem.* 1992, *96*, 3812.

Hoshino, A., Manabe, N., Fujioka, K., Suzuki, K., Yasuhara, M. and Yamamoto, K. (2007). Use of Fluorescent Quantum Dots Bioconjugates for Cellular Imaging of Immune Cells, Cell Organelle Labeling, and Nanomedicine: Surface Modification Regulates Biological Function, Including Cytotoxicity. *J. Artif. Organs*, Vol. 10, No. 3, pp. 149-157.

Huang DBPPV-CdSe-ZnS Quantum-Dot Light-Emitting Diodes. *IEEE Photonics Technol. Lett.*, Vol, C.Y., Su, Y.-K., Wen, T.-C., Guo, T.-F., and Tu, M.-L. (2008). Single-Layered Hybrid. 20, No. 4, pp. 282-284.

Huynh, W.U., Peng, X., Alivisatos, A.P. (1999). Preparation and Characterization of CdSe Nanoparticles Prepared by Using Ultrasonic Irradiation. *Adv. Mater.*, Vol. 11, pp. 923-938.

Huynh, W.U., Dittmer, J.J., Alivisatos, A.P. (2002). Hybrid Polymer-Nanorod Solar Cell. *Science*, Vol. 295, No. 5564, pp. 2425-2427.

Invitrogen – a Provider of Essential Life Science Technologies (2010). http://www.invitrogen.com

Jaiswal J.K.; Mattoussi H.; Mauro J.M.; Simon S.M. *Nature Biotechnol.* 2003,21, 47.

Jamieson, T., Bakhshi, R., Petrova, D., Pocock, R., Imani, M., Seifalian, A.M. (2007). Biological Applications of Quantum Dots. *Biomaterials* Vol. 28, pp. 4717-4728.

Ji, X., Zheng, J., Xu, J., Rastogi, V.K., Cheng, T.Ch., DeFrank, J.J. and Leblanc, R.M. (2005). (CdSe)ZnS Quantum Dots and Organophosphorus Hydrolase Bioconjugate as Biosensor for Detection of Paraoxon. *J. Phys. Chem. B*, Vol. 109, pp. 3793-3799.

Johnson, F.A., and Loudon, R. (1964). *Proc. Roy. Soc.* A, Vol. 281, 274-277.

Kim, S., Fisher, B., Eisler, H.-J., Bawendi, M. (2003). Type-II quantum dots: Te/CdSe(core/shell) and CdSe/ZnTe(core/shell) heterostructures. *J Am Chem Soc* Vol. 125, pp. 11466–11567.

Kim, S., Bawendi, M.G. (2003). Oligomeric Ligands for Luminescent and Stable Nanocrystal Quantum Dots. *J Am Chem Soc*, Vol. 125, pp. 14652–14653.

Kirchner, C., Leidl, T., Kudera, S. (2005). Cytoxicity of Colloidal CdSe and CdSe/ZnS Nanoparticles. *Nano Lett.*, Vol. 5(2), pp. 331-338.

Klude, M., Passow, T., Heinke, H. and Hommel, D. (2002). Electro-Optical Characterization of CdSe Quantum Dot Laser Diode. *Phys. Status Solidi (b)*, Vol.229, No.2, pp. 1029-1052.

Kongkanand, A., Tvrdy, K., Takechi, K., Kuno, M, and Kamat, P.V. (2008). Quantum Dots Solar Cells. *J. Am. Chem. Soc.* Vol. 130, 4007-4015. (2008).

Kortan, A.R.; Hull, R., Opila, R.L., Bawendi, M.G., Steigerwald, M.L., Carroll, P.J., Brus, L.E. (1990). Nucleation and Growth of Cadmium Selenide on Zinc Sulfide Quantum Crystallite Seeds, and Vice Versa, in Inverse Micelle Media. *J. Am. Chem. Soc.* Vol. 112, pp. 1327-1332.

Kuno, M., Fromm, D.P., Hamann, H.F., Gallagher, A., Nesbitt, D.J. (2001). "On"/"off" Fluorescence Intermittency of Single Semiconductor Quantum Dots. *J. Chem. Phys.* Vol. 115, pp. 1028-1031.

Korsunskaya, N.E., Markevich, I.V., Torchinskaya, T.V. and Sheinkman, M.K. (1980a). Photosensitivity Degradation Mechanism in CdS:Cu Single Crystals , *phys. stat. sol (a),* Vol. 60, pp. 565-572.

Korsunskaya, N.E., Markevich, I.V., Torchinskaya, T.V. and Sheinkman, M.K. (1980b). Electrodiffusion of shallow donors in CdS crystals, *J.Phys.C. Solid St.Phys.,* Vol. 13, pp. 2975 -2978.

Korsunskaya, N.E., Markevich, I.V., Torchinskaya, T.V. and Sheinkman, M.K. (1982). Recharge-enhanced transformations of donor-acceptor pairs and clusters in CdS *J. Phys. Chem. Solid.* Vol. 43, pp. 475-479.

Kozielski, M., Muhle, M., Z. Blaszczak, Z. (2004). *J. Molecul. Liquid.* Vol. 111, pp. 1-5.

Larson, D.R., Zipfel, W.R., Williams, R.M., Clark, S.W., Bruchez, M.P., Wise, F.W., Webb, W.W. (2003). Water-Soluble Quantum Dots for Multiphonon Fluorescence Imaging in Vivo. *Science*, Vol. 300, pp. 1434-1436.

Lee, LY., Ong, S.L., Hu, J.Y., Ng, W.J., Feng, Y.Y., X.L. Tan, X.L. (2004). Use of Semiconductor Quantum Dots for Photostable Immunofluorescence Labeling of Cryptosporidium parvum. *Appl Environ Microbiol*, Vol. 70, pp. 5732-5736.

Liu,Y., Qiu, H.Y., Xu, Y., Wu, D., Li, M.J., J.X. Jiang, J.X. and G.Q. Lai, G.Q. (2007). Synthesis and Optical Properties of CdSe nanocrystals and CdSe/ZnS Quantum Dots. *J. Nanopart. Res.*, Vol. 9, pp. 745-747.

Liang, J.G., Huang, S., Zeng, D., He, Z., Ji, X. and Yang, H. (2006). Highly Luminescent CdTe Quantum Dots Prepared in Aqueous Phase as an Altenative Fluorescent Probe for Cell Imaging. *Talanta*, Vol. 69, pp. 126-129.

Liboff, R.L., Greenberg, J. (2001). The Hexagon Quantum Billiard. *J. Stat. Phys.* Vol. 105, pp. 389-402

Liboff, R.L. (1994). The Polygon Quantum Billiard Problem. *J. Math. Phys.* Vol. 35, No.2, pp. 596-607

Lopez-Luke, T., Wolcott, A., Xu, L.P., Chen, S.W., Wcn, Z.H., Li, J.H., De La Rosa, E. and Zhang, J.Z. (2008). Conjugating Luminescent CdTe Quantum Dots with Biomolecules. *J. Phys. Chem.* C, Vol. 112, pp. 1282-1287.

Lou, X., Weng, W.J., Du, P.Y., Shen, G. and Han, G.R. (2004). Synthesis and Optical Properties of CdSe Nanocrystals and CdSe/ZnS Quantum dots. *Rare Met. Mater. Eng.*, Vol. 33, pp. 291-299.

Madelung, O. (Ed.). (1992). *Semiconductors, Data in Science and Technology*. Springer-Verlag, Berlin.

Malik, M.A., O'Brien, P. and Revaprasadu, N. (2005). Precursor Routes to Semiconductor Quantum Dots. *Phos. Sulfur Silicon Relat. Elem.*, Vol. 180, pp. 689-712.

Mattoussi, H., Radzilowski, L.H., Dabbousi, B.O., Fogg, D.E., Schrock, R.R., Thomas, E.L., Rubner, M.F., Bawendi, M.G. (1999). Composite Thin Films of CdSe Nanocrystals and a Surface Passivating/Electron Transporting Block Copolymer. *J. Appl. Phys.* 1999, Vol. 86, 4390-4399.

Mattoussi, H., Mauro, J.M., Goldman, E.R., Anderson, G.P., Sundar, V.C., Mikulec, F.V. (2000). Self-Assembly of CdSe-ZnS Quantum Dots Bioconjugates Using an Engineered Recombinant Protein. *J Am. Chem Soc.*, Vol.122, pp.12142–12150.

Medintz IL, Uyeda HT, Goldman ER, Mattoussi H. *Nat Mater* 2005;4:435–46.

Meulenberg, R.W., Jennings, T., Stroue, G.F. (2004). Compressive and Tensile Stress in Colloidal CdSe Semiconductor Quantum Dots. *Phys. Rev. B*, Vol. 70, No. 23, 235311.

Miyazaki S, Yamaguchi H, Takada M, Hou WM, Takeichi Y, Yasubuchi H. *Acta Pharm Nordica* 1990;2:401–6.

Murcia, M.J.; Shaw, D.L.; Long, E.C.; Naumann, C.A. (2008). Fluorescence Correlation Spectroscopy of CdSe/ZnS Quantum Dots Optical Bioimaging Probes with Ultra-Thin Biocompatible Coating. *Opt. Commun.*, Vol. 281, No. 7, pp. 1771-1780.

Murray, C.B., Norris, D.J., Bawendi, M.G. (1993). Synthesis and Characterization of Nearly Monodisperse CdE (E = Sulfur, Selenium, Tellurium) Semiconductor Nanocrystallites. *J Am.Chem.Soc.*, Vol. 115, pp. 8706-8715.

Murray, C.B., Kagan, C.R., Bawendi, M.G. (2000). Synthesis and Characterization of Monodisperse Nanocrystals and Close-Packed Nanocrystal Assemblies. *Annu. Rev. Mater. Sci.*, Vol. 30, pp. 545-610.

Murray, C.B., Sun, S., Gaschler, W., Doyle, H., Betley, T.A., C.R. Kagan, C.R. (2001). Colloidal synthesis of nanocrystals and nanocrystal superlattices. *IBM J. Res. Dev.*, Vol. 45, pp. 47-56.

Nakamoto, K. (1997). *Infrared and Raman Spectra of Inorganic and Coordination Compounds*, Part A, John Wiley &Sons, Inc., N.Y.

Nann, T. and Riegler, J. (2002). Monodisperse CdSe Nanorods at Low Temperatures. *Chem. Eur. J.*, Vol. 8, No. 20, pp. 4791-4795.

Nazzal, A.Y., X. Y. Wang, X.Y., Qu, L.H., Yu, W., Wang, Y.Z., Peng, X.G., and Xiao, M. (2004). *J. Phys. Chem. B* Vol. 108, pp. 55075511.

Nordell, K.J., Boatman, E.M., Lisensky, G.C. (2005). A Safer, Easier, Faster Synthesis for CdSe Quantum Dot Nanocrystals. *J. Chem.Educ.*, Vol. 82, pp. 1697-1699.

Norris, D.J., Bawendi, M.G. Measurement and Assignment of the Size-Dependent Optical Spectrum in CdSe Quantum Dots. (1996). *Phys. Rev. B*, 53, 16338.

Norris, D.J., Efros, Al.L., Rosen, M. and Bawendi, M.G. (1996). Size Dependence of Exciton Fine Structure in CdSe Quantum Dots. *Phys.Rev. B*, Vol.53, No. 24, 16347.

Oda, M., Tsukamoto, J., Hasegawa, A., Iwami, N., K. Nishiura, Hagiwara, I., Amdo, N., Horiuchi, H. and Tani, T. (2006). *J. Luminecs.*, Vol. 119–120, pp. 570-573.

Parak, W.J., Gerion, D., Zanchet, D., Woerz, A.S., Pellegrino, T., Micheel, Ch., Williams, Sh.S., Seitz, M., Bruehl, R.E., Bryant, Z., Bustamante, C., Bertozzi, C.R. and Alivisatos, A.P. (2002). Conjugation of DNA to Silanized Colloidal Semiconductor Nanocrystalline Quantum Dots. *Chem. Mater.*, Vol. 14, pp. 2113-2119.

Park, J., An, K., Hwang, Y., Park, J.E.G., Noh, H., Kim, J., Park, J., Hwang, N.M. and Hyeon, T. (2004). Ultra-large Scale Synthesis of Monodisperse nanocrystals. *Nat. Mater.*, Vol. 3, pp. 891-895.

Park, J., Lee, K.H., Galloway, J.F. and Searson, P.C. (2008). Synthesis of Cadmium Selenide Quantum Dots from a Non-Coordinating Solvent: Growth Kinetics and Particle Size Distribution. *J. Phys. Chem.* C, Vol. 112, pp. 17849-17854.

Parungo, C.P., Ohnishi, S., Kim, S.W., Kim, S., Laurence, R.G., Soltesz, E.G. (2005). Intraoperative Identification of Esophageal Sentinel Limph Nodes Using Near-Infrared Fluorescence Imaging. *J Thorac. Cardiovasc Surg.*, Vol. 129, pp. 844-850.

Pathak, S., Choi, S.K., Arnheim, N., M.E. Thompson, M.E. (2001). Hydroxylated Quantum Dots as Luminescent Probes for in Situ Hybridization. *J. Am. Chem. Soc* . Vol. 123, pp. 4103-4104.

Pellegrino T, Manna L, Kudera S, Liedl T, Koktysh D, Rogach AL, *Nano Lett* 2004;4:703–7.

Peng, X., Schlamp M.C., Kadavanich A.V., Alivisatos A.P. (1997). Epitaxial Growth of Highly Luminescent CdSe/CdS Core/Shell Nanocrystals with Photostabiliy and Electronic Accessibility. *J Am Chem Soc.*, Vol. 119, pp.7019–7029.

Peng, Z.A., and Peng X. (2001). Mechanisms of Shape Evolution of CdSe Nanocrystals. *J. Am. Chem. Soc.*, Vol. 123, pp. 1389-1395.

Ping Yang, Masanori Ando, Norio Murase. Encapsulation of Emitting CdTe QDs Within Silica Beads to Retain Initial Photoluminescence Efficiency. *Journal of Colloid and Interface Science*, Vol. 316, pp. 420–427.

Portney, N.G., and Ozkan, M. (2006). Nano-Oncology: Drug Delivery, Imaging and Sensing. *Anal. Bioanal. Chem.*, Vol. 384, pp. 620-630.

Qu, L.H., Peng, Z.A., Peng, X.G. (2001). Synthesis Conditions for Semiconductor CdSe Nanocrystals in Organic Solvents. *Nano Lett*, Vol. 1, pp. 333-337.

Qu, L., Peng, X.G. (2002). Control of Photoluminescence Properties of CdSe Nanocrystals in Growth. *J. Am. Chem. Soc,* Vol. 124, pp. 2049-2055.

Rakovich, Yu.P., J.F. Donegan, S.A. Filonovich, M.J.M. Gomes, D.V. Talapin, A.L. Rogach, A. Eychmuller, A. (2003). *Physica E,* Vol. 17, pp. 99 - 100.

Roberti, T.W., Cherepy, N.J., and Zhang, J.Z. (1998). *J. Chem. Phys.* Vol. 108, pp. 2143-2150.

Rosenthal, S.J., McBride, J., Pennycook, S.J. and Feldman, L.C. (2007). Synthesis, surface studies, composition and structural characterization of CdSe, core/shell and biologically active nanocrystals. *Surf. Sci. Rep.*, Vol. 62, pp. 111-157.

Rowe, B. W. , Pas, S. J. , Hill, A. J. , Suzuki, R., Freeman, B.D., Paul, D.R. (2009). *Polymer* Vol. 50, pp. 6149-6152.

Rusakov, K.I., Gladyshchuk, A.A., Rakovich, Yu.P., Donegan, J.F., Filonovich, S.A., Gomes, M.J.M., Talapin, D.V., Rogach, A.L., and Eychmüller, A. (2003). *Optics and Spectroscopy*, Vol. 94, pp. 859-863.

Salgueiriño-Maceira, V., Correa-Duarte, M.A., Spasova, M., Liz-Marzán, L.M., M. Farle, M. (2006). Composite Silica Spheres with Magnetic and Luminescent Functionalities. *Adv. Funct. Mater.*, Vol. 16, pp. 509-514.

Selvan, S.T., Li, C.L., Ando, M., Murase, N. (2004). Synthesis of Highly Photoluminescent Semiconductor nanoparticles by Aqueous Solution. *Chem. Lett.*, Vol. 33, pp. 434-435.

Selvan, S.T., Tan, T.T., Ying, J.Y. (2005). Robust, Non-Cytotoxic, silica-Coated CdSe Quantum Dots with Efficient Photoluminescence. *Adv. Mater.*, Vol. 17, pp. 1620-1625.

Shelby, M.D., and Wilkes, G.L. (1998). *Polymer* Vol. 39 No. 26, pp. 6767–6779.

Schiff, L.I. (1968). *Quantum Mechanics*, 3rd ed., McGraw-Hill, Inc., N.Y.

Schmid, M., S. Crampin, S., Varga, P. (2000). STM and STS of bulk electron scattering by subsurface objects. *J. Electron Spectr. and Rel. Phenomena*, Vol. 109, pp. 71-84

Smith, A.M. & Nie, Sh. (2004). Chemical analysis and cellular imaging with quantum dots. *Analyst*, Vol. 129, No. 8, pp. 672-677.

Sundar, V.C., Eisler, H.J., Bawendi, M.G. (2002). Room-Temperature, Tunable Gain Media from Novel II–VI Nanocrystal–Titania Composite Matrices. *Adv. Mater* 2002, Vol. 14, pp. 739-743.

Tanaka, A., Onari, S., Arai, T. (1992). Raman Scattering from CdSe Microcrystals Embedded in a Geramante Glass Matrix. *Phys. Rev. B*, Vol. 45, 6587.

Tashiro, A., Nakamura, H., Uehara, M., Ogino, K., Watari, T., Shimizu, H. and Maeda, H. (2004). マイクロリアクターを用いたCdSeナノ粒子の合成 (in Japanese) *Kagaku Kogaku Ronbunshu*, Vol. 30, pp. 113-116.

Temple , P.A. & Hathaway, C.E. (1973). *Phys. Rev. B*, Vol. 7, pp. 3685-3691.

Tessler, N., Medvedev, V., Kazes, M., Kan, S.H., U. Banin, U. (2002). Efficient Near-Infrared Polymer Nanocrystal Light-Emitting Diodes. *Science*, Vol. 295, p. 1506.

Torchynska, T.V., Diaz Cano, A., M. Dybic, S. Ostapenko, M. Morales Rodrigez, S. Jimenes Sandoval, Y. Vorobiev, C. Phelan, A. Zajac, T. Zhukov, T. Sellers, T. (2007). *phys. stat. sol. (c)*, 4, pp. 241-244.

Torchynska, T.V., Douda, J., Ostapenko, S., S. Jimenez-Sandoval, C. Phelan, A. Zajac, T. Zhukov, Sellers, T. (2008). *J. Non-Crystal. Solids*, Vol. 354, pp. 2885-2890.

Torchynska, T.V. (2009a). Interface States and Bio-Conjugation of CdSe/ZnS Core-Shell Quantum Dots. *Nanotechnology*, Vol. 20, 095401.

Torchynska, T.V., Douda, J., Calva, P.A., Ostapenko, S.S., and Peña Sierra, R. (2009b). Photoluminescence of Bioconjugated Core-Shell CdSe/ZnS Quantum Dots. *J. Vac. Sci. &Technol. B*, Vol. 27(2), pp. 836-841.

T.V. Torchynska, J. Douda, R. Pena Siera, (2009c). Photoluminescence of CdSe/ZnS core/shell quantum dots of different sizes, *phys. stat. sol. (c)* Vol. 6, pp. 143-147.

Torchynska, T.V., Quintos Vazquez, A.L., Pena Sierra, R., Gazarian, K., Shcherbyna, L. (2010). Modification of Optical Properties at Bioconjugation of Core-Shell CdSe/ZnS Quantum Dots. *J. of Physics, Conference Ser.*, Vol. 245, 012013.

Vega Macotela, L.G., Douda, J., Torchynska, T.V., Peña Sierra, R. and Shcherbyna, L. (2010a). Transformation of Photoluminescence Spectra at the Bioconjugation of Core-Shell CdSe/ZhS Quantum Dots. *Phys. Stat. Sol C*, Vol. 7, pp. 724-727.

Vega Macotela, L.G., Torchynska, T.V., Douda, J. and Peña Sierra , R. (2010b). Variation of Raman spectra of CdSe/ZnS quantum dots at the bioconjugation *phys.stat.solid. (c),* Vol. 7, pp. 1192-1195.

Vorobiev, Y.V., Vieira, V.R., Horley, P.P., Gorley, P.N., González-Hernández, J. (2009). Energy spectrum of an electron confined in the hexagon-shaped quantum well. *Science in China Series E: Technological Sciences,* Vol. 52, No. 1, pp. 15-18, ISSN 1006-9321

Vorobiev, Y.V., Gorley, P.N., Vieira, V.R., Horley, P.P., González-Hernández, J. Torchynska, T.V., Diaz Cano, A. (2010). Effect of boundary conditions on the energy spectra of semiconductor quantum dots calculated in the effective mass approximation. *Physica E,* Vol. 42, No. 9, pp.2264-2267, ISSN 1386-9477

Vorobiev, Y.V., Vieira, V.R., Ribeiro, P., Gorley, V., Horley, P.P., González-Hernández, J., and Torchynska, T. (2011) Energy Spectra of an Electron in a Pyramid-shaped Quantum Dot in Effective Mass Approximation with Even Mirror Boundary Conditions. *Proceedings of 3rd WSEAS Conference on Nanotechnology,* WSEAS Press, pp. 127-131, ISBN: 978-960-474-276-9, Cambridge, England, February 20 - 22 de 2011.

Walker, G.W., Sundar, V.C., Rudzinski, C.M., A.W. Wun, A.W., Bawendi, M.G., and Nocera, D.G. (2003). Quantum-dot Optical Temperature Probe. *Appl. Phys. Lett.* Vol. 83, No. 17, pp. 3555-3558.

Wang YA, Li JJ, Chen HY, Peng XG. (2002). *J Am Chem Soc.,* Vol. 124, pp. 2293–2298.

Wang, S., Jarrett, B.R., Kauzlarich, S.M., and Louie, A.Y. (2007). Core/Shell Quantum Dots with High Relaxivity and Photoluminescence for Multimodality Imaging. *J. Am. Chem. Soc.* Vol. 129, pp. 3848-3847.

William, W.Yu., Emmanuel Chang, Rebekah Drezek, Vicki L.C. (2006). Water Soluble Quantum Dots for Biomedical Applications. *Biochemical and Biophysical Research Communications,* Vol. 348, pp. 781–786.

Wolcott, A., Gerion, D., Visconte, M., Sun, J., Schwartzberg, Ad., Chen, Sh., and Zhang, J.Z. (2006). Silica Coated CdTe Quantum Dots Functionalized with Thiols for Bioconjugation to IgG Proteins. *J. Phys. Chem. B,* Vol. 110, p.5779-5789.

Wu, X.Y., Liu, H.J., Liu, J.Q., Haley, K.N., Treadway, J.A., J.P. Larson, J.P. (2002). Immunofluorescent Labelling of Cancer Marker Her2 and Other Cellular Targets with Semiconductor Quantum Dots. *Nat Biotechnol,* 21, 41-46.

Yang, L., Li, Y. (2006). Simultaneous Detection of *Escherichia coli* 0157:H7 and *Salmonella* Typhimurum Using Quantum Dots as Fluorescence Labels. *Analyst,* Vol. 131, pp. 394-401.

Yoon, J.H., Chae, W.S., Im, S.J. and Kim, Y.R. (2005). Mild Synthesis of Ultra-Small CdSe Quantum Dots in Ethylenediamine Solution. *Mater. Lett.,* Vol.59, pp. 1430-1433.

Yu, K., Zaman, B., Singh, S., Dashan, W. and Ripmeester, J.A. (2005). Colloidal CdSe Nanocrystals from Tri-n-Octyl *J. Nanosci. Nanotechnol.* Vol. 5, pp. 659-668.

Yu, W.W., Wang, A., Peng, X. (2003). Formation and Stability of Size-, Shape-, and Structure-Controlled CdTe Nanocrystals: Ligand Effects on Monomers and Nanocrystals. *Chem. Mater.,* Vol. 15(22), 4300-4308.

Zenkevich, E.I., Blaudeck, T., Shulga, A.M., Cichosb, F., C. von Borczyskowski, C. (2007). Identification and Assignment of Porphyrin CdSe Hetero-Nanoassemblies. *J. Luminescence,* Vol. 122–123, pp. 784–788.

Zhang, C.Y., Yeh, H.C., Kuroki, M.T., T.H. Wang., T.H. (2005). Quantum-Dot Based Nanosensor for RRE IIB RNA-Rev Peptide. *Nat. Mater.*, Vol. 4, pp. 826–831.

Zhao, J., Bardecker, J.A., Munro, A.M., Liu, M.S., Niu, Y., Ding, I.-K., Luo, J., Chen, B., Jen, A.K.-Y., and Ginger, D.S. (2006). Efficient CdSe/CdS Quantum Dot Light-Emitting Diodes Using a Thermally Polymerized Hole Transport Layer. *Nano Lett.*, Vol. 6, pp. 463-467.

11

Cross Cultural Principles for Bioethics

Mette Ebbesen
University of Aarhus
Denmark

1. Introduction

Ethics in relation to the practice of medicine had continuity from the time of Hippocrates (ca. 460-377 BC) to the 1970s focusing on the physician-patient relationship and moral obligations of beneficence and nonmaleficence. In the 1970s developments such as the gene splicing method and in vitro fertilization (IVF) created concerns about the adequacy of these long-established moral obligations (Beauchamp & Childress, 2009, p. 1). In addition to technological developments, historically, horrifying medical experimentation in concentration camps (the Nuremberg trials in the late 1940s) and the following Helsinki Declaration on the protection of human subjects had influence on the establishment of ethics committees worldwide and a shift toward focusing on the moral obligation of respecting informed consent of research subjects (Andersen, 1999, pp. 11-15; Beauchamp & Childress, 2009, pp. 1, 117; Ebbesen, 2009).

The discipline of bioethics or biomedical ethics[1] was established in the 1970s and various professions are involved such as ethics consultants, health care professionals, medical doctors, biomedical researchers, philosophers, theologians, and politicians. This essay, however, focuses on bioethics as an academic philosophical discipline and on empirical investigation of the ethics of the biomedical profession (Ebbesen, 2009).

Most research within the academic philosophical discipline of bioethics focus on theoretical reflections on the adequacy of ethical theories and principles. The principles of biomedical ethics of the American ethicists Tom L. Beauchamp & James F. Childress (2009) is an example. Beauchamp & Childress examined "considered moral judgements and the way moral beliefs cohere" and found that the general principles of beneficence, nonmaleficence, respect for autonomy, and justice play a vital role in biomedical ethics (Beauchamp & Childress, 2009, p. 13). They believe that these principles are an analytical framework and a suitable starting point for biomedical ethics (Beauchamp & Childress, 2009, p. 12). However, Beauchamp & Childress state that these four principles are not only specific for biomedical ethics; the principles form the core part of a cross cultural (universal) common morality. Beauchamp & Childress appeal to the common morality normatively by saying that the common morality establishes moral standards for everyone and failing to accept these standards is unethical. And, they appeal to the common morality descriptively by saying that it can be studied empirically whether the common morality is actually present in all cultures (Beauchamp & Childress, 2009, p. 4).

---

[1] In this essay the concepts of bioethics and biomedical ethics are used interchangeable to describe the analysis and discussion of ethical problems of biomedicine.

There is debate on whether the principles and method of Beauchamp & Childress are specific American and whether they can be used outside America, for instance in Europe and Asia. This essay examines these issues by introducing the theory of Beauchamp & Childress, by reviewing a Danish empirical study where Danish oncologists and Danish molecular biologists were interviewed, and lastly by outlining future perspective for broader empirical studies.

2. The common morality

Beauchamp believes that people from different cultures share some moral rules in common. These moral rules are for instance "Tell the truth", "Do not kill", "Rescue persons who are in danger", and "Do not steal". These moral rules are not implemented the same way in all cultures, however, the norms themselves are cross cultural. According to Beauchamp, these rules are justified by more abstract general principles. There is a transparent connection between these rules and the more general principles. For example the moral rule of "Tell the truth" is justified by the general principle of respect for autonomy, the rule "Do not kill" is justified by the principle of nonmaleficence, the rule "Rescue persons who are in danger" is justified by the principle of beneficence, and lastly, the moral rule "Do not steal" is justified by the principle of justice. One rule can be justified by more than one principle; hence there is a non-linear connection between rules and principles. This shared, universal system of rules and principles constitutes what Beauchamp calls moral in the narrow sense or the common morality (Beauchamp, 1997, p. 26). He defines the common morality as "the set of norms shared by all persons committed to the objectives of morality. The objectives of morality, I will argue, are those of promoting human flourishing by counteracting conditions that cause the quality of people's lives to worsen" (Beauchamp, 2003, p. 260). Beauchamp is aware that not everybody accepts or lives up to the demands of the common morality. This is not because these persons have a different morality; it is simply because they are immoral. Hence, the common morality is not just a morality that differs from other moralities (Beauchamp, 2003, p. 260). The common morality is "applicable to all persons in all places, and all human conduct is rightly judged by its standards" (Beauchamp, 2003, p. 260). Hence, the common morality provides an objective basis for moral judgment.

The moral rules and principles of the common morality are often so unspecific and content-thin that they only provide a basic guideline or orientation for addressing specific moral problems, for instance as to whether treatment without patient content is a moral acceptable enterprise (Beauchamp, 1997, p. 27). Practical moral problems of this kind require that the unspecific content-thin rules and principles of the common morality are made specific and implemented. Since answers to practical moral problems and the balancing of different values do often vary from one culture to another, specification and implementation of norms and principles are often done in different ways in different cultures. The universal system of rules and principles of the common morality does then form the basis or the starting point for this implementation (Beauchamp, 1997, p. 27-28). Beauchamp does not ignore that moral decision-making and practices vary from one culture to another, but they do not vary so much that the common morality is called into question. This plurality of moral decision-making and moral practices constitutes what Beauchamp calls moral in the broad sense introducing the concept of moral differences (Beauchamp, 1997, p. 27). Beauchamp believes that while the common morality or morality in the narrow sense "contains only general moral standards that are conspicuously abstract, universal, and content-thin" morality in the broad sense presents "concrete, nonuniversal, and content-rich norms" (Beauchamp, 2003, p. 261). Morality in the broad sense implements "the many responsibilities, aspirations, idealism, attitudes, and sensitivities that spring from cultural traditions, religious traditions, professional practice, institutional rules and the like" (Beauchamp, 2003, p. 261). Hence, Beauchamp argues that multiculturalism is not in opposition to universal ethical principles and he defends multiculturalism as a form of universalism (personal communication).

3. The four basic principles of the common morality

Beauchamp defends a moral framework of four clusters of moral principles which form the core part of the common morality. These four principles are: respect for autonomy (respecting the decision-making capacities of autonomous persons), nonmaleficence (avoiding the causation of harm), beneficence (providing benefits and balancing benefits, burdens, and risks), and justice (fairness in the distribution of benefits and risks). To interpret a principle is to tell what the principle is about and Beauchamp argues that the four principles are interpreted differently in different cultures. In figure 1 the four basic principles of the common morality are presented.

Respect for autonomy

- "As a negative obligation: Autonomous actions should not be subjected to controlling constraints by others" (Beauchamp & Childress, 2009, p. 104).
- "As a positive obligation, this principle requires both respectful treatment in disclosing information and actions that foster autonomous decision making" (Beauchamp & Childress, 2009, p. 104). Furthermore, this principle obligates to "disclose information, to probe for and ensure understanding and voluntariness, and to foster adequate decision making" (Beauchamp & Childress, 2009, p. 104).

The Principle of Beneficence

- One ought to prevent and remove evil or harm
- One ought to do and promote good (Beauchamp & Childress, 2009, p. 151).

The Principle of Nonmaleficence

- "One ought not to inflict evil or harm", where harm is understood as "thwarting, defeating, or setting back some party's interests" (Beauchamp & Childress, 2009, pp. 151-152).

The Principle of justice

Beauchamp & Childress do not think that a single principle can address all problems of distributive justice (Beauchamp & Childress, 2009, p. 241). They defend a framework for allocation that incorporates both utilitarian and egalitarian standards. A fair health care system includes two strategies for health care allocation: 1) a utilitarian approach stressing maximal benefit to patients and society, and 2) an egalitarian strategy emphasising the equal worth of persons and fair opportunity (Beauchamp & Childress, 2009, pp. 275, 281).

Fig. 1. **The four basic principles of the common morality.** A brief formulation of the four ethical principles: respect for autonomy, beneficence, nonmaleficence, and justice (Beauchamp & Childress, 2009; Ebbesen, 2009).

4. Managing complex cases of biomedicine

The four ethical principles of respect for autonomy, beneficence, nonmaleficence, and justice can be used when managing complex or problematic cases of biomedicine. When the principles are used in biomedicine it is often necessary to make the principles specific for that actual case. A specification of a principle is to narrow its scope and making it action-guiding. Beauchamp & Childress explain specification as "a process of reducing the indeterminate character of abstract norms and generating more specific, action-guiding content" (Beauchamp & Childress, 2009, p. 17). Specification involves a fine-tuning of the range and scope of the principle by increasing information about that specific situation (what time, where, what persons are involved, and so forth). Each principle is prima facie binding, which means that it "must be fulfilled unless it conflicts, on a particular occasion, with an equal or stronger obligation" (Beauchamp & Childress, 2009, p.15). If principles conflict they can be justifiably overridden which is the act of balancing (meaning that none of the principles are absolute). Balancing principles tells about their weight and strength, when balancing two principles, one principle is infringed by another (Beauchamp & Childress, 2009, pp. 19-20). Beauchamp & Childress list six conditions that must be met to justify the infringement of one prima facie principle by another (figure 2). Beauchamp & Childress state that physicians' acts of balancing and specifying ethical principles often involve "sympathetic insight, humane responsiveness, and the practical wisdom of evaluating a particular patient's circumstance and needs" (Beauchamp & Childress, 2009, p. 22).

1. "Good reasons can be offered to act on the overriding norm rather than on the infringed norm".
2. "The moral objective justifying the infringement has a realistic prospect of achievement".
3. "No morally preferable alternative actions are available".
4. "The lowest level of infringement, commensurate with achieving the primary goal of the action, has been selected".
5. "Any negative effects of the infringement have been minimized"
6. "All affected parties have been treated impartially" (Beauchamp & Childress, 2009, p. 23).

Fig. 2. **Conditions constraining balancing.** Conditions that must be met to justify infringement of one prima facie norm in order to adhere to another (Beauchamp & Childress, 2009; Ebbesen, 2009).

5. Empirical justification of the common morality

The Danish physician and philosopher Soeren Holm states that the four principles of Beauchamp & Childress are developed from American common morality and that they reflect certain aspects of American society and therefore they are limited to America and unsuited for Europe (Holm, 1997). Two Danish ethicists Jacob Rendtorff and Peter Kemp present a European alternative to Beauchamp & Childress' principles. Rendtorff & Kemp state that there are four ethical principles specifically suited for managing problematic cases of biomedicine in Europe, namely the principles of autonomy, dignity, integrity, and vulnerability (Rendtorff & Kemp, 2000). However, I believe that ethical principles always do contain obligations such as 'you ought to respect ...'. What Rendtorff & Kemp call principles do not contain obligations. Hence, strictly speaking, they cannot be considered as principles but as ethical concepts which can be reformulated into ethical principles. This can be done the following way: 'Respect for autonomy', Respect for dignity', and so forth. Beauchamp does also argue that the so-called principles of Rendtorff & Kemp are not principles at all. For instance, Beauchamp considers integrity is a virtue and vulnerability as a property or condition of persons. Furthermore, he thinks that the concept of dignity is one of the most obscure concepts of bioethics, since nobody knows what dignity is. Moreover, as can be seen above, Beauchamp does not believe in specific European ethical principles (personal communication).

Beauchamp states that empirical research could prove him (or Rendtorff & Kemp) wrong. The hypothesis to be tested is that all persons committed to the objective of morality adhere to the common morality (and thereby to the four ethical principles, which form the basis of the common morality) (Beauchamp, 2003, p. 264). First, persons should be screened to test whether they are committed to the objectives of morality (which "are those of promoting human flourishing by counteracting conditions that cause the quality of people's lives to worsen" (Beauchamp, 2003, p. 260)). Persons not committed to morality should then be excluded from the study. Next, it should be tested "whether cultural or individual differences emerge over the (most general) norms believed to achieve best the objectives of morality" (Beauchamp, 2003, p. 264). Beauchamp writes: "Should it turn out that the individuals or cultures studied do not share the norms that I hypothesize to comprise the common morality, then there is no common morality of the sort I claim and my particular hypothesis has been falsified" (Beauchamp, 2003, p. 264).

If it turns out that other general norms than the ones proposed by Beauchamp are shared across cultures, then the empirical study proves the presence of a common morality, however, of another sort than the one proposed by Beauchamp. Such an empirical study does not tell whether the norms of the common morality are adequate or in need of change. This is a normative question and not an empirical one (Beauchamp, 2003, p. 265). Beauchamp appeals to the common morality in both normative and nonnormative ways. The common morality has normative force meaning that it sets up moral standards for everyone and failing to accept these standards is unethical. Nonnormatively, Beauchamp claims that it can be studied empirically whether the common morality is present in all cultures. So, claims about the existence of the common morality can be justified empirically and analysis of the adequacy of the common morality involves normative investigation (Beauchamp, 2003, p. 265).

6. A Danish empirical study

One of the aims of a Danish empirical study where oncologists and molecular biologists were interviewed was to test whether there is a difference in the ethical considerations or principles at stake between the two groups. Since this study explores part of Beauchamp's hypothesis, he followed this study personally. This study was based on 12 semi-structured interviews with three groups of respondents: a group of oncology physicians working in a clinic at a public hospital and two groups of molecular biologists conducting basic research, one group employed at a public university and the other in private biotechnological company. The interview texts were transcribed word-for-word and analysed using a phenomenological hermeneutical method for interpreting interview texts inspired by the theory of interpretation presented by the French philosopher Paul Ricoeur. There were three steps in the data analysis. First, the texts were read several times in order to grasp their meaning as a whole. Next, themes were formulated across the whole interview material. And lastly, the themes were reflected on in relation to the literature which helped to revise, widen, and deepen the understanding of the texts (Ricoeur, 1976; Ebbesen & Pedersen 2007[a]).

The results of the study are summarised shortly. This empirical study indicated that oncology physicians and molecular biologists employed in a private biopharmaceutical company had the specific principle of beneficence in mind in their daily work. Both groups seemed motivated to help sick patients. According to the study, molecular biologists explicitly considered nonmaleficence in relation to the environment, the researchers' own health, and animal models; and only implicitly in relation to patients or human subjects. In contrast, considerations of nonmaleficence by oncology physicians related to patients or human subjects. Physicians and molecular biologists both considered the principle of respect for autonomy as a negative obligation in the sense that informed consent of patients should be respected. Molecular biologists stressed that very sick patients might be constrained by the circumstances to make a certain choice. However, in contrast to molecular biologists, physicians experienced the principle of respect for autonomy as a positive obligation because the physician, in dialogue with the patient, offers a medical prognosis evaluation based upon the patients' wishes and ideas, mutual understanding, and respect. Finally, this study disclosed a utilitarian element in the concept of justice as experienced by molecular biologists from the private biopharmaceutical company and egalitarian and utilitarian characteristics in the overall conception of justice as conceived by oncology physicians. Molecular biologists employed at a public university were, in this study, concerned with just allocation of resources; however, they did not support a specific theory of justice (Ebbesen & Pedersen 2007[b], 2008[a], 2008[b]).

This study showed that the ethical principles of respect for autonomy, beneficence, nonmaleficence, and justice as formulated by Beauchamp & Childress were related to the ethical reflections of the Danish oncology physicians and the Danish molecular biologists, and hence that they are important for Danish biomedical practice. Apparently, no empirical studies have investigated specifically the importance of the four principles previously; therefore, this empirical study contributes to an enhanced understanding of Beauchamp & Childress' theory from a new point of view. It could be objected, however, that the study did not centre on respondents who had already been screened to assure that they are morally committed, as Beauchamp recommend. According to Beauchamp, a way of screening whether persons are committed to morality is to test whether they are committed to the principle of nonmaleficence since this principle can be seen as the most basic principle of morality (personal communication). All respondents included in the study valued nonmaleficient behaviour.

7. Perspectives

Beauchamp & Childress believe that their four basic ethical principles are included in the cross-cultural common morality (Beauchamp & Childress, 2009). However, as described above, some of Beauchamp & Childress' opponents state that their theory has been developed from the American common morality and that it reflects certain characteristics of American society. Therefore, the theory might not be useful in other societies. Nevertheless, the results of the Danish empirical study demonstrate that the theory is related to Danish biomedical practice.

Future perspectives of the Danish empirical study are to explore whether Beauchamp & Childress' principles are cross-cultural and thereby have a universal perspective. This could be done by investigating whether there is a difference in the ethical considerations and principles at stake between physician oncologists working in different cultural settings (e.g. Scandinavian, Southern European, Asian, and American cultures). For instance, in Japan the principle of respect for autonomy is said to be more family oriented than in America (Fan, 1997). What is needed is a qualitative investigation of Japanese culture. This future study might show that Beauchamp & Childress' principles need reformulation to be used in specific cultural settings.

8. References

Andersen S (1999). What is bioethics? (In Danish). In: Bioethics. Jensen KK, Andersen S (eds.), pp. 11-18. Denmark: Rosinante Forlag A/S.

Beauchamp TL (1997). Comparative studies: Japan and America. In Kazumasa Hoshino (ed.). Japanese and Western bioethics, pp. 25-47. The Netherlands: Kluwer Academic Publishers.

Beauchamp TL (2003). A defense of the common morality. Kennedy Inst Ethics J 13(3):259-74.

Beauchamp TL, Childress JF (2009). Principles of biomedical ethics. 6th ed. Oxford: Oxford University Press.

Ebbesen M, Pedersen BD (2007[a]). Using empirical research to formulate normative ethical principles in biomedicine. Med Health Care Philos 10(1):33-48.

Ebbesen M, Pedersen BD (2007[b]). Empirical investigation of the ethical reasoning of physicians and molecular biologists – the importance of the four principles of biomedical ethics. Philos Ethics Humanit Med 2:23.

Ebbesen M, Pedersen BD (2008[a]). The principle of respect for autonomy - concordant with the experience of physicians and molecular biologists in their daily work? BMC Med Ethics 9:5.

Ebbesen M, Pedersen BD (2008[b]). The role of ethics in the daily work of oncology physicians and molecular biologists – results of an empirical study. Bus Prof Ethics J 27(1):19-46.

Ebbesen, M (2009). Bioethics in theory and practice. Ph.D. thesis. Denmark: University of Aarhus.

Fan R (1997). A report from East Asia. Self-determination vs. family-determination: Two incommensurable principles of autonomy. Bioethics 11(3&4):309-322.

Holm S (1995). Not just autonomy - the principles of American biomedical ethics. J Med Ethics 21(6):332-338.

Rendtorff J, Kemp P (2000). Basic ethical principles in European bioethics and biolaw. Vol. 1: autonomy, dignity, integrity and vulnerability. Denmark: Centre for ethics and law.

Ricoeur P (1976). Interpretation theory: discourse and the surplus of meaning. Texas: The Texas Christian University Press.

12

Pulse Wave Analysis

Zhaopeng Fan, Gong Zhang and Simon Liao
University of Winnipeg
Canada

1. Introduction

Cardiovascular refers to the Cardio (heart) and vascular (blood vessels). The system has two major functional parts: central circulation system and systemic circulation system. Central circulation includes the pulmonary circulation and the heart from where the pulse wave is generated. Systemic circulation is the path that the blood goes from and to the heart. (Green 1984) Pulse wave is detected at arteries which include elastic arteries, medium muscular arteries, small arteries and arterioles. The typical muscular artery has three layers: tunica intima as inner layer, tunica media as middle layer, and tunica adventitia for the outer layer. (Kangasniemi & Opas 1997) The material properties of arteries are highly nonlinear. (langewouters et al. 1984) It depends on the contents of arterial wall: how collagen, elastin and protein are located in the arteries. Functional and structural changes in the arterial wall can be used as early marker for the hypertensive and cardiac diseases.

Blood flow is the key to monitor the cardiovascular health condition since it is generated and restrict within such system. Currently the most widely used method for haemodynamic parameters detecting is invasive thermo-dilution method. Impedance-cardiography is the most commonly used non-invasive method nowadays; however, it is too complex for clinical routine check. Pulse wave analysis is an innovative method in the market to do fast and no burden testing (Zhang et al. 2008)

Pulse is one of the most critical signals of human life. It comes directly from heart to the blood vessel system. As pulse transmitted, reflections will occur at different level of blood vessels. Other conditions such as resistance of blood flow, elastic of vessel wall, and blood viscosity have clear influence on pulse. Pathological changes affect pulse in different ways: the strength, reflection, and frequency. So pulse provides abundant and reliable information about cardiovascular system.

Pulse can be recorded to a set of time series data and represented as a diagraph which is called pulse waveform or pulse wave for short.

Gathering pulse at wrist by finger has been a major diagnosis method in China since 500 BC. Physicians used palpation of the pulse as a diagnostic tool during the examination. In 300AD, "Maijing" categoried pulse into 24 types and became the first systematic literature about the pulse. Grecian started to notice the rhythm, strength, and velocity at 400BC. Struthius described a method to watch the pulse wave by putting a leaf on the artery, which is considered as early stage of pulse wave monitoring. In 1860, Etienne Jules Mary invented a level based sphygmograph to measure the pulse rate. It is the first device can actually record the pulse wave. Frederick observed normal radial pressure wave and the carotid wave to find the normal waveform and the differences between those waveforms. (Mahomed 1872) He figured out the special effect on the radial waveform caused by the high blood pressure. It helps to learn the natural history of essential hypertension.(Mahomed 1877) The effects of arterial degeneration by aging on the pulse wave were also shown on his work.(Mahomed 1874) His researches have been used in the life insurance field. (Postel_Vinay 1996)

The analysis was based on the basic mathematic algorithms in nineteenth century: dividing the wave into increasing part and decreasing part, calculating the height and area of the wave. Calculus, hemodynamic, biomathematics and pattern recognition techniques has been used in pulse wave analysis by taking advantage of Information Technology. However, utilizing the classic pulse theory with current techniques is still a big challenge.

2. Pulse wave analysis methods

2.1 Research data source

With informed consent, 517 sets of testing data were collected from 318 subjects. The ages of subjects range from 1 to 91 years (mean ± SD, 55 ± 20). 87 subjects were chosen from normal people (mean ±SD, 51 ±17) and the rest were recorded from patients in Department of Cardiology at Shandong Provincial Hospital in China (mean ± SD, 62 ±13). Normal people were assigned to the control group corresponding to the patients group. All medical records were collected in order to do research on each risk factor. Risk factor groups, including smoking group (mean ±SD, 66.089±13.112) and diabetes group (mean ±SD, 64±11.941), are created based on the risk factors from medical records.

2.2 Pulse wave factors

Using pulse data directly is unreliable since any change of haemodynamic condition has effects on pulse wave data. But there are still many researches for pulse wave analysis because the pulse data is much easier and safer to get than most other signals. With considering related conditions, pulse wave factors analysis can achieve higher accuracy.

Most recent researches give positive results with comparing pulse wave factors analysis and standard methods. Pathophysiological Laboratory Netherlands did study on continuous cardiac output monitoring with pulse contour during cardiac surgery (Jansen 1990). Cardiac output was measured 8 to 12 times during the operation with pulse contour and thermodilution. The result shows linear regression between two methods. The cardiac output calculated by pulse wave factors is accurate even when heart rate, blood pressure, and total peripheral resistance change.

To reduce the effects of other factors, pulse wave factors had been tested among different groups. Rodig picked two groups of patients based on ejection fraction: 13 patients in group 1 with ejection fraction greater than 45% and 13 patients in group 2 with ejection fraction less than 45%. Both pulse wave factors and thermodilution technique had been used to calculate the cardiac output 12 times during the surgery. The mean differences for CO did not differ in either group (Rodig 1999). The differences became significant when systemic vascular resistance increased by 60% and early period after operation. It suggested that pulse wave factors analysis is a comparable method during the surgery. Calibration of the device will help to achieve more accurate result.

The patients with weak pulse waveform or arrhythmia should always avoid using the result of pulse wave factors as the major source since it become unreliable in such environment.

Early Detection of cardiovascular diseases is one of the most important usages for pulse wave monitoring. The convenience noninvasive technique makes it extremely suitable for widely use at community levels. Factors derived from pulse wave analysis have been used to detect hypertension, coronary artery diseases. For example, losing the diastolic component is the result of reduced compliance of arteries. (Cohn 1995) Pulse wave is suggested to be early marker for those diseases and guide for health care professions during the therapy.

Pulse wave were used to be analyzed in two ways: point based analysis, area based analysis. Point based analysis is usually designed for specific risk factor. It picks up top, bottom points from different components of the waveform or derivative curve. Then the calculation is done regarding to the medical significant of those points. Stiffness Index is a well-known factor in this category.

Arteries stiffen is a consequence of age and atherosclerosis. Two of the leading causes of death in the developed world in nowadays, myocardial infarction and stroke, are a direct consequence of atherosclerosis. Arterial stiffness is an indicator of increased cardiovascular disease risk. Among many new methods applied to detect arterial stiffness, pulse wave monitoring is a rapidly developing one.

Arterial pulse is one of the most fundamental life signals in medicine, which has been used since ancient time. With the help of new information technology, pulse wave analysis has been utilized to detect many aspects of heart diseases especially the ones involving arterial stiffness.

Total arterial compliance and increased central Pulse Wave Velocity (PWV) are associated with arterial wall stiffening. They are recognized as the dominant risk factors for cardiovascular disease. The contour of the peripheral pressure and volume pulse affected by the vascular aging on the upper limb is also well-known. The worsen artery stiffness with an increase in pulse wave velocity is cited as the main reason for the change of pulse contour.

PWV is the velocity of the pulse pressure. The blood has speed of several meters per second at the aorta and slow down to several mm per second at peripheral network. The PWV is much faster than that. Normal PWV has the range from 5 meters per second to 15 meters per second. (O'Rourke & Mancia 1999)

Since pulse pressure and pulse wave velocity are closely linked to cardiovascular morbidity, some non- invasive methods to assess arterial stiffness based on pulse wave analysis have been introduced. However, these methods need to measure the difference of centre artery pulse and the reflected pulse wave, which is a complicated process. On the other hand, the Digital Volume Pulse (DVP) may be obtained simply by measuring the blood volume of finger, which becomes a potentially attractive waveform to analyze.

Millasseau et al have demonstrated that arterial stiffness, as measured by peripheral pulse wave analysis, is correlated with the measurement of central aortic stiffness and PWV between carotid and femoral artery, which is considered as a reliable method in assessment of cardiovascular pathologic changes for adults. They introduced the Stiffness Index (SI), which was derived from the pulse wave analysis for artery stiffness assessment and was correlated with PWV ($r=0.65$, $P<0.0001$). It is an effective non-invasive method for assessing artery stiffness.

Pulse Wave Velocity is the golden standard for arterial stiffness diagnosis. Researches show that Stiffness Index has equivalent output as PWV. It uses the reflection of the pulse as the second source to get the time difference without additional sensors which make it more applicable to the Home Monitoring System. As shown in figure 1, the systolic top shows the time that pulse reach the finger; diastolic top represents the time that pulse reflection reach the finger. The distance that pulse goes through has direct relationship with the height of the subject. SI can be calculated by $h/\Delta t$.

Area Based analysis specialized in the blood volume monitoring such as Cardiac Output (CO). The attempt for getting cardiac output from pulse wave started more than one hundred years ago (Erlanger 1904). The pulse wave is the result of interaction between stroke volume and arteries resistance. Building the model of arterial tree helped the calculation of CO from pulse wave. The simplest model used in clinic contains single resistance. Other elements should be involved in the calculation including capacitance element, resistance element (Cholley 1995).

Not all models have reliable results, even some widely used one can only work in specific environment. Windkessel Model consists of four elements: left ventricle, aortic valve, arterial vascular compartment, and peripheral flow pathway. Testing of the model in normotensive and hypertensive subjects shows that the model is only valid when the pressure wave speed is high enough with no reflection sites exist (Timothy 2002).

Cardiac Index (CI) is an important parameter related to the CO and body surface area. Tomas compared the CI value among pulmonary artery thermodilution, arterial thermodilution and pulse wave analysis for critically ill patients. The mean differences among three methods are within 1.01% and standard derivation are within 6.51%. (Felbinger 2004) The pulse wave factors provide clinically acceptable accuracy.

In addition to long term monitoring, pulse wave analysis is also useful for emergency environment. Cardiac Function can be evaluated within several seconds.

2.1.1 Stiffness Index

The pulse wave sensor detects the blood flow at the index finger and tracks the strength of the flow as pulse wave data. To record the pulse wave, the patients were comfortably rested with the right hand supported. A pulse wave sensor was applied to the index finger of right hand. Only the appropriate and stable contour of the pulse wave was recorded.

As shown in Figure, the first part of the waveform (systolic component) is result of pressure transmissions along a direct path from the aortic root to the wrist. The second part (diastolic component) is caused by the pressure transmitted from the ventricle along the aorta to the lower body. The time interval between the diastolic component and the systolic component depends upon the PWV of the pressure waves within the aorta and large arteries which is related to artery stiffness. The SI is an estimate of the PWV about artery stiffness and is obtained from subject height (h) divided by the time between the systolic and diastolic peaks of the pulse wave contour. The height of the diastolic component of the pulse wave relates to the amount of pressure wave reflection.

SI is highly related to the pulse rate because it is calculated by the time interval between systole and diastole. Younger people with high pulse rate can get a relative high score than older people with slow pulse rate. Adjustment based on pulse rate can be applied on SI calculation.

The testing results based on age are shown in Figure and Figure, which indicate that the adjusted SI is more sensitive than SI.

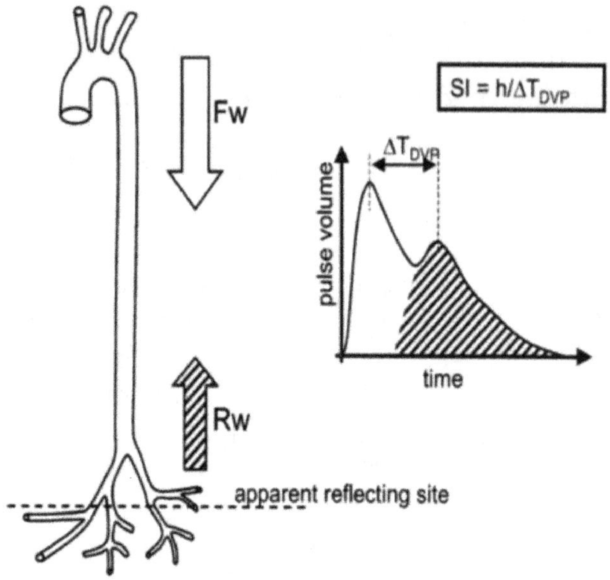

Fig. 1. Stiffness index is related to the time delay between the systolic and diastolic components of the waveform and the subject's height

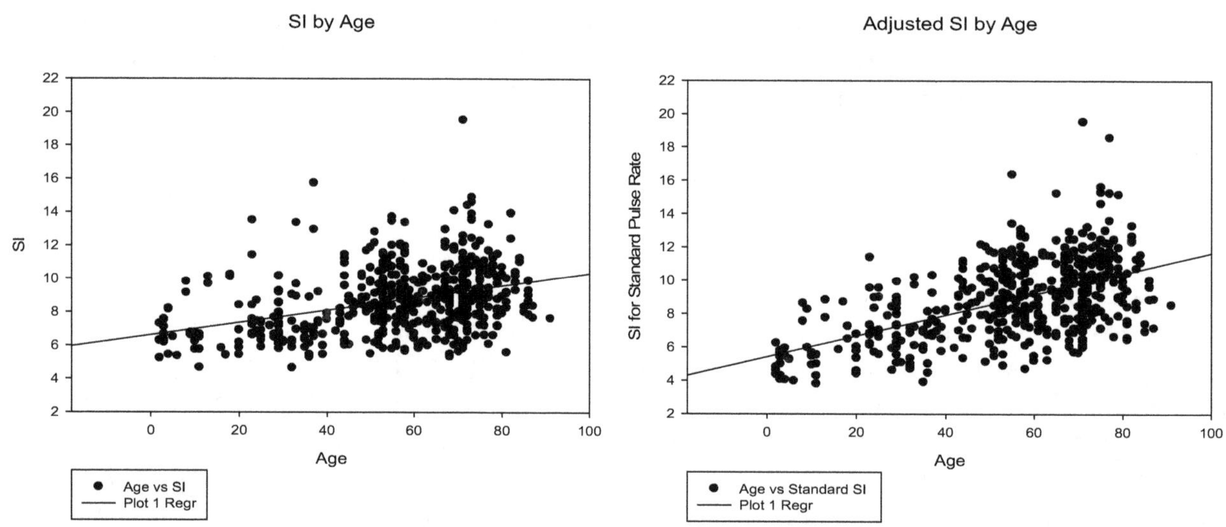

Fig. 2. Correlation for Stiffness Index and age (r=0.275, p = 9.833E-019). A closer relationship could be found between adjusted Stiffness Index and age. (r=0.536, p=7.279E-040)

In order to test the sensitivity of primary factor SI, we compare it with the collected data from different groups.

SI is much higher in patients group (SI: 9.576±2.250) than that of control group (SI: 7.558±1.751). On the other hand, it has positive correlation with age for both groups. All people in patients group came from the Department of Cardiology at Shandong Provincial Hospital and most of them have atherosclerosis which is the main reason for arterial stiffness. This result shows that the SI is a significant factor in pulse wave analysis to detect the degree of arterial stiffness.

Risk factor groups are very import in this research. Diabetes group (SI: 9.975±2.174) and smoking group (SI: 10.039±2.587) have even higher SI than patients group as a whole. SI is reliable for research to detect risk factors.

By analyzing with different factors, SI is found to be correlated with age, weight, and systolic blood pressure. With the comparison of patients and control groups, we find that SI has less correlation with age for patients with heart disease. However, when people have other risk factors such as smoking and diabetes, SI has no longer visible correlation with age. It also indicates that SI is sensitive to cardiovascular diseases and risk factors. People who have cardiovascular diseases or risk factor will have higher than normal SI. In general, illness and risk factors will have more impact on SI. This makes SI a perceptible indication in diagnosing arterial stiffness.

SI can be affected by the cardiac condition as we described before. The adjusted SI can only rectify influence of heart rate in a certain level. Other abnormal cardiac conditions, such as heart failure, will disturb the pulse wave form in different ways. A basic judgment of cardiac condition will make SI more catholicity.

2.1.2 Cardiac Output

The pulse contour method for calculation of cardiac output can be done based on the theory of elastic cavity (Liu & Li, 1987).

- Blood flow continuous equation:

$$
\begin{aligned}
Q_{in} &= Q_{out} + \frac{dV}{dt_1} \\
Q_{out} &+ \frac{dV}{dt_2} = 0
\end{aligned}
\tag{1}
$$

where Q_{in} is the volume of blood flowing into the artery and Q_{out} is the volume of blood flowing into the vein. t_1 and t_2 are the systolic and diastolic period, respectively.

- Equation between pressure remainder and blood flow:

$$
Q_{out} = \frac{p - p_v}{R} \tag{2}
$$

where p is the arterial pressure, p_v is the venous pressure, and R indicates the peripheral resistance of cardiovascular system.

- Arterial pressure volume equation:

$$
AC = \frac{dV}{dp} \tag{3}
$$

where AC is a constant that depends on the arterial compliance.

Based on the above three equations, the analytic equation of elastic cavity can be calculated:

$$
\begin{aligned}
Q_{in} &= AC\frac{dp}{dt_1} + \frac{p - p_v}{R} \\
AC\frac{dp}{dt_2} &+ \frac{p - p_v}{R} = 0
\end{aligned}
\tag{4}
$$

Computing the integral of Equation (4):

$$S_v = AC\left(p_s^* - p_d\right) + \frac{A_S}{R}$$
$$AC\left(p_d - p_s^*\right) + \frac{A_d}{R} = 0 \tag{5}$$

where S_v is the stroke volume during a heartbeat. We refer to Figure 4 for A_s, A_d, p_s, and p_d. Cardiac Output is highly correlated to age, weight, and systolic blood pressure. It shows the working status of the heart while SI shows the degree of arterial stiffness. We can also find that many subjects in patients group have abnormal Cardiac Output (CO: 4.567±1.309). But there is no significant correlation between SI and CO. Therefore, CO is a good complement of SI for analyzing cardiovascular condition.

2.3 Waveform analysis

The calculation based on the points with special meanings is very sensitive in the detection of risks. It uses simple algorithm to achieve the balance of performance and accuracy. But it's difficult to evaluate the overall cardiovascular condition only with several risk factors. The pulse is produced by the cooperation of heart, blood vessel, micro circulation and other parties. The more information included the more accurate classification we can get. This research used some sample wave forms to represent the different categories. A wave form belongs to a category if it's more similar to the wave form in that category than any other wave forms.

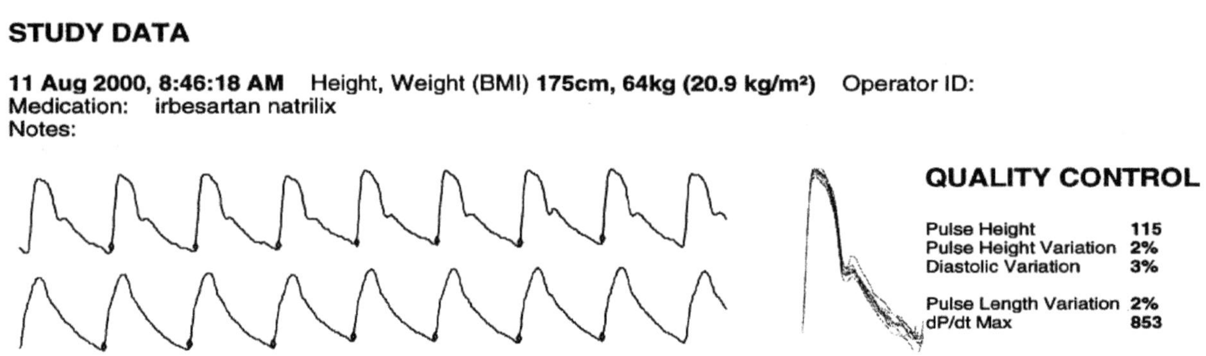

Fig. 3. Variation for continue waveforms. (O'Rourke 2001)

Pulse wave is relatively stable under the testing condition: subject setting in a quite environment and keeping calm. The pulse wave analysis result is highly repeatable in this condition. Actually the similarity of pulse waveforms doesn't change a lot under similar cardiovascular health condition even the heart rate and pulse strength changed, so waveform analysis can fit in different scenarios other than specific testing environment.
There are several classification system for the pulse wave. In the paper "Characteristics of the dicrotic notch of the arterial pulse wave in coronary heart diease", Tomas treat the notch as the indicator and classify pulse wave into four categories as following:

- Class I: A distinct incisura is inscribed on the downward slop of the pulse wave
- Class II: No incisura develops but the line of descent becomes horizontal
- Class III: No notch is present but a well-defined change in the angle of descent is observed
- Class IV: No evidence of a notch is seen

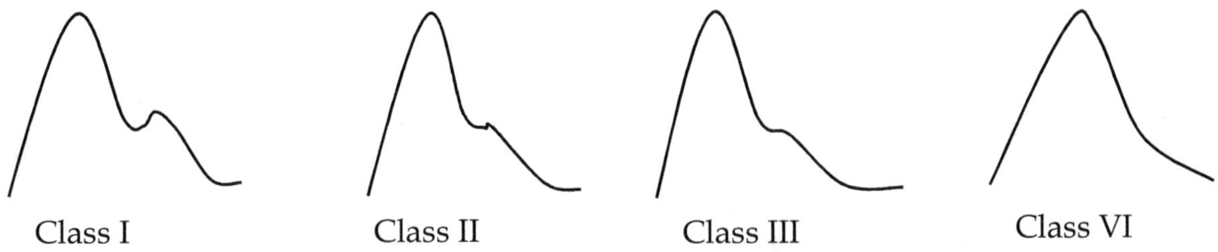

Fig. 4. Four classes of waveform based on dicrotic notch

This classification focus on the notch of the wave form which is considered as the indicator of arterial stiffness. Bates evaluates continues wave forms to include other possible diseases. He gave detail description of the pulse wave and discussed the cause of each pulse wave type. Possible diseases were also provided in his research.

Pulse type	Physiological cause	Possible disease
small & weak	decreased stroke volume	heart failure, hypovolemia, severe aortic stenosis
	increased peripheral resistance	
large & bounding	increased stroke volume	fever, anaemia, hyperthyroidism, aortic regurgitation, bradycardia, heart block, atherosclerosis
	decreased peripheral resistance	
	decreased compliance	
bisferiens	increased arterial pulse with double systolic peak	aortic regurgitation, aortic stenosis and regurgitation, hypertropic cardiomyopathy
pulsus alternans	pulse amplitude varies from peak to peak, rhythm basically regular	left ventricular failure

Table 1. Possible diseases which can be diagnosed based on the different types of cardiovascular pulse shapes (Bates 1995).

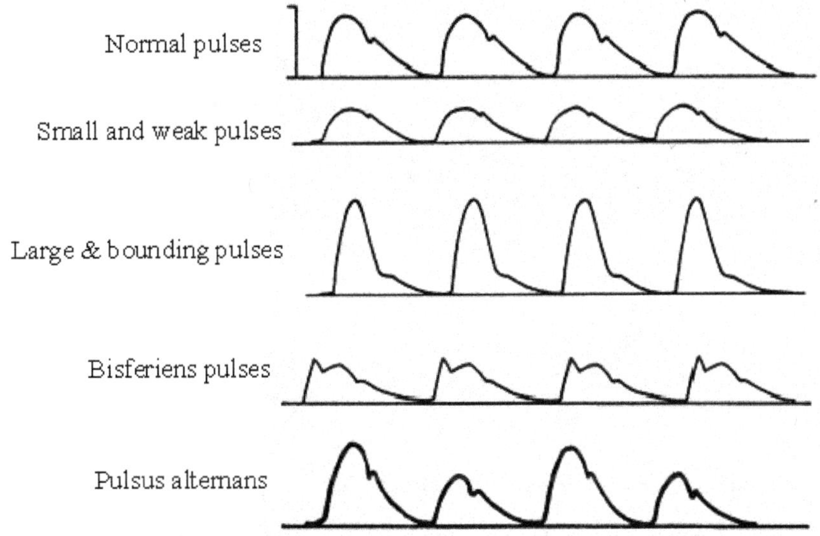

Fig. 5. Pulse wave classification from Bates

In order to get more precise information from the wave form, researchers take the traditional pulse diagnosis as the reference and mapping the characters of pulse diagnosis with the pattern of wave form. It can be used to detect certain cardiovascular risk as well as the classification. For example, acute anterior myocardial infarction will have a sharp systolic component and very small diastolic component which suggests poor blood supply.

2.2.1 Fourier transform and wavelet

Fourier Transform and Wavelet Transform have been used to perform the basic analysis on the pulse waveform. Fourier transform is a basic and important transform for linear analysis which usually transfers the signal from time domain (signal based on time) to frequency domain (the transform depends on frequency).

The Fourier theory states that any continuous signals or time serial data can be expressed as overlay of sine waves with different frequencies. This process can help signal analysis because the sine wave is well understood and treated as simple function in both mathematics and physics. Fourier transform calculates the frequency, amplitude, and phase based on this theory. Significant features could be detected by Fourier transform from similar time series data with big differences in frequency domain.

The Fourier transform can be treated as a special calculus formula that expresses the qualified function into sine basis functions. The function with the lowest frequency is called the fundamental. It has the same repetition rate of the periodic signal under evaluation. The frequency of other functions is integer times of the fundamental frequency.

Inverse Fourier transform can be used to recover the time series signal after the analysis on frequency domain is done.

With comparing the original waveform and transform data, some special features can be detected in the frequency domain.

The regular waveform from a normal subject has data nearly U shape distributed in the frequency domain. Lower frequencies and higher frequencies get bigger values and the slop goes smoothly from negative to positive. The peak value at lower frequency side is almost 50% bigger than the peak value at higher frequency side. The data become inconspicuous for frequencies between10 and 190 Hz. The higher values in time domain will result in the higher value in frequency domain.

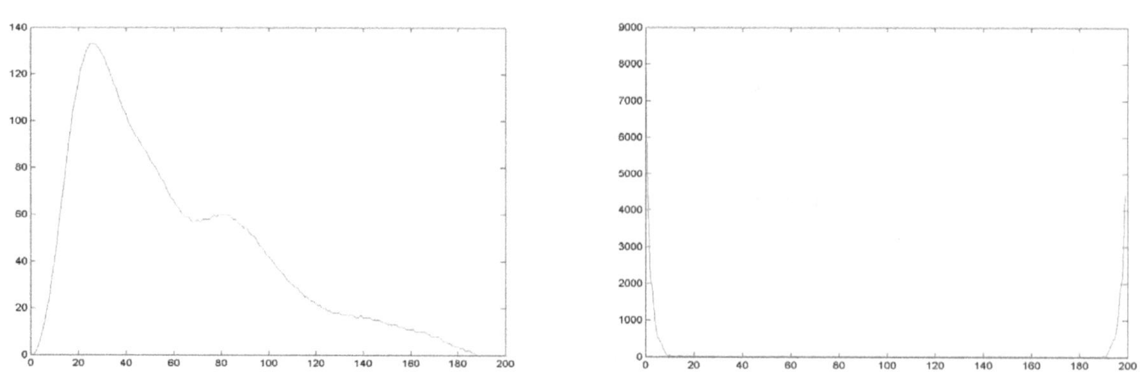

Fig. 6. Fourier Transform for a typical pulse waveform

Patients with old myocardial infarction often have obtuse systolic component and weak diastolic component due to the abnormal cardiac function. The diastolic component has a round top and much wider than the normal waveform. This feature will generate a local maximum value at around 7Hz and 193Hz. This feature can be used to detect the cardiac function diseases which cause slow change rate at pulse waveform.

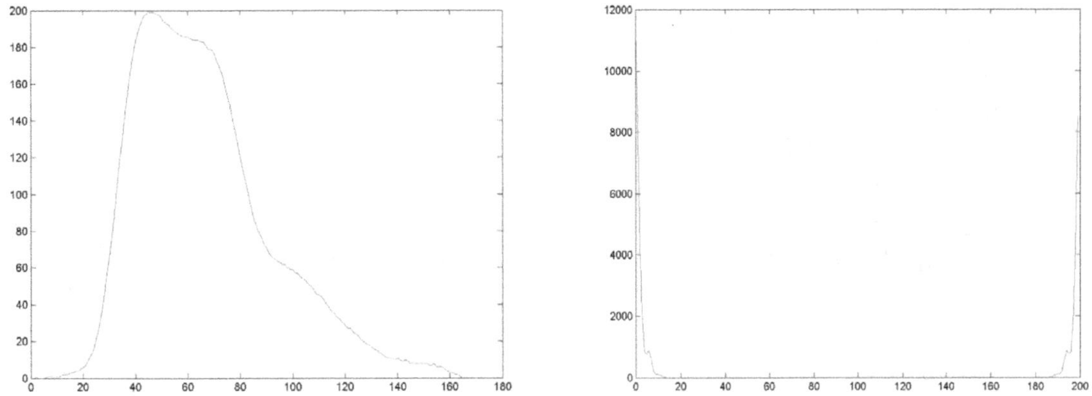

Fig. 7. Typical waveform of old myocardial infarction and their Fourier Transform

In a group of 100 selected testing data (50 normal waveform and 50 typical waveforms for old myocardial infarction), 48 testing data has local maximum at around 7Hz and 52 has smooth U shape distribution at frequency domain. 6 normal waveforms have been classified to old myocardia infarction by mistake and 8 typical myocardia infarction waveforms were not detected. Some possible reasons for mistake in the test:

1. Big wide diastolic component may cause the local maximum value in frequency domain.
2. Slow heart rate
3. Unstable pulse
4. Incomplete waveforms caused by device

The shape of diastolic component is important to arterial stiffness analysis. But it's difficult to get the corresponding features at frequency domain because the diastolic part is relatively small and can be easily affected by systolic part in FFT. The features for arterial stiffness can not be derived directly from the Fourier transform.

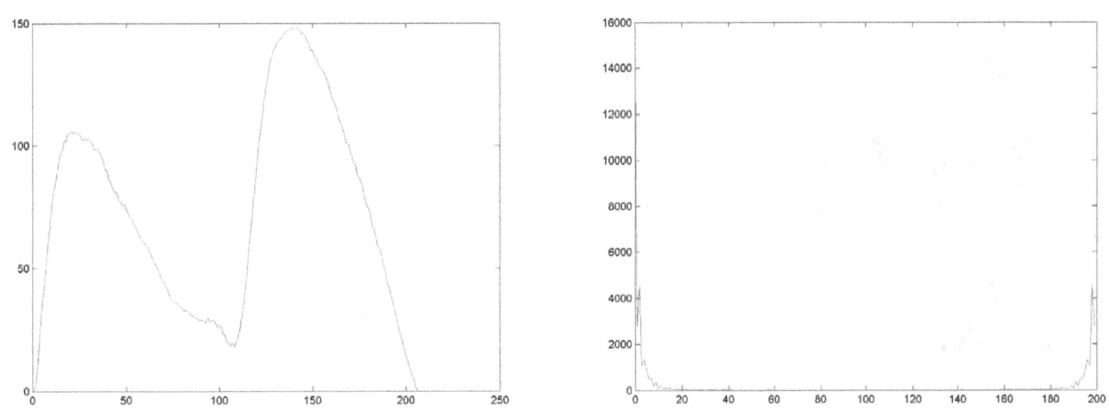

Fig. 8. Arrhythmia cause the second pulse arrives in advanced while the first pulse waveform is not complete yet. FFT shows that multi local maximum values appear at both higher frequency end and lower frequency end.

Arrhythmia is a common abnormal electrical activity in cardiovascular system. The heart rate might go too fast or too slow which will cause the waveforms change shape among continuous pulses. This feature can be captured in both time domain and frequency domain. The basic feature in time domain is time variance among continuous pulses exceeding the average level. The incomplete waveforms and merged waveforms often result in the pulse detection fails which is also a sign of arrhythmia. Eight typical arrhythmia waveforms have been identified from testing data and the patients do have arrhythmia history on file.
Features from FFT are helpful to detect some disease or certain cardiac condition, but it's difficult to achieve high accuracy by frequency domain analysis only.
Wavelet transform is well known for localized variations of power analysis. It uses the time and frequency domains together to describe the variability. Wavelet functions are localized in space while Fourier sine and cosine functions are not.

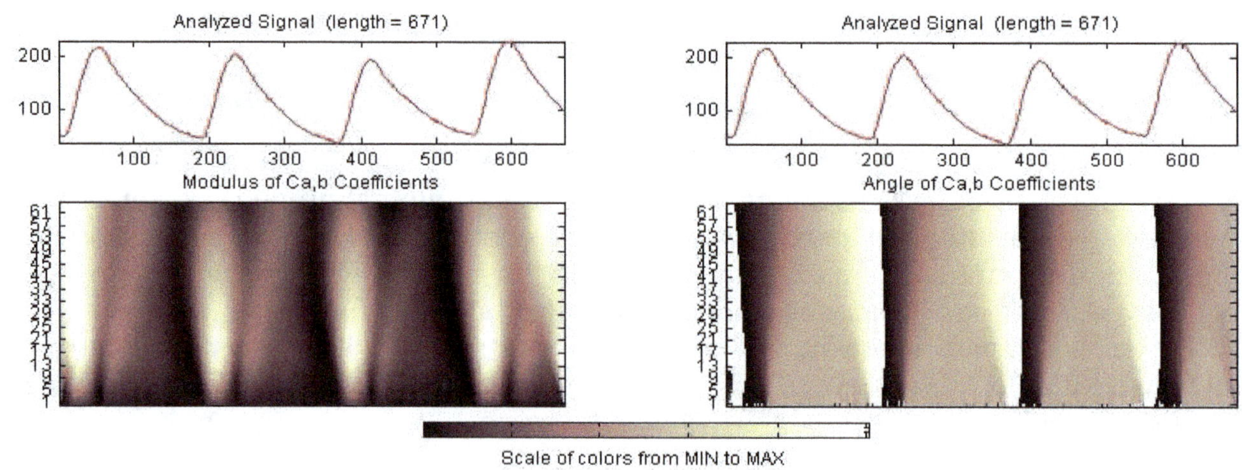

Fig. 9. Wavelet transform for pulse wave with no diastolic component.

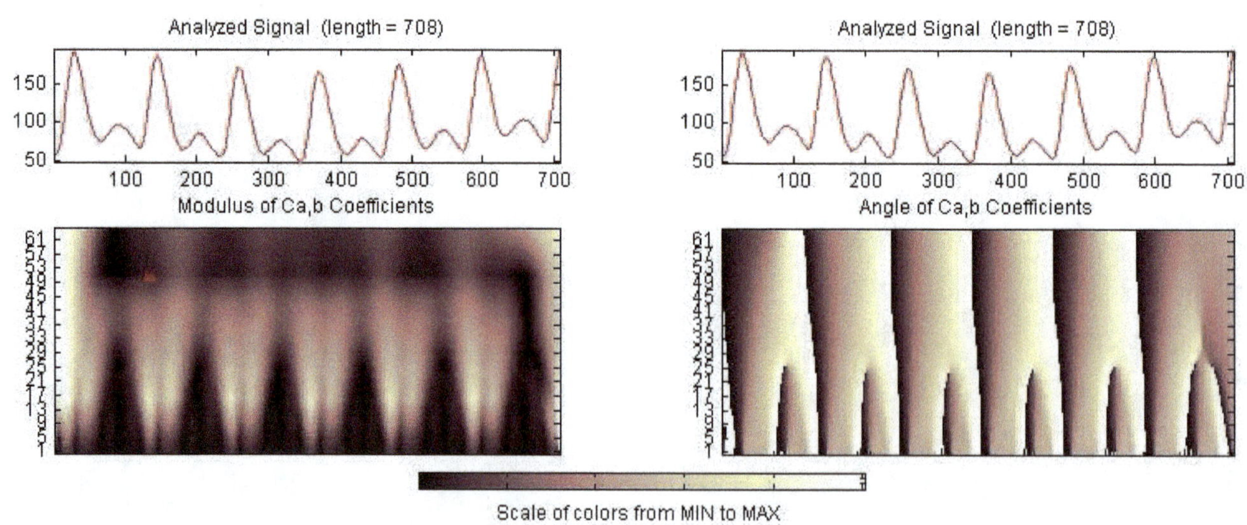

Fig. 10. Wavelet transform for pulse wave with clear diastolic component.

The algorithm can extract information from many kinds of data including audio and images especially in geophysics fields. It has been used to analyze tropical convection (Weng 1994),

the El Niño–Southern Oscillation (Gu 1995), atmospheric cold fronts (Gamage 1993), central England temperature (Baliunas 1997), the dispersion of ocean waves (Meyers 1993), wave growth and breaking (Liu 1994), and coherent structures in turbulent flows (Farge 1992).
Wavelet provides multi-resolution analysis to the source data that make the result more adequate for feature detection.
Fig. 9. and Fig. 10 show the difference between pulse wave with diastolic component and pulse wave without diastolic component. Diastolic component can be easily detected by value variance among adjacent points. It has significant impact on slope changes of continuous values. It also generates additional peak values at Wavelet transform result.

2.2.2 Waveform similarity

Since pulse data is two dimensional time serial data, the mining techniques for time serial data can be applied on it. The waveforms can be categorized based on the similarity between testing waveform and well classified sample waveforms. Because the waveforms have same structure: taller systolic component with lower diastolic component following, the similarity calculation can achieve high accuracy. It can be measured by the total distance of corresponding points between sample waveform and testing waveform warping.

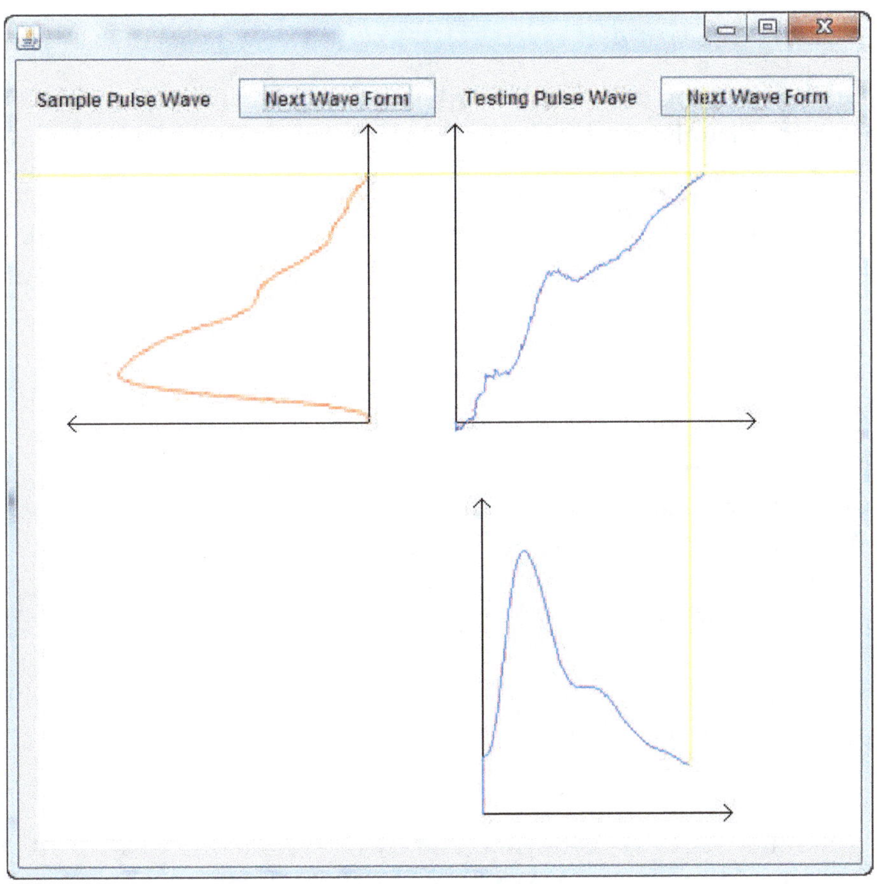

Fig. 11. Demonstration for waveform difference comparison

One of the most fundamental concepts in the nonlinear pattern recognition is that of 'time-warping' a reference to an input pattern so as to register the two patterns in time. The DTW proposed by Sakoe and Chiba (1971) is one of the most versatile algorithms in speech recognition. Figure shows the basic idea about the time warping.

The majority application for DTW was speak recognition in the early research period. (Sakoe 1978) It achieve higher recognition rate with lower cost than most other algorithms. Medical data has been analyzed with DTW recently. ECG is one of the most common signals in health care environment, so most researches focus on ECG signal analysis.

DTW was applied to ECG segmentation first since segmenting the ECG automatically is the foundation for abnormal conduction detection and all analysis tasks. DTW based single lead method achieve smaller mean error with higher standard deviation than two-lead Laguna's method. (Vullings 1998)

DTW

A sample waveform is denoted as $\{x_i(j)\ , I \leq j \leq J\}$, and an unknown frame of the signal as $\{x(i), I \leq i \leq I)$. The purpose of the time warping is to provide a mapping between the time indices i and j such that a time registration between the waveforms is obtained. We denote the mapping by a sequence of points c = (i,j), between i and j as (Sakoe and Chiba 1978)

$$M = \{c(k),\ \ 1 \leq k \leq K\} \tag{6}$$

where c(k) = (i(k), j(k)) and $\{ x(i), 1 \leq i \leq I \}$ is testing data, $\{ x_t(j), 1 \leq j \leq J \}$ is the template data. Warping function finds the minimal distance between two sets of data:

$$d\big(c(k)\big) = d\big(i(k),\ \ j(k)\big) = \big\|x\big(i(k)\big) - x_t\big(j(k)\big)\big\|_2 \tag{7}$$

The smaller the value of d, the higher the similarity between x(i) and $x_t(j)$

The optimal path minimize the accumulated distance D_T

$$D_T = \min_{\{M\}} \sum_{k=1}^{K} d\big(c(k)\big)w(k) \tag{8}$$

Where w(k) is a non-negative weighting coefficient.

To find the optimal path, we use

$$D\big(c(k)\big) = d\big(c(k)\big) + \min\ \ \Big(D\big(c(k-1)\big)\Big) \tag{9}$$

Where $D\big(c(k)\big)$ represents the minimal accumulated distance

There's two restrictions for warping pulse wave

1. Monotonic Condition: $i(k\text{-}1) \leq i(k)$ and $j(k\text{-}1 \leq j(k)$
2. Continuity condition : $i(k) - i(k\text{-}1) \leq 1$ and $j(k) - j(k\text{-}1) \leq 1$

The symmetric DW equation with slope of 1 is

$$\mathrm{D}\big(\mathrm{c(k)}\big) = \mathrm{d}\big(\mathrm{c(k)}\big) + \min\begin{pmatrix} D\big(i(k-1), j(k-2)\big) + \ 2d(i(k), j(k-1)) \\ D\big(i(k-1), j(k-1)\big) + \ 2d(c(k)) \\ D\big(i(k-2), j(k-1)\big) + \ 2d(i(k-1), j(k)) \end{pmatrix} \tag{10}$$

The optimal accumulated distance is normalized by (I+J) for symmetric form.

To implement this algorithm, I designed three classes: TimeSeriesPoint, TimeSeries, and DTW. TimeSeriesPoint can hold an array of double values which means the algorithm can process signals from multiple sensors or leads. The number of signals is defined as the dimensions of the time series data. The get function will return the value for a specific signal based on the input dimension. There are also some utility methods to return the data array, hash the value, or check the equivalence to other TimeSeriesPoint.

TimeSeries is a collection of TimeSeriesPoints. A list of labels and a list of time reading are provided for the time series data to mark the time and special points. Label and time reading can be retrieved for each point by the method getLabel(int n) and getTimeAtNthPoint(int n). The size of the TimeSeries is the number of TimeSeriesPoints stored in the data structure. Method getMeasurement(int pointIndex, int valueIndex) is provided to find the value of specific signal at the given time point.

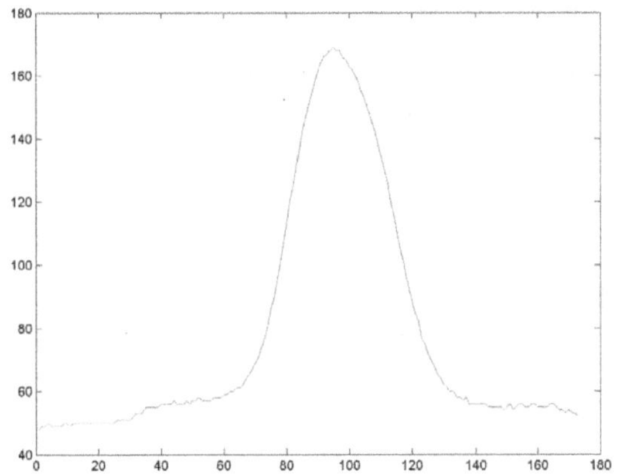

Fig. 12. Pulse wave form from a patient with acute anterior myocardial infarction

The above pulse wave was taken from a male patient at department of cardiology. He had a history of myocardial infarction for 8 years and came to the clinic again for angina pectoris. His cardiac function was rated as NYHA level IV and had to sleep in bed.

The waveform is a typical one with poor cardiac function. The systolic part is very sharp and narrow that suggests very low Cardiac Output. The diastolic component is lost since the weak pulse. Blood vessel condition is not measurable because the cardiac function is in an accurate stage.

The characteristics of this pulse wave can be summarized as following:

- Low pulse pressure
- Low cardiac output
- At least half of the waveform is around the base line
- Sharp and narrow systolic component
- No diastolic component

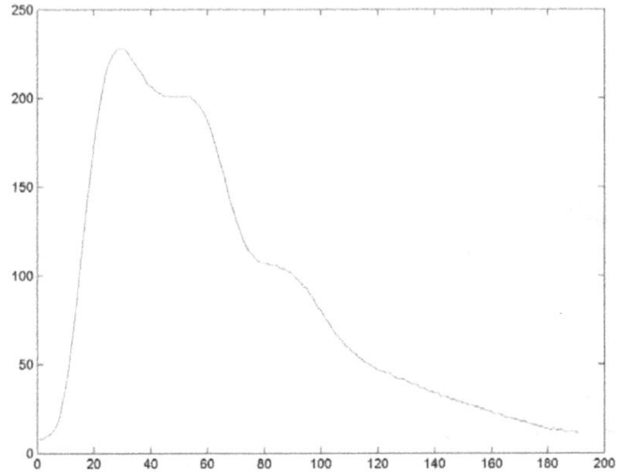

Fig. 1. Pulse wave for patient with Old myocardial infarction and degenerative valvular disease

The above pulse wave is collected from a patient with old myocardial infarction and degenerative valvular disease. He has chest distress and ictal thoracalgia for eighteen years. Gasping happened for the recent 6 months and the pain increased in intensity for the last 3 months. The patient also has mitral regurgitation and tricuspid regurgitation that make him difficult to finish some daily activities. His cardiac function is rated NYHA IV.

The waveform has regular shape with diastolic component. The systolic part becomes broader than usual which might because of the compensatory blood supply after myocardial infarction. The waveform has multiple peak values after systolic top should be the result of old myocardial infarction and degenerative valvular disease.

With review of similar waveforms and medical history, waveforms in this category have

- The waveforms have a broader systolic component
- The diastolic component could have different shape depends on the arteries condition.
- The cardiac output usually has normal values.

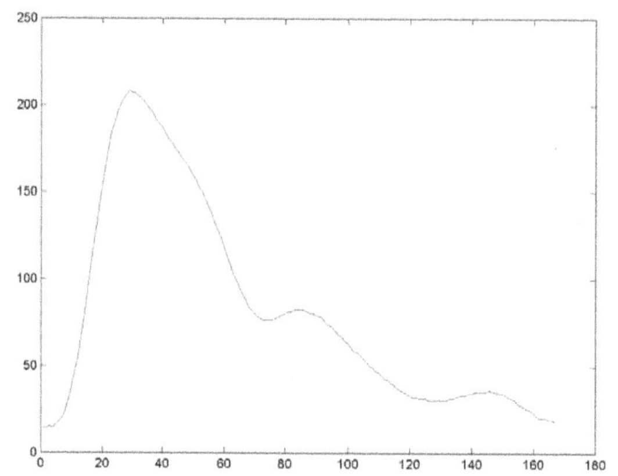

Fig. 2. Pulse wave for a patient with Ventricular aneurysm

This pulse wave belongs to a 57 years old male patient. Coronary angiography shows that arteriostenosis at left anterior descending artery reduce 40% - 50% of the artery's capacity. The first diagonal branch and leftcircumflex also have arteriostenosis. Ventricular aneurysm occupies 30% chambers of the heart.

The systolic part of waveform doesn't have very clear features. The diastolic component goes vertical direction longer than normal waveform. A little uplift could be observed at the end of diastolic component.

There are eight patients with Ventricular aneurysm in the pulse database and 6 of them have pulse wave belong to this category.

- Major significance in diastolic part, give more weight when calculating distance
- Having extra step to check the end of diastolic component will help to identify the waveform

A fifteen years old male patient took the pulse wave test after admission in hospital. He had palpitation for eight years and had oliguresis, edema of lower extremity for recent 3 months. He had fast heart rate which could reach 140/min. The heart border expanded to left and the pulse was weak. Cardiac ultrasonic shows that left ventricle had spherical expansion. The interventricular septum and ventricular wall were thin. The cardiac output and cardiac index decreased.

This class of waveform is characterized by separated systolic component and diastolic component. The pulse pressure decreased to a very low lever before the diastolic component and the diastolic part is relatively bigger.

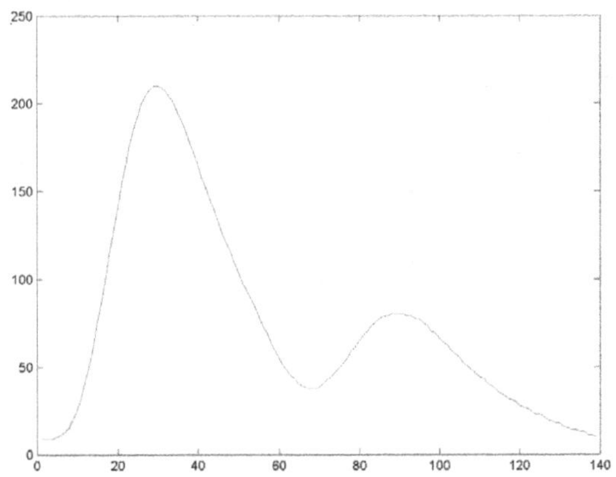

Fig. 3. Pulse wave for Dilated cardiomyopathy

3. Pulse wave monitoring system

Analysis techniques have strength on different areas. Pulse wave factors have good detection rate for cardiovascular risks. Waveform analysis is more suitable for over all evaluation and cardiovascular health classification. The combination of both strategies is the model proposed in this thesis.

The monitoring system is designed to adapt this model. Single test data can provide some hints of subject's health condition. If showing the history data of the subject together, the trend line of the health condition is much more valuable for subject's treatment. Considering the similar pulse data with medical records gives additional support for decision making.

The system includes four modules to handle the data acquisition, transfer and local storage. The four modules are (Figure): Electrocardiogram Sensor, Pulse Oximeter Sensor, Non Invasive Blood Pressure Sensor, a computer or mobile device collecting vital signs and transmitted to Control Center.

Since patients have various risk at different time periods, whole day model will be established during the training period. Usually some measurements are significantly lower at night such as systolic blood pressure, diastolic blood pressure, pulse rate etc. The system will create different criteria for risk detection based on training data. This solution gives continuous improvements at server side for both individual health condition analysis and overall research on pulse wave.

Control Center accepts two types of data: real time monitoring data and offline monitoring data. Real time monitoring aims at detecting serious heart condition in a timely manner. Real time data are bytes (value ranged from 0 – 255) transferred in binary format in order to reduce bandwidth consuming. The standard sampling rate is 200 points per second and can be reduced to 100 or 50 points per second based on the performance of the computer or portable device. Once the connection is initialized, device will send data every second which means up to 200 bytes per channel. The maximum capacity of real time data package contains 3-lead ECG and 1 pulse wave data. A modern server can easily handle more than one hundred connections with high quality service at the same time.

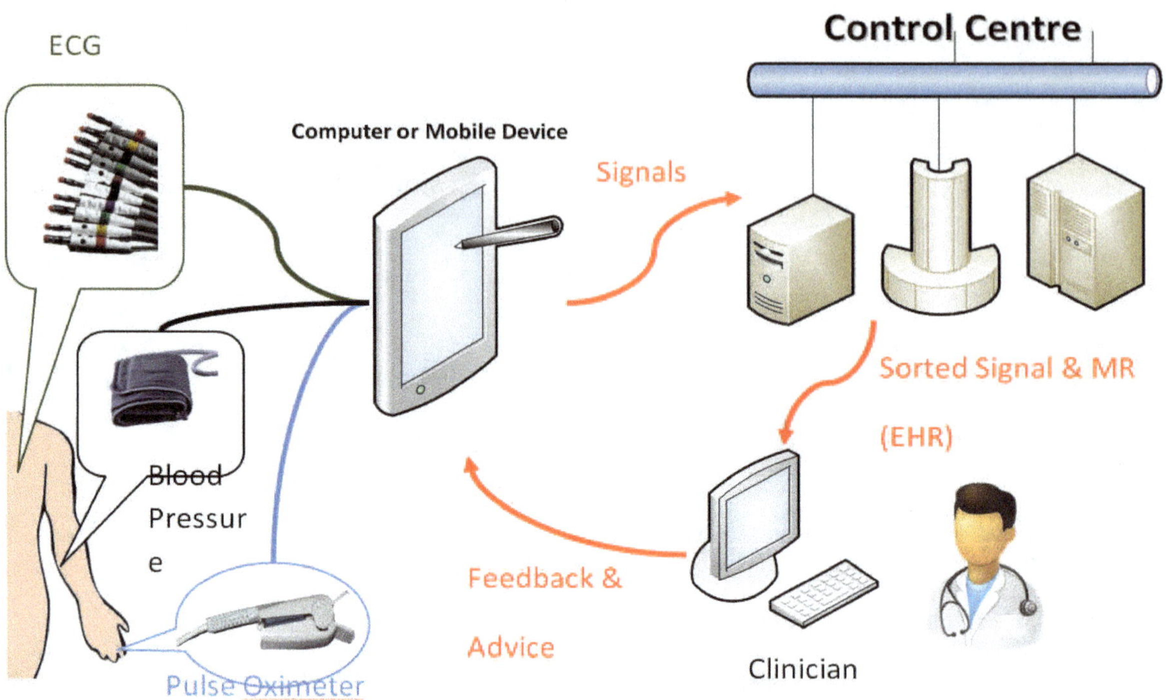

Fig. 4. Remote Monitoring System using pulse oximeter, ECG, and Blood pressure

Control Center has Distributed Structure to improve the Quality of Service. The Gateway is responsible for load balance and server management. It accepts connection requests and forwards them to different servers. Local server will receive high priority for the connections which means servers are likely to serve local users first. Those servers which can work individually, will process the messages in detail. We can easily maintain servers in the system and problem with one server will not affect the system in this way. Servers will select typical and abnormal monitoring data with the statistic logs (monitoring time, maximum, minimum, average of monitoring values, etc) and upload back to data center for future references. Data center has ability to trace the usage of specific user based on the routing records.

The abnormal ECG or Pulse Wave forms will be detected at server side. Actions might be taken after the data is reviewed by medical professionals. Control center will contact the relatives or emergency department in some predefined situations.

Offline data will be generated at client side regarding to the usage. It also includes the typical and abnormal monitoring data with the statistic logs. The system provides a web based application for user to manage monitoring records. Users can easily find out their health condition among specific time period with the help of system assessment. Doctors' advice may add to the system when review is done.

Research verifies that the medical data is more valuable if they can be analyzed together. Data transfer and present layers follows the Electronic Health Record standard. The monitoring network not only backup data, analyze them in different scales, but also provide the pulse data on the cloud to convenience users accessing their pulse records anytime from home, clinic and other places.

4. References

Alan, S.; Ulgen, MS.; Ozturk, O.; Alan, B.; Ozdemir, L. & Toprak, N. (2003). Relation between coronary artery disease, risk factors and intima-media thickness of carotid artery, arterial distensibility, and stiffness index. *Angiology* 2003;54:261-267.

Baliunas, S., P. Frick, D. Sokoloff, and W. Soon, 1997: Time scales and trends in the central England temperature data (1659–1990): A wavelet analysis. *Geophys. Res. Lett.*, 24, 1351–54.

Bates, B. (1995) *A Guide to Physical Examination, 6th edition*, J.B. Lippingcott Company, Philadelphia, USA.

Berton, C. & Cholley, B. (2002). Equipment review: New techniques for cardiac output measurement - oesophageal Doppler, Fick principle using carbon dioxide, and pulse contour analysis. *Critical Care* 2002, 6:216–221

Cain, ME.; Ambos, D.; Witkowski, FX. & Sobel, BE. (1984). Fast-Fourier transform analysis of signal-averaged electrocardiograms for identification of patients prone to sustained ventricular tachycardia, *Circulation* 69 (1984), pp. 711–720.

Cholley, BP.; Shroff, SG.; Sandelski, J.; Korcarz, C.; Balasia, BA.; Jain, S.; Berger, DS.; Murphy, MB.; Marcus, RH. & Lang, RM. (1995). Differential effects of chronic oral antihypertensive therapies on systemic arterial circulation and ventricular energetics in African-American patients. *Circulation*. 1995;91:1052–1062.

Cohn, JN.; Finkelstein, SM.; McVeigh, GE. et al. Noninvasive pulse wave analysis for the early detection of vascular disease. *Hypertension* 1995;26:503–8.

Dar, O.; Riley, J.; Chapman, C.; Dubrey, SW.; Morris, S.; Rosen, SD.; Roughton, M. & Cowie, MR. (2009). A randomized trial of home telemonitoring in a typical elderly heart failure population in North West London: results of the Home-HF study. *Eur J Heart Fail*. 2009 Mar;11(3):319–325

Eguchi, K.; Kuruvilla, S.; Ogedegbe, G.; Gerin, W.; Schwartz, JE. & Pickering, TG. (2009). What is the optimal interval between successive home blood pressure readings using an automated oscillometric device? *Journal of Hypertension*, 27, 1172-1177.

Erlanger, J. & Hooker, D. R. (1904). *Johns Hopk. Hosp. Rep.* 12, 357.

Farge, M., 1992: Wavelet transforms and their applications to turbulence. *Annu. Rev. Fluid Mech.*, 24, 395–457.

Felbinger, TW.; Reuter, DA.; Eltzschig, HK.; Bayerlein, J. & Goetz, AE. (2005). Cardiac index measurements during rapid preload changes: a comparison of pulmonary artery thermodilution with arterial pulse contour analysis. *J Clin Anesth* 2005;17:241-8

Gamage, N., and W. Blumen, 1993: Comparative analysis of lowlevel cold fronts: Wavelet, Fourier, and empirical orthogonal function decompositions. *Mon. Wea. Rev.*, 121, 2867–2878.

Green, JF. (1984) Mechanical Concepts in Cardiovascular and Pulmonary Physiology. *Lea & Febiger*, Philadelphia, Pennsylvania, USA.

Gu, D., and S. G. H. Philander, 1995: Secular changes of annual and interannual variability in the Tropics during the past century. *J. Climate*, 8, 864–876.

Hast, J. (2003) "Self-mixing interferometry and its applications in non invasive pulse detection," Ph.D. dissertation, Department of Electrical and Information Engineering, University of Oulu, Finland, 2003.

Huang, B. & Kinsmer, W. (2002) "ECG frame classification using Dynamic Time Warping," Proc. IEEE Canadian Conference on Electrical & Computer Engineering, 2002.

Kangasniemi, K. & Opas, H. (1997). Suomalainen lääkärikeskus 1. Toinen painos. WSOY, Porvoo (In Finnish).

Langewouters, G J.; Wesseling, KH. & Goedhard, W J A (1984) The static elastic properties of 45 human thoracic and 20 abdominal aortas in vitro and the parameters of a new model. *Journal of Biomechanics* 17: 425–435.

Liu, P. C., 1994: Wavelet spectrum analysis and ocean windwaves. Wavelets in Geophysics, E. Foufoula-Georgiou and P. Kumar, Eds., *Academic Press*, 151–166.

Mahomed, F. A. (1872). The physiological and clinical use of the sphygmograph. *Medical Times Gazette* 1, 62—64.

Mahomed, F. A. (1874). The aetiology of bright's disease and the prealbuminuric stage. *Med Chir Trans* 57:197-228

Mahomed, F. A. (1877). On the sphygmographic evidence of arterio-capillary fibrosis. *Trans Path Soc* 28:394-397

Meyers, S. D., B. G. Kelly, and J. J. O'Brien, 1993: An introduction to wavelet analysis in oceanography and meteorology: With application to the dispersion of Yanai waves. *Mon. Wea. Rev.*, 121, 2858–2866.

O'Rourke, MF & Mancia, G. (1999) Arterial stiffness. *J Hypertens*. 1999;17:1–4.

O'Rourke, M.; Pauca, A. & Jiang, X-J. (2001) Pulse wave analysis. *Br J Clin Pharmacol*. 2001; 51: 507–522.

Persell, SD.; Dunne, AP.; Lloyd-Jones, DM. & Baker, DW. (2009) Electronic health record-based cardiac risk assessment and identification of unmet preventive needs. *Med Care* 47:418–424, 2009

Postel-Vinay, MC. (1996) Growth hormone- and prolactin-binding proteins: soluble forms of receptors. *Horm Res* 45:178–181

Rödig, G.; Prasser, C.; Keyl, C.; Liebold, A. & Hobbhahn, J. (1999). Continuous cardiac output measurement: pulse contour analysis vs thermodilution technique in cardiac surgical patients. *Br J Anaesth* 1999; 82: 525–30

Sakoe, H. & Chiba, S. (1978). Dynamic Programming Optimization for Spoken Word Recongition, *IEEE Transactions on Signal Processing*, Vol. 26, pp 43- 49.

Spencker, S.; Coban, N.; Koch, L.; Schirdewan, A. & Muller, D. (2009). Potential role of home monitoring to reduce inappropriate shocks in implantable cardioverter-defibrillator patients due to lead failure. *Europace* 2009;11:483-8.

Timothy, SM.; Barbara, ES; Joseph, L. & Izzo, Jr (2002) Validity and Reliability of Diastolic Pulse Contour Analysis (Windkessel Model) in Humans. *Hypertension* 2002; 39:963-8

Vullings, H.; Verhaegen, M. & Verbruggen, H. (1998) "Automated ECG segmentation with dynamic time warping," in Proc. 20th Ann. Int. Conf. IEEE Engineering in Medicine and Biology Soc., Hong Kong, 1998, pp. 163–166.

Weng, H., and K.-M. Lau, 1994: Wavelets, period doubling, and time-frequency localization with application to organization of convection over the tropical western Pacific. *J. Atmos. Sci.*, 51, 2523–2541.

Zhang, G.; Kong, X. & Liao, S. (2008). "Pulse wave analysis for cardiovascular information monitoring in patients with chronic heart failure: effects of COQ10 treatment" Montreal: Bio-engineering 2008

13

Fine Biomedical Imaging Using X-Ray Phase-Sensitive Technique

Akio Yoneyama[1], Shigehito Yamada[2] and Tohoru Takeda[3]
[1]*Advanced Research Laboratory, Hitachi Ltd.*
[2]*Congenital Anomaly Research Center, Kyoto University*
[3]*Allied Health Sciences, Kitasato University*
Japan

1. Introduction

X-ray imaging is widely used for non-destructive observations of the inner structures of samples in many fields, such as biological, clinical, and industrial ones. The transparency of X-rays is much higher than that of visible light, and therefore the spatial distribution of X-ray intensity passing through a sample (radiography) can visualize the mass-density distribution inside the sample. However, X-ray intensity barely changes when passing through samples consisting of a light element, such as carbon, oxygen, or nitrogen, because of the extremely high transmittance of X-rays. Therefore, the sensitivity of absorption-contrast X-ray imaging is not sufficient for carrying out fine observations of samples such as biological soft tissues and organic materials. Contrast agents, including heavy elements such as iodine, and long exposure to X-rays are ordinarily used to improve sensitivity. However, these supplementary methods may cause allergic reactions and expose subjects to extremely high X-ray dosages.

A fundamental solution to this problem is use of the phase information of X-rays. X-rays are electromagnetic waves having very short wavelength and are mainly characterized by their amplitude and phase. When they pass through samples, their amplitude is decreased and the phase is shifted. In the hard X-ray region, the cross-section of phase shift for light elements is about 1000 times larger than that of absorption (Momose & Fukuda, 1995). Therefore, phase-contrast X-ray imaging, which uses phase shift caused by the sample as image contrast, provides a way of conducting fine observations of biomedical samples without the need for contrast agents or excessive X-ray dosages.

For phase-shift detection, it is essential to convert the phase shift into the change in X-ray intensity because we can only detect the intensity of X-rays by using current-detecting devices. Many conversion methods, such as interferometry with an X-ray crystal interferometer (Momose & Fukuda, 1995; Momose, 1995; Takeda et al., 1995), diffractometry with a perfect analyzer crystal (Davis et al., 1995; Ignal and Beliaevskaya, 1995; Chapman et al., 1997), a propagation-based method with a Fresnel pattern (Snigirev et al., 1995; Wilkins et al., 1996), and Talbot interferometry with a Talbot grating interferometer (Momose et al., 2003; Weitkamp et al., 2005), have been developed recently. The principle difference between these methods is in the detection of physical values; that is, interferometry detects the phase shift directly, while the other methods detect the first or second spatial derivation of the phase shift.

Therefore, interferometry has the highest sensitivity and is suitable for radiographic and three-dimensional (3D) observation of samples requiring high density resolution, such as biomedical soft tissues. On the other hand, the other methods have a large dynamic range of density and are suitable for observation of samples including regions with large differences in density, such as bone and soft tissues (Yoneyama et al., 2008).

Among these methods, interferometry and diffractometry are two major techniques for biomedical imaging, and 2D and 3D observations of various biomedical samples have been performed using synchrotron radiation. Note that Talbot interferometry using a conventional X-ray source has been studied actively for clinical use recently (Momose, 2009; Donath et al., 2010), because it has the advantage of cone-beam and/or polychromatic X-rays being useable.

Early X-ray interferometric imaging (XII) was achieved by using a monolithic crystal X-ray interferometer having three wafers cut from one silicon ingot (Bonse & Hart, 1965). Radiographic observations of rat cerebella (Momose & Fukuda, 1995), metastatic liver tumors in humans (Takeda et al., 1995), and cancerous breast tissues (Takeda et al., 2004) were conducted. The high sensitivity of XII enables differences in biological soft tissues such as cancers and normal tissues to be visualized. Phase-contrast X-ray computed tomography was also achieved in combination with general computed tomography (Momose et al., 1995). Non-destructive 3D observations of small columnar samples of various biological soft tissues were made (Momose et al., 1996; Takeda et al., 2000). To broaden the scope of interferometry to biomedical applications such as *in vivo* observations, imaging systems fitted with a two-crystal X-ray interferometer (Becker & Bonse, 1974) have been developed (Yoneyama et al., 1999, 2002, 2004a). The latest version of the system has a 60 × 40-mm field of view at an X-ray energy of 17.8 keV (Yoneyama et al., 2004a), and it enables 3D observations with a density resolution of less than 1 mg/mm^3. By using this system, *in vivo* radiographic observation of blood flow in a rat liver (Takeda et al., 2004a), *in vivo* 3D observation of a tumor implanted in nude mice (Takeda et al., 2004b; Yoneyama et al., 2006), and quantitative analysis of β-amyloid plaques in brains extracted from Alzheimer's disease model mice (Noda-Saita et al., 2006) were successfully performed.

Diffractometry was expanded and termed diffraction-enhanced imaging (DEI) for fine biomedical observations (Chapman et al., 1997). With this method, observations of breast cancer tissues (Pisano et al., 2000), articular cartilage (Mollenhauer et al., 2002; Ando et al., 2004), and amyloid plaques in the brain of a mouse model of Alzheimer's disease (Connor et al., 2009) were performed. The results showed that DEI had a higher sensitivity than that of conventional radiography and computed tomography. In addition, many developments in DEI (recently known by the more generic name of analyzer-based imaging (ABI)) have also been actively studied, and three images of a sample depicting refraction, ultra-small-angle scatter, and absorption have been obtained recently (Oltulu et al., 2003; Wernick et al., 2003; Rigon et al., 2007). To shorten the measurement time and lower the X-ray dose, a new derivative method using two diffraction beams (forward and normal) was also developed, and a fine tomographic image of breast cancer was obtained (Sunaguchi et al., 2010). In addition, high-energy DEI was developed to extend the dynamic range of density, and an obtained image of an electrical cable showed clearly not only the core and ground wire made of copper but also the isolator and outer jacket made of polymer (Yoneyama et al., 2009).

In this chapter, we will describe the principle of phase-contrast X-ray imaging, two major methods for detecting X-ray phase-shift (XII and DEI), imaging systems for XII and DEI, and examples of fine 2D and 3D images of pathological soft tissues and mice embryos.

2. Principle, methods, and imaging system

2.1 Principle of phase-contrast imaging

When X-rays pass through a sample, their amplitude is decreased by absorption and their phase is shifted as shown in Fig. 1 (a). In the hard X-ray region, the refractive index n of the sample is written as

$$n = 1 - \delta - i\beta \tag{1}$$

$$\delta = \frac{\lambda^2 r_e}{2\pi} \sum_i N_i (Z_i + f'_i) \tag{2}$$

$$\beta = \frac{\lambda^2 r_e}{2\pi} \sum_i N_i f''_i, \tag{3}$$

where r_e is the classical electron radius, λ is the wavelength of the X-ray, N_i is the atomic density of element i, Z_i is the atomic number of element i, and f'_i and f''_i are the real and imaginary parts respectively of the anomalous scattering factor of element i. By using these constituents of the refractive index, the X-ray intensity change $\ln(I/I_o)$, caused by amplitude decrease in a uniform-density sample, is given by

$$\ln\left(\frac{I}{Io}\right) = -\frac{4\pi\beta t}{\lambda} \tag{4}$$

and the phase-shift $d\theta$ is given by

$$d\theta = \frac{2\pi\delta t}{\lambda}, \tag{5}$$

where t is the thickness of the sample. Conventional absorption-contrast X-ray imaging uses $\ln(I/I_o)$ as image contrast while phase-contrast X-ray imaging uses $d\theta$. Therefore, the sensitivity ratio between absorption- and phase-contrast imaging is given by the ratio of β to δ. The calculated sensitivity ratios (δ/β) to atomic number for various X-ray energies are plotted in Fig. 1(b). The results show that the ratio of light elements, such as hydrogen, oxygen, nitrogen, and carbon, runs to about 1000 times. Thus, the sensitivity of phase-contrast X-ray

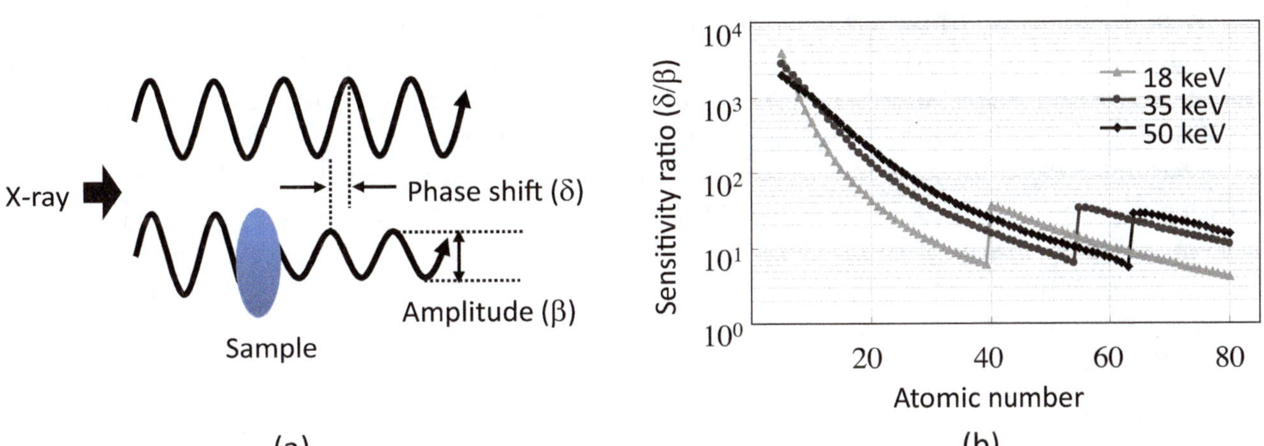

Fig. 1. (a) Interaction between X-ray and sample. When X-ray passes through sample, its amplitude is decreased and phase is shifted. (b) Sensitivity ratios between phase- and absorption-contrast imaging. Ratios increase to about 1000 for light elements.

imaging for light elements is about 1000 times higher than that of absorption-contrast X-ray imaging in principle. The high sensitivity of phase-contrast X-ray imaging provides many advantages for biomedical observations. First, fine observations of samples consisting of light elements, such as biological soft tissues and organic materials, can be performed in a short measurement time. Second, the usage of contrast agents is not required, and therefore the density distribution in a sample can be measured independently without considering reactions to contrast agents. Third, δ is almost proportional to the electron density of samples and the square of X-ray energy while β changes abruptly near the energy of the absorption edges; density distribution in a sample can be measured without considering the influence of the difference of the X-ray energy.

Conventional X-ray computed tomography (CT) uses intensity change $\ln(I/I_o)$ in samples as input data for reconstruction calculations. When X-rays pass through samples having different density and element regions, $\ln(I/I_o)$ is written as

$$\ln\left(\frac{I}{Io}\right) = \frac{4\pi}{\lambda}\int \beta\, dz, \tag{6}$$

where the integration is carried out along the direction of the X-rays. On the other hand, phase-shift $d\theta$ caused by the sample is written as

$$d\theta = \frac{2\pi}{\lambda}\int \delta dz. \tag{7}$$

The difference between the two equations above is only in δ and β, which are the same as in the radiographic observations. Therefore, CT using phase-shift information can be carried out using the same algorithm of reconstruction as conventional X-ray CT. The sensitivity of phase-contrast CT is about 1000 times higher than that of conventional CT for the same reason as previously mentioned for radiographic observation. In addition, $d\theta$ is proportional to the sample electron density; the obtained tomograms then provide the electron density distribution of the sample.

2.2 Phase-detection methods

2.2.1 Interferometric method

A schematic view of a monolithic triple Laue-case X-ray interferometer (Bonse & Hart, 1965) used in early X-ray interferometric imaging is shown in Fig. 2(a). This interferometer is made of silicon crystal and is monolithically cut from one silicon ingot to have three thin crystal wafers. The incident X-ray is divided into two beams (object and reference beams) at the first wafer (S), and these beams are reflected at the second wafer (M) by Laue-case X-ray diffraction. The reflected beams are then superposed at the third wafer (A), and they generate two interference beams by similar X-ray diffraction. Thus, this interferometer acts as a Mach-Zehnder interferometer in the visible light region. The intensity of the interference beams, I_i, is given by

$$I_i = I_o + I_r + 2\sqrt{I_0 I_r}\,v\cos(d\theta), \tag{8}$$

where I_o is the intensity of the object beam, I_r is that of the reference beam, v is the absolute value of the complex degree of coherence, and $d\theta$ is the phase shift caused by the sample placed in the path of the object beam. Therefore, $d\theta$ can be detected by measuring the interference intensity changes.

To obtain a quantitative phase map showing the spatial distribution of $d\theta$, a sub-fringe method, such as Fourier transfer (FT) (Takeda et al., 1982) and fringe scanning (FS) (Bruning et al., 1974), is required. The former method is traditionally used in *in vivo* observations as it is used to detect phase shifts from only one interference pattern. The latter method, which requires multiple interference images to calculate phase shift, has a wide dynamic range of density and high spatial resolution compared to that of FT. Therefore, this method is normally used for fine observations of static samples such as formalin-fixed biomedical soft tissues.

To broaden the scope of X-ray interferometric imaging in biomedical applications such as *in vivo* observations, a large-area field of view and suppression of the thermal disturbance caused by a sample's heat are indispensable. However, the monolithic X-ray interferometer cannot cope with these requirements because the field of view is limited by the size of the silicon ingot from which the interferometer was cut, and the sample cannot be set apart from the optical components of the interferometer due to the geometrical limitations. To overcome these limitations, a two-crystal X-ray interferometer consisting of two silicon-crystal blocks each having two crystal wafers has been developed (Fig. 2 (b)) (Becker & Bonse, 1974). By dividing the crystal block of the interferometer into two blocks, the field of view can be extended by four times or more. In addition, the distance between the crystal blocks and the sample can be kept long; the thermal influence, such as deformation of the crystal wafers caused by the sample's heat, is negligible and can be applied for the observation of living samples. On the other hand, a relative rotation between the blocks changes the X-ray phase very sensitively, and therefore rotational stabilization of the subnano-radian order is necessary for performing fine observations.

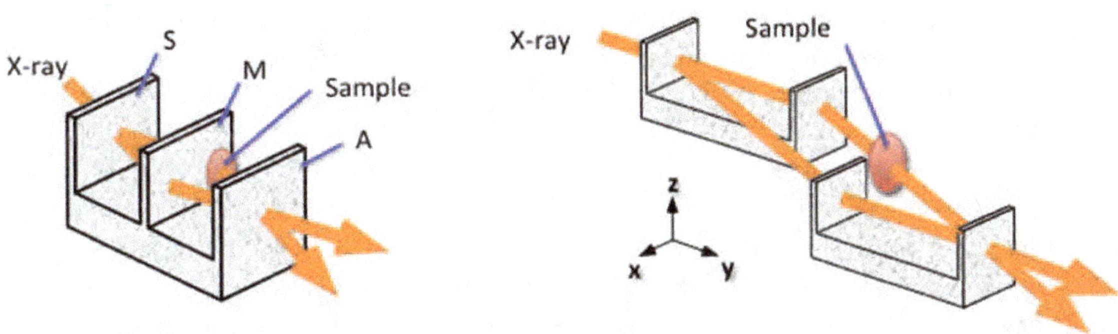

Fig. 2. (a) Monolithic triple Laue-case X-ray interferometer and (b) skew-symmetric two-crystal X-ray interferometer.

2.2.2 Diffraction-enhanced method

When X-rays pass through a sample, their optical paths (propagation direction) diverge slightly due to refraction by the sample as shown in Fig. 3(a). This refraction angle, *ds*, is given by

$$ds = \frac{\lambda}{2\pi}\frac{d\theta}{dx}, \quad (9)$$

where $d\theta/dx$ is the spatial differential of the phase shift. Therefore, phase shift $d\theta$ can be obtained by calculating the integral of *ds*. The *ds* can be detected using the X-ray diffraction of the perfect crystal placed downstream of the sample for analyzing. The intensity of the diffracted X-ray changes depending on the incidence angle to the crystal around the Bragg angle, θ_B, as shown in Fig. 3(b). This curve is called a rocking curve, and its full width at half maximum (FWHM) is a few arc seconds for a perfect silicon crystal. In addition, the slopes near the angles θ_L or θ_H, where the diffracted intensity is half the maximum, are very steep. Therefore, the intensity of the diffracted X-ray can be made almost proportional to *ds* by adjusting the analyzer crystal to θ_L or θ_H. Namely, the crystal functions as an angular analyzer of the *ds*, and the *ds* can be very sensitively detected as changes in the intensity of the diffracted X-ray.

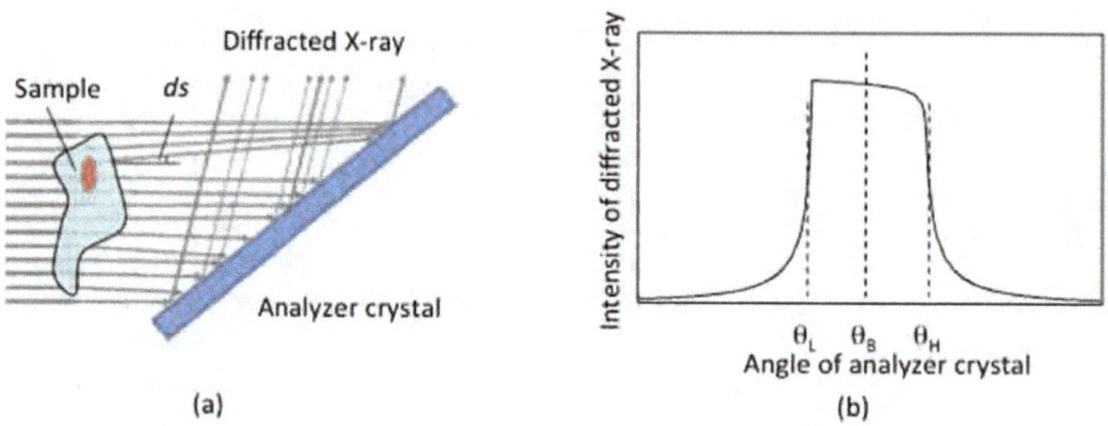

Fig. 3. (a) Diffraction-enhanced method and (b) diffracted X-ray intensity (rocking curve) obtained by rotating analyzer crystal (calculation).

To obtain a correct phase map without the effect of the X-ray absorption by the sample, measurement methods using multiple diffraction images taken at different crystal angles are required. One measurement method is diffraction-enhanced imaging using two (i.e., "T") images (DEIT) (Chapman et al., 1997). The *ds* is calculated as

$$\mathrm{ds(x,z)} = \frac{I_H(x,z,)R(\theta_H) - I_L(x,z,)R(\theta_L)}{I_H(x,z,)\left(\frac{dR}{d\theta}\right)(\theta_H) + I_L(x,z,)\left(\frac{dR}{d\theta}\right)(\theta_L)}, \tag{10}$$

where $R(\theta)$ is the reflectivity of the analyzer crystal and I is the intensity of the diffracted X-ray. Only two images are needed, so this method is suitable for quick measurements such as *in vivo* observations. However, if the *ds* is larger than the FWHM of the rocking curve, the intensity of the diffracted X-ray shows an incorrect value because the angular point on the rocking curve is far from the peak, where the *ds* is not proportional to the diffracted intensity. Therefore, the dynamic range of density of DEIT is not as wide as that of the method obtained by scanning the analyzer crystal throughout the rocking curve, i.e., diffraction-enhanced imaging using many (i.e., "M") images (DEIM) (Koyama et al., 2004). The *ds* in DEIM is calculated as

$$\mathrm{ds(x,z)} = \frac{\sum_{k=1}^{n} \theta_k I_k(x,z)}{\sum_{k=1}^{n} I_k(x,z)}, \tag{11}$$

where θ_k is the angle of the analyzer crystal and I_k is the intensity of the diffracted X-ray at θ_k. The scanning angular range depends on the spatial density changes in the sample. For samples with large spatial density changes, a large range is required to obtain correct images. A long measurement time is required to obtain the images, but the dynamic range is not limited by the angular width of the total reflection of the analyzer crystal.

2.3 Imaging system

2.3.1 Crystal X-ray interferometric imaging (XII) system

A schematic view of an XII system (Yoneyama et al., 2004a; Yoneyama et al., 2005) fitted with a skew-symmetric two-crystal X-ray interferometer (STXI) is shown in Fig. 4. The system consists of an asymmetric crystal, an STXI, positioning tables for the STXI, a sample positioner, and a phase shifter. The imaging system has been set up at beamline BL-14C2 (at the Photon Factory in Tsukuba, Japan) to use the X-ray synchrotron radiation emitted from a vertical wiggler. The X-ray is monochromatized by a Si (220) double-crystal monochromator (not shown), enlarged horizontally by the Si (220) asymmetric crystal, and irradiated onto the first block of the STXI. One interference image generated by the STXI is taken with the charge-coupled device (CCD)-based low-noise X-ray imager for detecting the phase map of the sample. The other image is used in the feedback system stabilizing the X-ray phase fluctuation. The main specifications of the imaging system are shown in Table 1.

To attain subnano-radian mechanical stability of the STXI for fine observation, the positioning tables of the STXI are simplified as much as possible, made robust against vibration, and driven by laminated piezoelectric translator (PZT) actuators. In addition, the drift rotation is suppressed by the feedback system, which controls the PZT's expansion so as to cancel the movement of the X-ray interference pattern caused by the drift rotation between the crystal blocks of the STXI (Yoneyama et al., 2004b). Due to these features, mechanical stability (standard deviation) within 0.04 nrad was achieved, enabling fine observations of biomedical samples to be obtained.

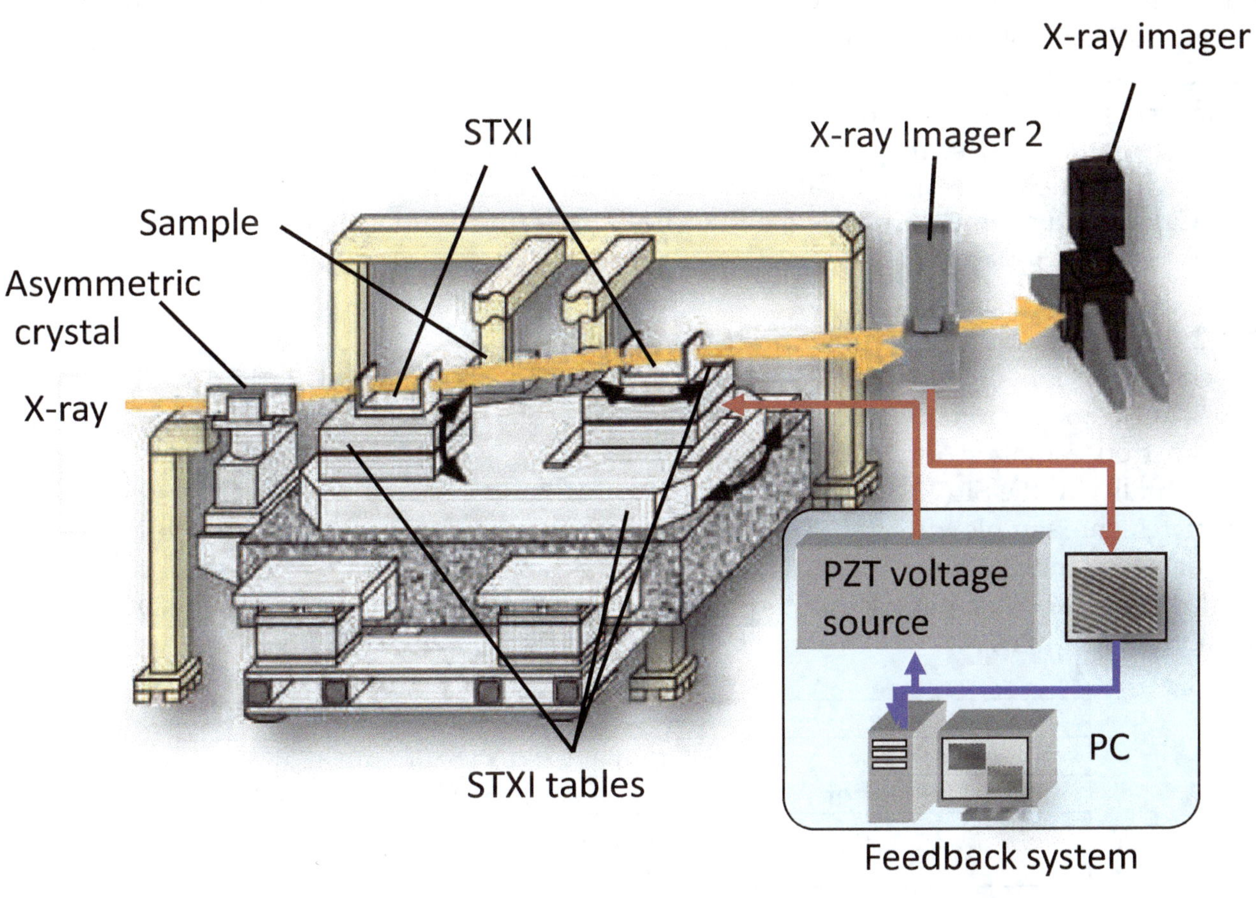

Fig. 4. Schematic view of XII system using two-crystal X-ray interferometer.

X-ray energy	17–52 keV
Field of view	60×30 mm at 17 keV; 25×30 mm at 35 keV
Spatial resolution	Approx. 50 μm
Density resolution	Approx. 1 mg/cm3 for 3D measurement for 2 hours

Table 1. Main specifications of XII system.

The X-ray imager consists of a scintillator that converts X-rays into visible light, a relay-lens system that transfers the light from the scintillator to a camera, and a full-frame-type CCD camera (Momose et al., 2001). The field of view of this imager is 36 × 36 mm, composed of 2048 × 2048 pixels of 18-μm square, and the image-transfer period is about 3 s for a full image. Gd_2O_2S (GOS) was used to fabricate the scintillator. The GOS thickness is 30 μm, and its absorption ratio is 78 and 20% for 17.8- and 35-keV X-rays, respectively. The CCD camera is cooled with water instead of an air fan to avoid any mechanical vibration.

A sample is placed in the object beam path using a sample positioner composed of vertical and horizontal linear tables and a rotational table with the horizontal axis. Each table is driven by stepping motors operated by remote control. A plastic wedge used as a phase-shifter is also positioned by another positioner with the same structure as the sample positioner. Each positioner is attached to rails installed on the frame and can move perpendicular to the interfering beam so that it can be roughly adjusted and the samples can be exchanged. The frame stands independently of the STXI table so as to prevent vibration caused by the motion of the positioner from disturbing the interference.

Interference images for the FS method are taken by scanning the wedge vertically at even intervals. For 3D observation, the sample is rotated perpendicularly to the beam path for 180 degrees by using the rotational table of the sample positioner. The phase-contrast tomograms are obtained as follows.

1. Calculate the phase map from the obtained interference images by the FS method.
2. Unwrap the phase map and then generate a sinogram from it.
3. Calculate the tomograms using a filter-back projection with a Shepp-Logan filter (Shepp & Logan, 1974).

2.3.2 Diffraction-enhanced imaging (DEI) system

A schematic view of a DEI system (Yoneyama et al., 2008) is shown in Fig. 5. The system consists of an asymmetric crystal, an analyzer crystal, and an X-ray imager. The X-ray synchrotron radiation emitted from the storage ring is monochromatized and enlarged horizontally by the Si (220) symmetric crystal in the same way as in the XII system, and it irradiates the sample directly. The X-ray beam that has passed through the sample is diffracted by the Si (220) analyzer crystal placed downstream of the sample and is detected by the same X-ray imager used in the XII system. The main specifications of the DEI system are shown in Table 2.

X-ray energy	17–70 keV
Field of view	60×30 mm at 17 keV; 8×30 mm at 70 keV
Spatial resolution	Approx. 50 μm
Density resolution	More than a few mg/cm3 for 3D measurement for 2 hours

Table 2. Main specifications of DEI system.

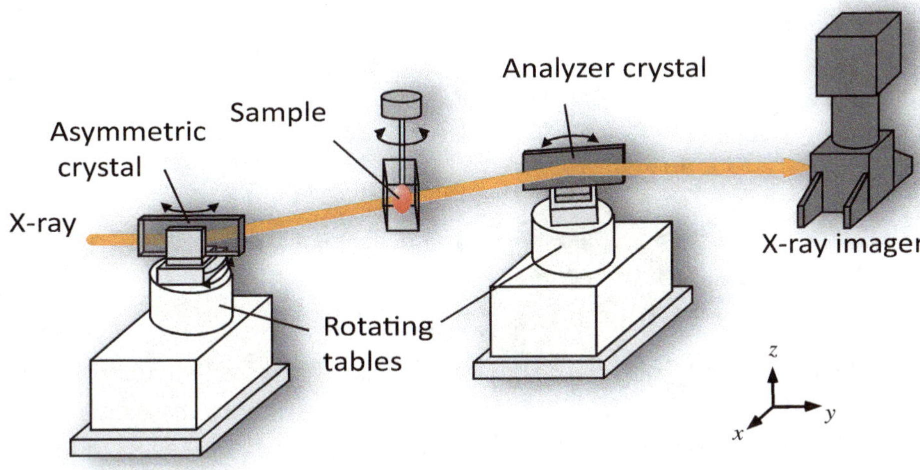

Fig. 5. Schematic view of DEI system using Si (220) diffraction.

The asymmetric and analyzer crystals are mounted on a precise rotational mechanism consisting of a vertical rotational table and a tilt table. Each table is driven by a stepping motor remotely, and the rotational resolutions are 0.05 and 8 µrad for horizontal and tilt rotation, respectively. By using these precise tables, the drift rotation of the analyzer crystal can be made negligible. The sample is positioned by a sample positioner composed of vertical linear tables and a rotational table with the vertical axis. For 3D observation, the sample is rotated vertically for 180 degrees by using the rotational table. The tomograms are obtained as follows.

1. Calculate the *ds* map from obtained diffracted X-ray images by using equation (10) or (11).
2. Calculate the phase map by using

$$d\theta = \frac{2\pi}{\lambda} \int ds(x,z)\, dx.$$

3. Generate a sinogram from the phase map.
4. Calculate the tomograms using a filter-back projection with a Shepp-Logan filter.

2.4 Comparison of imaging performance

Figure 6 shows the phase maps of a formalin-fixed rat liver obtained using (a) XII, (b) DEIT, (c) DEIM, and (d) conventional radiography (absorption contrast). Each image was 24-mm wide and 25-mm high. The X-ray energy was set to 17.8 keV, and the total X-ray dose for obtaining the images was adjusted to remain at the same level by changing the exposure time. The sample was put in a sample cell filled with formalin to prevent rapid phase shifts caused by a large density difference between the sample and its surrounding environment. The fringe number for FS in XII was set at 3, and 11 diffraction images were used for DEIM. Large blood vessels with a diameter of ~1 mm can be clearly seen in phase maps (a) to (c), but not in (d), because the phase shift of saline solution injected in blood vessels is different from that of the surrounding liver tissues (Takeda et al., 2002). Blood vessels with a diameter of less than 100 µm can be seen in (a), but not in (b) and (c). In addition, phase maps (b) and (c) include many horizontal noise lines caused by the integral calculation of *ds* along the x-axis (horizontal direction in the figures). As shown here, the radiographic image quality of XII is better than that of DEIM and DEIT because DEI has no sensitivity in the vertical direction.

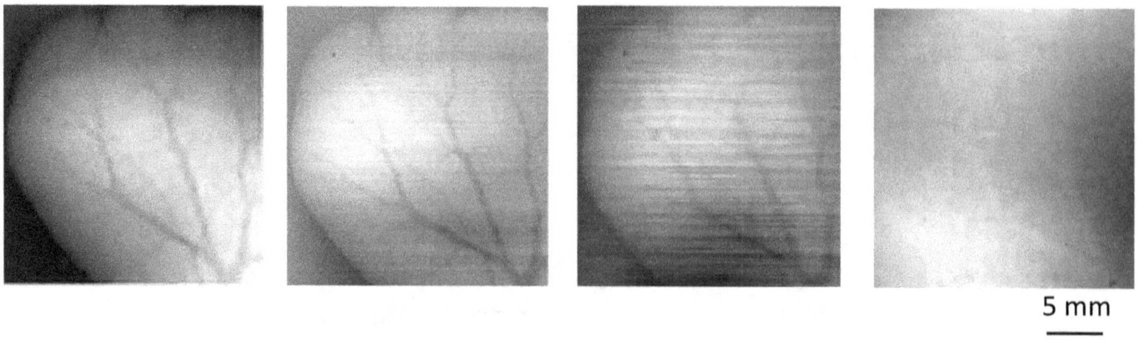

(a) (b) (c) (d)

Fig. 6. Phase maps of rat liver obtained using (a) XII, (b) DEIT, (c) DEIM, and (d) conventional radiography. Large blood vessels with a diameter of ~1 mm can be clearly seen in every phase map, but blood vessels with a diameter of less than 100 μm can only be seen in (a).

Figure 7 shows 3D images and tomograms of a formalin-fixed rat kidney obtained using (a) XII, (b) DEIT, and (c) DEIM. The X-ray energy was set at 35 keV, and the X-ray dose was adjusted to remain at the same level in the same way as in radiographic imaging. The sample was rotated in the sample cell filled with formalin to decrease artifacts caused by a large density difference between the sample and its surrounding environment. The image quality of (a) is better than that of (b) and (c); soft tissues such as blood vessels, medullas, and cortexes are clearly visible in (a), while the details of tissues cannot be distinguished in (b) and (c).

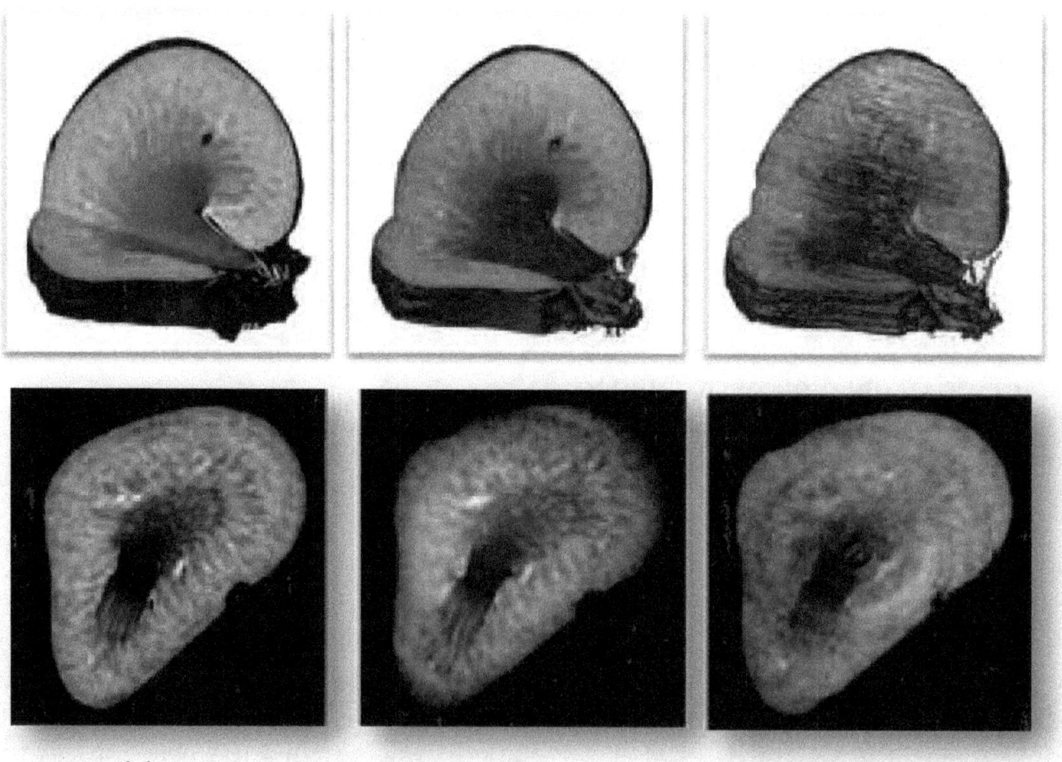

(a) (b) (c)

Fig. 7. 3D images and tomograms of rat kidney obtained using (a) XII, (b) DEIT, and (c) DEIM, with 35-keV X-ray beam. Soft tissues such as blood vessels, medullas, and cortexes are clearly visible in (a), while only cortexes can be distinguished in (b) and (c).

The density resolutions of XII, DEIT, and DEIM for X-ray intensities at the sample position are shown in Fig. 8. The density resolutions were calculated from the standard deviation of the relative refractive index in the background regions in each obtained tomogram. The X-ray energy was set at 35 keV, and typical total exposure times to obtain one data set for one projection were 1.5, 3, 7.5, 15, and 30 s. To conduct the comparison correctly, the same phantom consisting of polyethylene tubes filled with saline solution was used with each imaging system. As expected from the observations of the kidney, this result shows that the sensitivity of XII was the highest among these methods. In addition, the sensitivity of DEIM is about one fifth that of DEIT because all the images (including those obtained at the angles far from the Bragg condition) were used to calculate the *ds* for a wider dynamic range of density. Note that images obtained by DEIT and DEIM include many horizontal noise lines as shown in Fig. 6, and therefore it is thought that the relative difference of the density resolution between XII and DEIs is larger in 3D observations.

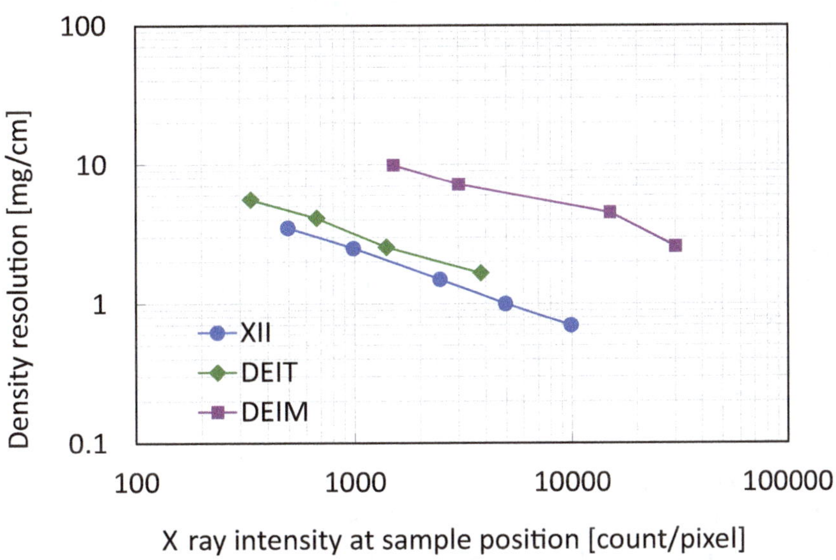

Fig. 8. Density resolution of XII, DEIT, and DEIM at each X-ray intensity.

A 3D image of a formalin-fixed rat tail obtained using DEIM with a 35-keV X-ray beam is shown in Fig. 9. The bone, disc, and hair are clearly visible. The density between the disc and the muscle was very different; therefore, the phase shift caused by the tail was too large and could not be detected correctly using either XII or DEIT. DEIM has lower sensitivity than the other methods, but it has a wide dynamic range of density and enables observation of a sample having regions with large differences in density.

3. Application for observation of pathological samples

Current biomedical research commonly uses various imaging techniques, such as X-ray CT, magnetic resonance imaging (MRI), positron emission tomography (PET), optical imaging, and supersonic imaging, to visualize the inner structures of objects (Wu & Tseng, 2004; Weissleder, 2006; Grenier et al., 2009; Hoffman & Grambhir, 2007). Micro-imaging techniques require high spatial resolution of the micrometer order and high contrast resolution, especially for basic biomedical research with small animals. For example, micro-X-ray CT with a conventional X-ray tube has spatial resolution of a few micrometers, but the contrast resolution is significantly low (Ritman, 2002).

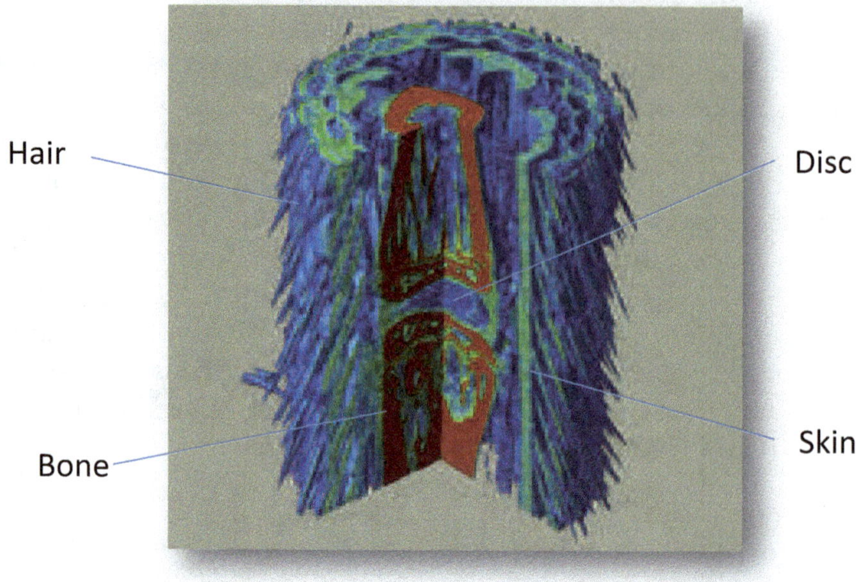

Fig. 9. 3D images of rat tail obtained using DEIM with 35-keV X-ray beam. Bone, disc, and hair are clearly visible.

X-ray interferometric imaging clearly depicts minute density differences within biological objects composed of low atomic number elements. Thus, this imaging technique was applied to observe biomedical objects, and detailed images that cannot be visualized by conventional X-ray imaging techniques was obtained. Here, we describe *ex-vivo* and *in-vivo* biomedical images obtained using XII.

3.1 Breast cancer imaging

A conventional X-ray mammogram is obtained as a projection image, and a lower X-ray energy of 18 keV is used to detect micro-calcification of more than 0.2 mm and soft tissue mass lesions of more than 2-3 mm. The phase-contrast X-ray imaging technique has high sensitivity to detect soft tissue lesions and enables the X-ray exposure for the patient to be decreased. The diagnosis of breast cancer is one of the most important targets of this technique.

An absorption-contrast X-ray image, phase map, and histological picture stained with hematoxylin-eosin of an invasive ductal breast cancer specimen are shown in Fig. 10. Breast tissue and its cancer, which is composed of fat, soft tissue, and micro-calcification, have a wide density difference. Therefore, to increase the dynamic range of density, a high X-ray energy of 51 keV was used in interferometric imaging of breast tissue specimens. In the phase map, the mosaic-like structure of breast cancer is clearly depicted, resembling the histological picture, whereas in the absorption-contrast image, the cancer and surrounding breast soft tissue are shown as homogeneous (Takeda et al., 2004c). The signal to noise ratio of the phase map at 51 keV on soft tissue against surrounding water was approximately 478-folds higher than that of the absorption X-ray image at 17.7 keV.

The phase map at 51 keV also had an excellent ability to enable differentiation of minute changes in the soft tissue density and detection of micro-calcifications of 0.036 mm that were undetected by the absorption-contrast X-ray technique. The phase map of the inner breast cancer structures matched well with pathological pictures. Therefore, XII might detect an extremely early stage of breast cancer, and thus it could improve the prognosis for the patient. In addition, the use of 51-keV X-ray energy markedly reduces the X-ray exposure of the patient. For example, to image a 50-mm-thick object, a 51-keV X-ray dose by XII would be less than 1/80 of the dose in conventional X-ray mammography.

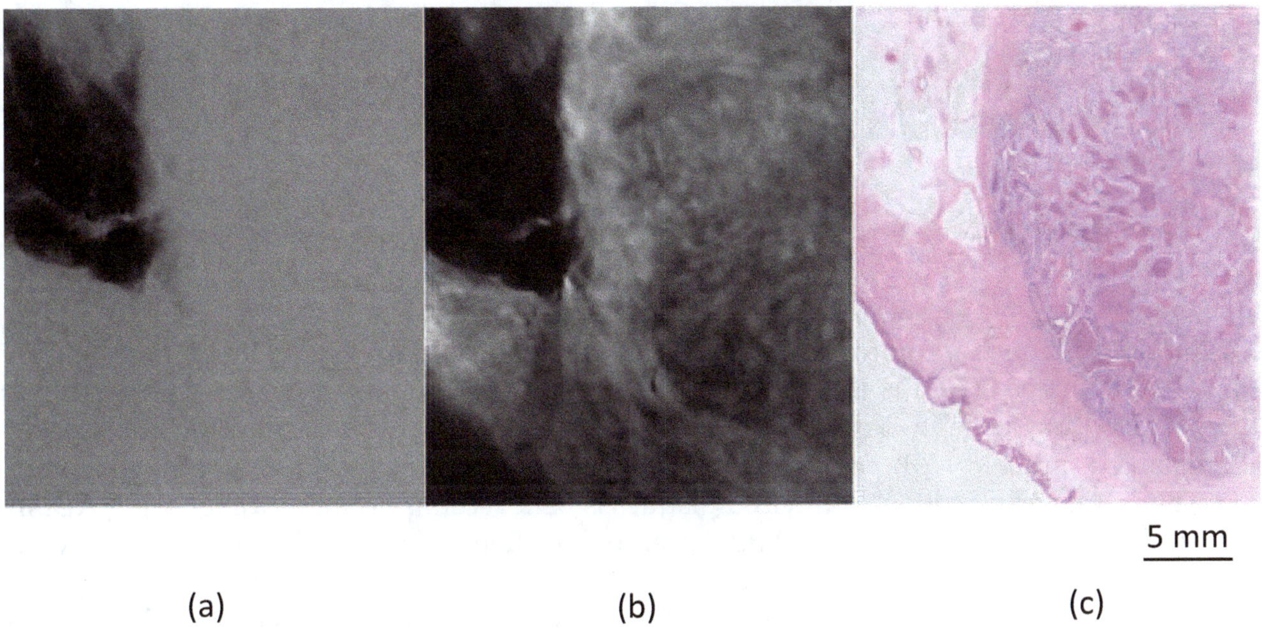

Fig. 10. (a) Absorption-contrast image, (b) phase map, and (c) pathological picture of 10-mm-thick formalin-fixed specimen of invasive ductal breast cancer.

3.2 Formalin-fixed colon cancer specimens from nude mice

Imaging of cancer is very important for diagnosis and determining a treatment strategy. In a conventional X-ray CT image, the absorption differences among cancer, fibrosis, necrosis, and normal tissues are difficult to detect because the differences in the linear attenuation coefficients of these tissues are very small. As mentioned earlier, XII enables visualization of the inner structures of human cancer specimens (Takeda et al., 2000) and animal cancer specimens (Momose et al., 1996; Takeda et al., 2004d), the brain (Beckmann et al., 1997), and the kidney (Wu et al., 2009) without contrast agents composed of heavy atomic elements. Here, we describe the images of cancer specimens obtained using XII at 35-keV X-ray energy.

The formalin-fixed specimens, approximately 12 mm in diameter, were of colon cancer that had been implanted in nude mice with a subsequent ethanol injection performed to examine the therapeutic effect of ethanol. Obtained sectional images clearly depicted the detailed inner structures of the subcutaneous implanted colon cancer mass, including cancer lesions, necrosis, mixed changes, surrounding tumor vessels, the subcutaneous thin muscle layer, subcutaneous tissue, and skin (Fig. 11). Cancer cells underwent necrosis in the central portion of the cancer mass due to the ethanol injection. In addition, the bulging of cancer from the thin muscle layer was well demonstrated. The pathological picture well resembled the phase-contrast sectional image. Thus, pathological information generated by the difference in density could be detected clearly. This indicates that quantitative evaluation could be easily performed using XII for new therapeutic applications.

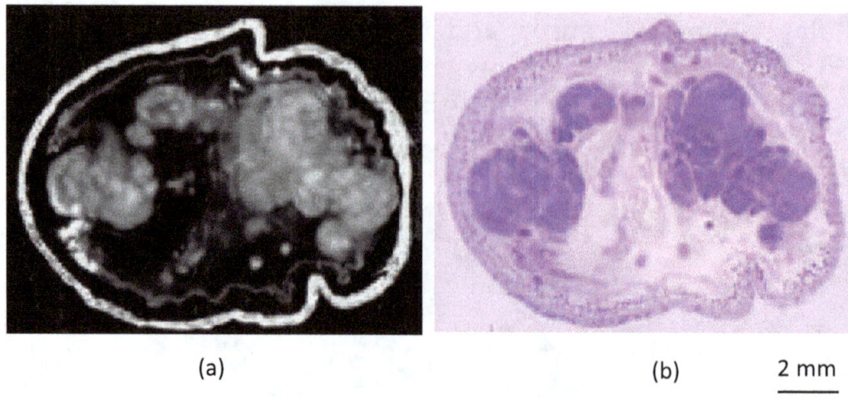

Fig. 11. (a) Phase-contrast X-ray CT and (b) pathological picture of colon cancer implanted in nude mouse.

3.3 Amyloid plaques in mouse model of Alzheimer's disease

Alzheimer's disease (AD) is the most common cause of dementia, and it is pathologically characterized by the deposition of amyloid plaques. Amyloid plaques, composed of densely aggregated β-amyloid (Aβ) peptides, are believed to play a key role in the pathogenesis of AD. Therefore, visualization of amyloid plaques is believed important for diagnosing AD. In this study, the brains from 12 PSAPP mice, an excellent AD model mouse for studying amyloid deposition, were imaged by XII at 17.8 keV X-ray energy.

Numerous bright white spots having high density were typically observed in the brains of 3 PSAPP mice at the age of 12 months, whereas no spots were depicted in an age-matched control mouse without the use of contrast agents. An example is shown in Fig. 12 (Noda-Saita et al., 2006). To confirm the identity of these bright spots, histological studies were performed after the observation. The bright spots were found to be identical to amyloid plaques. Finally, we performed quantitative analysis of Aβ spots in the brains of 3 PSAPP mice each at 4, 6, 9, and 12 months of age. The results showed that the quantity of Aβ spots clearly increased with age as shown in Fig. 13.

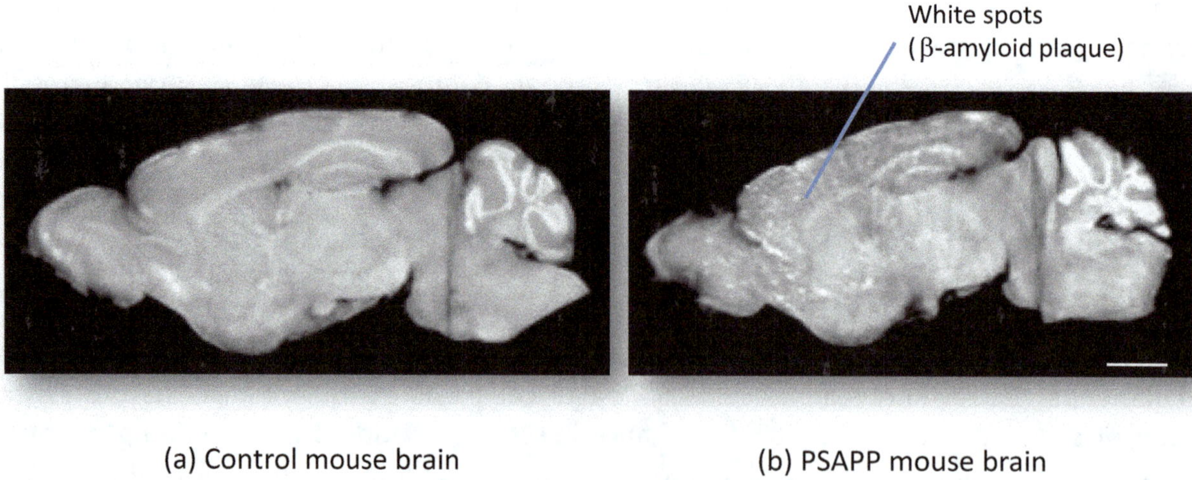

Fig. 12. Amyloid plaque in 12-month old mouse model of Alzheimer's disease. Identification of bright spots observed in brain of PSAPP mouse, but age-matched control mouse did not show such spots. Scale bars = 2 mm.

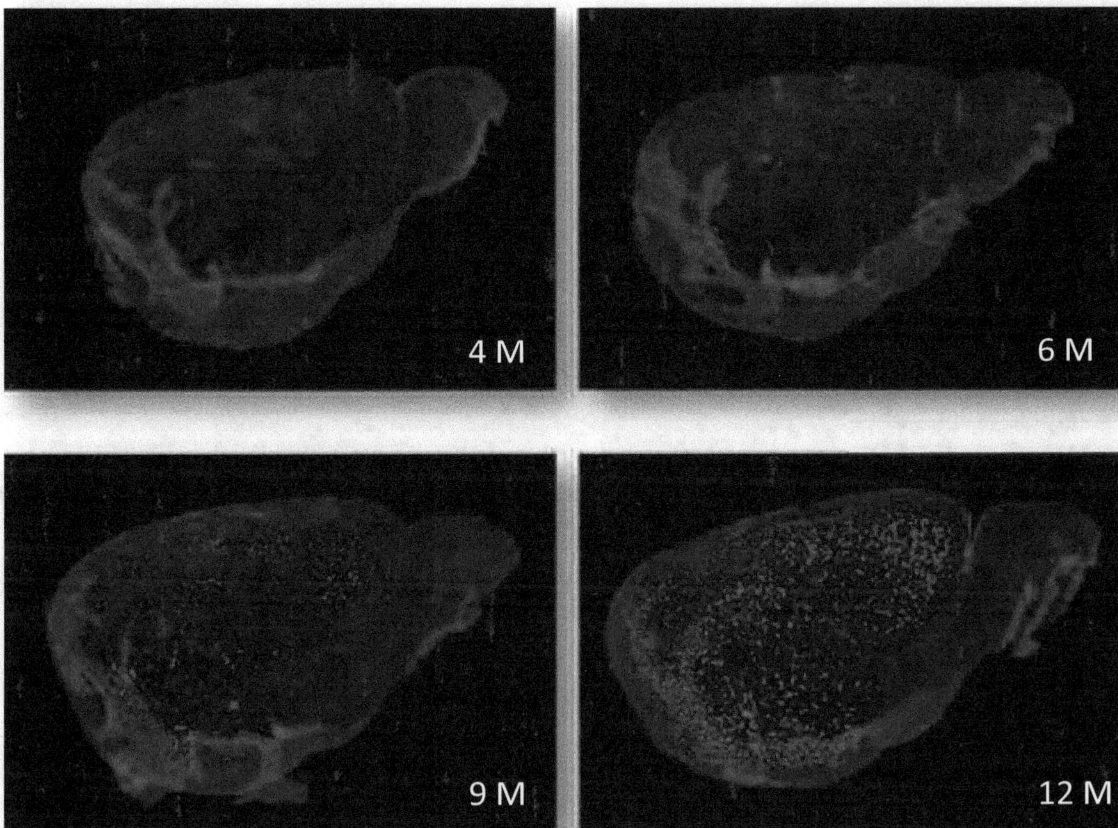

Fig. 13. Representative 3D images of Aβ spots (orange) in brain (cerebral cortex and hippocampus) of PSAPP mice at 4, 6, 9, and 12 months old.

3.4 Phase-contrast X-ray CT imaging of live mouse

In-vivo observation of a small animal disease model is very important for establishing a new diagnostic and/or treatment method in basic clinical research. With the benefit of a two-crystal interferometer, *in-vivo* imaging of a mouse implanted with colon cancer was achieved using the XII system (Takeda et al., 2004). Furthermore, sequential observation was performed to examine the treatment effect of paclitaxel as a cancer drug (Yoneyama et al., 2006).

A series of horizontal slice images obtained from a tumor following injection of paclitaxel is shown in Fig. 13. The tumor size did not change significantly, but the low density area (necrosis) near the center became larger gradually. A typical 3D image observed during the second day after cancer drug therapy started is shown in Fig. 14. The tumor was 10 mm in diameter and ~6 mm thick. The blue area indicates a low-density region and the green area indicates a high-density region.

These results showed that the phase-contrast X-ray CT enables us to perform detailed observation with high spatial resolution without harming the target, and therefore *ex-* and *in-vivo* visualization of biomedical objects is believed very useful for biomedical research.

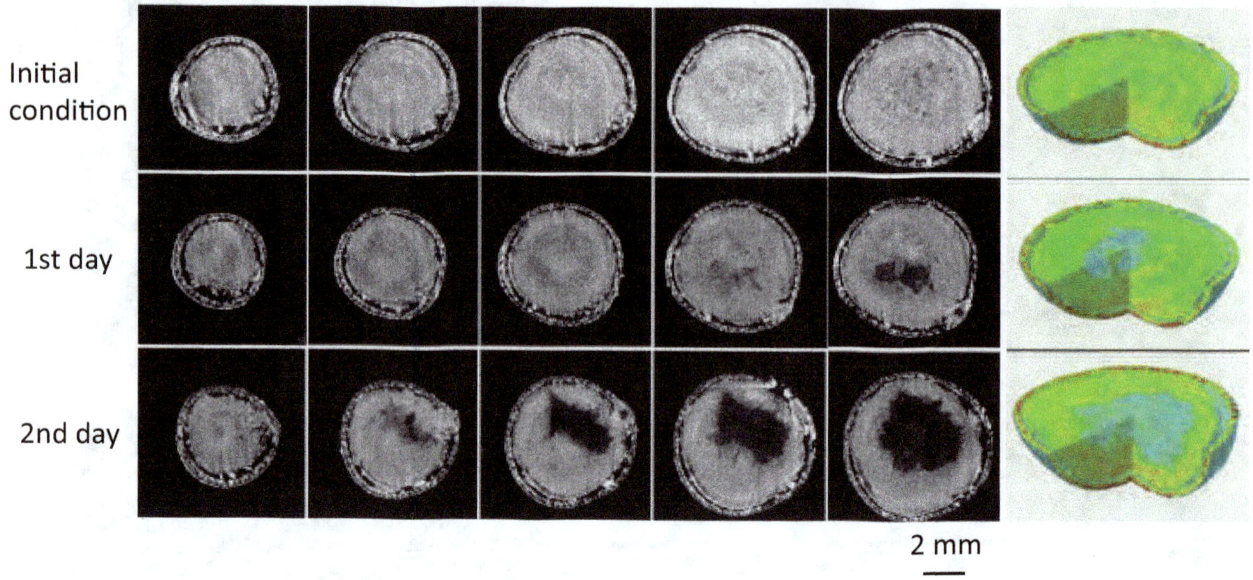

Fig. 14. Series of horizontal slice images of colon cancer and 3D in-vivo phase-contrast X-ray CT images taken before and after anti-cancer drug therapy started.

4. Application for embryo imaging

Embryos undergo complicated morphogenetic changes during the course of development. Classically, drawings and solid reconstruction were used to demonstrate the 3D changes of embryonic structures. The wax plate technique of reconstruction was used for embryology, and based on the reconstructed models, numerous accurate drawings of embryos were produced by hand (see Yamada et al., 2006). During the past 20 years, computer-assisted reconstruction of biological structures has become available, which has enabled the reconstruction of various 3D structures from serial sectional images. Non-destructive imaging technologies such as X-ray CT and magnetic resonance (MR) imaging, which were originally developed as non-invasive diagnostic tools in clinical medicine, have also been applied to the imaging and 3D reconstruction of tiny biological structures such as embryos. The MR microscopic technology has been widely used to scan and visualize relatively small samples, including mammalian embryos (Smith et al., 1996; Smith, 1999; Haishi et al., 2001; Yamada et al., 2010), but MR microscopy does not yield resolution or contrast high enough for millimetre-sized embryos. Conventional X-ray CT was also developed for microscopic observation of small structures, but it is not appropriate for soft tissues such as embryos.

Sequential images during mouse embryo development obtained by the DEI system are shown in Fig. 15. By using formalin-fixed mouse embryos, detailed observation of the internal organs can be made throughout the early to late stages of mouse embryonic development by tomographs, as well as of the external appearance by surface reconstruction. The developing bone structures do not affect the phase-contrast images (see E15.5 and E17.5 in Fig. 15).

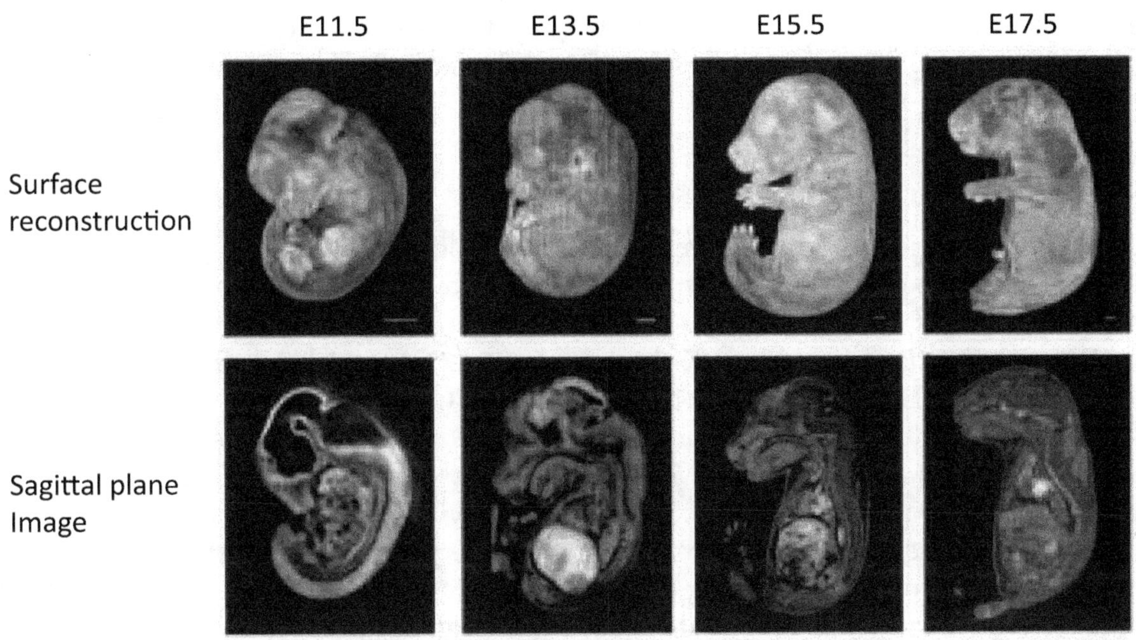

Fig. 15. Sequential images of mouse embryo development. Bars = 1 mm.

Embryo images obtained by the XII and DEI systems are shown in Fig. 16. Both systems can provide fine surface reconstruction and images of the internal structure. Images by the XII system seem to be better than those of the DEI system for the same embryo, although the scan time of DEI (1 hr) is much shorter than that of XII (4–5 hrs). The image sharpness can be affected by the direction of the rotation of the samples. Some precious samples were not glued directly on the stage but were embedded in agar, which was then fixed on the stage by an adhesive agent. Therefore, small deformation of the agar by gravity may affect the images by the XII system.

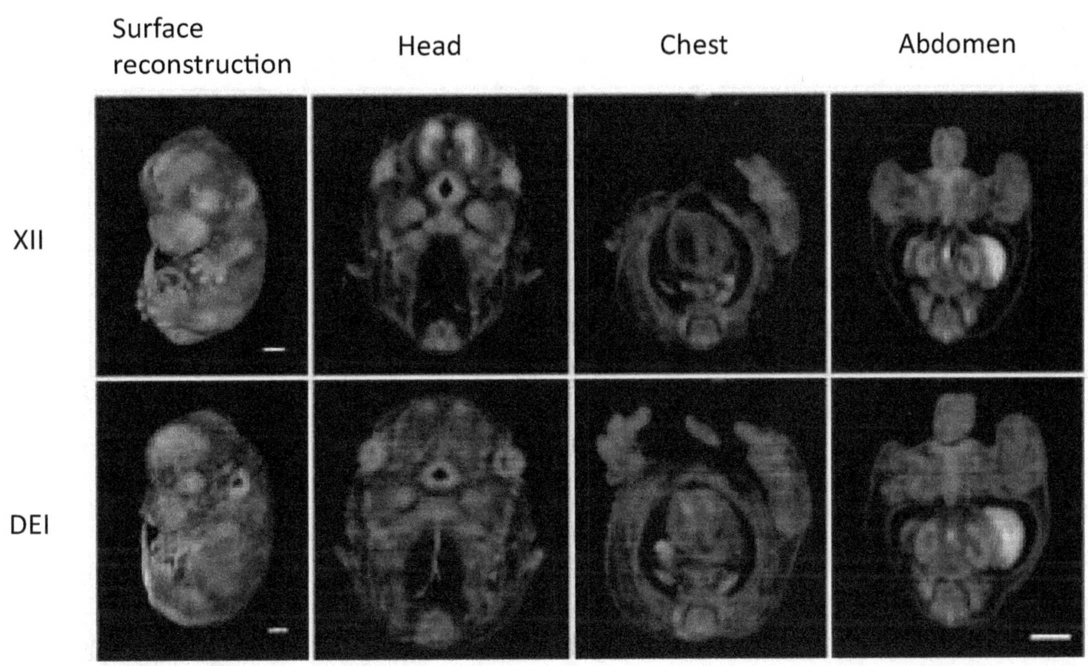

Fig. 16. Images by XII and DEI systems for E13.5 mouse embryo in Fig. 15. Bars = 1mm.

These images show that the phase-contrast X-ray CT has a wide enough field and high enough resolution for observation and analyses of morphological changes during embryo development.

5. Conclusion

Phase-contrast X-ray imaging is a novel imaging method using the X-ray phase shift caused by a sample as image contrast. The sensitivity of the method is much higher than that of the conventional method using X-ray absorption by the sample. To detect X-ray phase shift, many detection methods such as X-ray interferometric imaging (XII) and diffraction-enhanced imaging (DEI) have been developed. XII has the highest sensitivity (density resolution) and therefore is suitable for observations requiring high density resolution, such as visualization of β-amyloid plaques. DEI has a wide dynamic range of density and is thus suitable for observation of samples including regions with large differences in density, such as bone and soft tissues. Many fine observations of pathological soft tissues and mice embryos were performed by selecting the most suitable imaging method. The results show that phase-contrast X-ray imaging enables us to perform fine observation of biomedical and organic samples without extreme X-ray exposure or any supplemental agents.

6. Acknowledgments

We thank Dr. Y. Hirai of Saga Light Source, Dr. Y. Shitaka, Dr. K. Noda-Saita, Dr. N. Amino, Dr. M. Mori, and Dr. M. Kudoof of Astellas Pharma Inc. for experimental help and advice. We also thank Dr. K. Hyodo of the Photon Factory for his technical assistance at the beam line. The observations were carried out under Proposal Nos. 2002S2-001, 2005S2-001, and 2009S2-006 approved by the High Energy Accelerator Research Organization.
The experiment was approved by the Ethics Committee of the University of Tsukuba for the human sample, and the Medical Committee for the Use of Animals in Research of the University of Tsukuba and the Animal Ethical Committee of Astellas Pharma Inc. It conformed to the guidelines of the American Physiological Society for animal experiments.

7. References

Ando, M., Sugiyama, H., Kunisada, T., Shimao, D., Takeda, K., Hashizume, H., & Inoue, H. (2004). Construction of X-ray dark-field imaging with a view size of 80 mm square and first visualization of human articular cartilage of femoral head under a nearly clinical condition. *Jpn. J. Appl. Phys.*, 43, L1175-L1177

Becker, B. P. & Bonse, U. (1974). The skew-symmetric two-crystal X-ray interferometer. *J Appl. Cryst.*, 7, 593–598.

Beckmann, F., Bonse, U., Busch, F., & Gunnewig, O. (1997). X-ray microtomography using phase contrast for the investigation of organic matter. *J. Comput. Assist. Tomogr.*, 21, 539–553.

Bonse, U. & Hart, M. (1965). An X-ray interferometer. *Appl. Phys. Lett.*, 6, 155–156.

Bruning, J. H., Herriott, D. R., Gallagher, J. E., Rosenfeld, D. P., White, A. D., & Brangaccio, D. J. (1974). Digital wavefront measuring interferometer for testing optical surfaces and lenses. *Appl. Opt.*, 13, 2693–2703.

Chapman, D., Thomlinson, W., Johnston, R. E., Washburn, D., Pisano, E., Gmur, N., Zhong, Z., Menk, R., Arfelli, F., & Sayers, D. (1997). Diffraction enhanced x-ray imaging. *Phys. Med. Biol.*, 42, 2015–2025.

Connor, M. D., Benveniste, H., Dilmanian, F. A., Kritzer, M. F., Miller M. L., & Zhong, Z. (2009). Computed tomography of amyloid plaques in a mouse model of Alzheimer's disease using diffraction enhanced imaging. *Neuroimage,* 46, 908–914.

Davis, T. J., Gao, D., Gureyev, T. E., Stevenson, A. W., & Wilkins, S. W. (1995). Phase contrast imaging of weakly absorbing materials using hard X-rays. *Nature,* 373, 595–598.

Donath, T., Pfeiffer, F., Bunk O., Grünzweig, C., Hempel, E., Popescu, S., Vock, P., & David, C. (2010). Toward clinical X-ray phase-contrast CT: Demonstration of enhanced soft-tissue contrast in human specimen, *Investigative Radiology,* 45, 445–452.

Grenier, N., Sardanelli, F., Becker, C. D., Walecki, J., Sebag, G., Lomas, D. J., & Krestin, J. P. (2009). Development of molecular imaging in the European radiological community, *European Radiology,* 13, 655–656.

Haishi, T., Uematsu, T., Matsuda, Y., & Kose, K. (2001). Development of a 1.0 T MR microscope using a Nd-Fe-B permanent magnet. *Magn. Reson. Imaging,* 19, 875–880.

Hoffman, J. M. & Gambhir, S. S. (2007). Molecular imaging: the vision and opportunity for radiology in the future. *Radiology,* 244, 39–47.

Ingal, V. N. & Beliaevskaya, E. A. (1995). X-ray plane-wave topography observation of the phase contrast from a non-crystalline object. *J. of Physics* D, 28, 2314–2317.

Koyama, I., Hamaishi, Y., & Momose, A. (2004). Phase tomography using diffraction enhanced imaging. *AIP Conference Proceedings,* 705, 1283–1286.

Mollenhauer, J., Aurich, M. E., Zhong, Z., Muehleman, C., Cole, A. A., Hasnah, M., Oltulu, O., Kuettner, K. E., Margulis, A., & Chapman, L. D. (2002). Diffraction-enhanced X-ray imaging of articular cartilage. *Osteoarthritis and Cartilage,* 10, 163–171.

Momose, A. & Fukuda, J. (1995). Phase-contrast radiographs of nonstained rat cerebellar specimen. *Med. Phys.*, 22, 4, 375–380.

Momose, A. (1995). Demonstration of phase-contrast x-ray computed tomography using x-ray interferometer. *Nucl. Inst. and Meth. in Phys. Research* A, 352, 622–628.

Momose, A., Takeda, T., Itai, Y., & Hirano, K. (1996). Phase-contrast x-ray computed tomography for observing biological soft tissue. *Nature Med.*, 2, 473–47.

Momose, A., Takeda, T., Yoneyama, A., Koyama, I., & Itai, Y. (2001). Wide-area phase-contrast X-ray imaging using large X-ray interferometers. *Nucl. Instrum. Meth.,* A467-468, 917–920.

Momose, A., Kawamoto, S., Koyama, I., Hamaishi, Y., Takai, K., & Suzuki, Y. (2003). Demonstration of X-ray Talbot interferometry. *Jpn. J. Appl. Phys.*, 42, L866-L868.

Momose, A., Yashiro, W., & Kuwarara, H. (2009). Grating-based X-ray phase imaging using multiline X-ray source. *Jpn J. of Appl. Phys.,* 48, 076512.

Noda-Saita, K., Yoneyama, A., Shitaka, Y., Hirai, Y., Terai, K., Wu, J., Takeda, T., Hyodo, K., Osakabe, N., Yamaguchi, T., & Okada M. (2006). Quantitative analysis of amyloid plaques in a mouse model of Alzheimer's disease by phase-contrast X-ray computed tomography. *Neuroscience,* 138, 1205–1213.

Oltulu, O., Zhong, Z., Hasnah, M., Wernick, N. M., & Chapman, D. (2003). Extraction of extinction, refraction and absorption properties in diffraction enhanced imaging. *Journal of Physics* D, 35, 2152–2156.

Pisano, E. D., Johnston, R. E., Chapman, D., Geradts, J., Iacocca, M. V., Livasy, C. A., Washburn, D. B., Sayers, D. E., Zhong, Z., Kiss, M. Z., & Thomlinson, W. C. (2000). Human breast cancer specimens: Diffraction-enhanced imaging with histological correlation-improved conspicuity of lesion detail compared with digital radiography. *Radiology,* 214, 895–901.

Rigon, L., Arfelli, F., & Menk, R. H. (2007). Three-image diffraction enhanced imaging algorithm to extract absorption, refraction, and ultra small-angle scattering, *Appl. Phys. Lett.,* 90, 11, 114102.

Ritman E. L. (2002). Molecular imaging in small animals—roles for micro-CT. *Journal Cellular Biochemistry Supplement,* 39, 116–124.

Smith, B. R., Linney, E., Huff, D. S., & Johnson, G. A. (1996). Magnetic resonance microscopy of embryos. *Comput. Med Imaging Graph,* 20, 483–490.

Smith, B. R., Huff, D. S., & Johnson, G. A. (1999). Magnetic resonance imaging of embryos: an Internet resource for the study of embryonic development. *Comput. Med Imaging Graph,* 23, 33–40.

Snigirev, A., Snigirev, I., Kohn, V., Kuznetsov, S., & Schelokov, I. (1995). On the possibilities of x-ray phase contrast microimaging by coherent high-energy synchrotron radiation. *Rev. Sci. Instrum.,* 66, 5486–5492.

Sunaguchi, N., Yuasa, T., Huo, Q., Ichihara, S., & Ando, M., (2010). X-ray refraction-contrast computed tomography images using dark-field imaging optics. *Appl. Phys. Lett.,* 97, 15, 153701.

Takeda, M., Ina, H., & Kobayashi, S. (1982). Fourier-transform method of fringe pattern analysis for computer-based topography and interferometry. *J. Opt. Soc. Am.,* 72, 156–160.

Takeda, T., Momose, A., Itai, Y., Wu, J., & Hirano, K. (1995). Phase-contrast imaging with synchrotron X-rays for detecting cancer lesions. *Acad. Radiol.,* 2, 799–803.

Takeda, T., Momose, A., Hirano, K., Haraoka, S., Watanabe, T., & Itai, Y. (2000). Human carcinoma: Early experience with phase-contrast X-ray CT image with synchrotron radiation: Comparative specimen study with optical microscopy. *Radiology,* 214, 298–301.

Takeda, T., Momose, A., Wu, J., Yu, Q., Zeniya, T., Lwin, T. T., Yoneyama, A., & Itai, Y. (2002). Vessel imaging by interferometric phase-contrast x-ray technique. *Circulation,* 105, 1708–1712.

Takeda, T., Wu, J., Tsuchiya, Y., Lwin, T. T., Yoneyama, A., Itai, Y., & Itai, Y. (2004a). Vessel imaging by interferometric phase-contrast x-ray technique. *Proc. of 3rd Congress on Heart Disease,* 105, 143–146.

Takeda, T., Yoneyama, A., Wu, J., Lwin, T. T., Tsuchiya, Y., & Hyodo, K. (2004b). In-vivo imaging of cancer implanted in nude mice by two-crystal interferometer-based phase-contrast X-ray CT. *Jpn. J. Appl. Phys.,* 43, L1144-1146.

Takeda, T., Wu, J., Tsuchiya, Y., Yoneyama, A., Lwin, T. T., Aiyoshi, Y., Zeniya, T., Hyodo, K., & Ueno, E. (2004c). Interferometric X-ray imaging of breast cancer specimens at 51 keV X-ray energy. *Jpn. J. Appl. Phys.*, 43, 5652–5656.

Takeda, T., Wu, J., Tsuchiya, Y., Yoneyama, A., Lwin, T. T., Hyodo, K., & Itai, Y. (2004d). Interferometric phase-contrast X-ray CT image of VX2 rabbit cancer at 35 keV X-ray energy. *AIP Conference Proceedings,* 705, 1328–1331.

Weissleder, R. (2006). Molecular imaging in cancer. *Science,* 312, 1168–71.

Weitkamp, T., Diaz, A., & David, C. (2005). X-ray phase imaging with a grating interferometer. *Optics Express,* 13, 6296–6304.

Wernick, M. N., Wirjadi, O., Chapman, D., Zhong, Z., Galatsanos, N. P., Yang, Y., Brankov, J. G., Oltulu, O., Anastasio, M. A., & Muehleman, C. (2003). Multiple-image radiography. *Phys. Med. Biol.*, 48, 23, 3875–3895.

Wilkins, S. W., Gureyev, T. E., Gao, D., Pogany, A., & Steven, A. W. (1996). Phase-contrast imaging using polychromatic hard X-rays. *Nature,* 384, 335–338.

Wu, J. C., Tseng, J. R., & Gambhir, S. S. (2004). Molecular imaging of cardiovascular gene products. *J. Nucl. Cardiol.*, 11, 491–505.

Wu, J., Takeda, T., Lwin, T. T., Momose, A., Sunaguchi, N., Fukami, T., Yuasa, T., & Akatsuka, T. (2009). Imaging renal structures by X-ray phase-contrast microtomography. *Kidney International,* 75, 945–951.

Yamada, S., Uwabe, C., Nakatsu-Komatsu, T., Minekura, Y., Iwakura, M., Motoki, T., Nishimiya, K., Iiyama, M., Kakusho, K., Minoh, M., Mizuta, S., Matsuda, T., Matsuda, Y., Haishi, T., Kose, K., Fujii, S., & Shiota, K. (2006). Graphic and movie illustrations of human prenatal development and their application to embryological education based on the human embryo specimens in the Kyoto collection. *Dev. Dyn.*, 235, 468–477.

Yamada, S., Samtani, R. R., Lee, E. S., Lockett, E., Uwabe, C., Shiota, K., Anderson, S. A., & Lo, C. W. (2010). Developmental atlas of the early first trimester human embryo. *Dev. Dyn.*, 239, 1585–1595.

Yoneyama, A., Momose, A., Seya, E., Hirano, K., Takeda, T., & Itai, Y. (1999). Operation of a separated-type X-ray interferometer for phase-contrast X-ray imaging. *Review of Scientific Instruments*, 70, 4582–4586.

Yoneyama, A., Momose, A., Koyama, I., Seya, E., Takeda, T., Itai, Y., Hirano, K., & Hyodo, K. (2002). Large-area phase-contrast X-ray imaging using a two-crystal X-ray interferometer. *Journal of Synchrotron Radiation,* 9, 277–281.

Yoneyama, A., Takeda, T., Tsuchiya, Y., Wu, J., Lwin, T. T., Koizumi, A., Hyodo, K., & Itai, Y. (2004a). A phase-contrast X-ray imaging system—with a 60×30 mm field of view—based on a skew-symmetric two-crystal X-ray inteferometer. *Nucl. Inst. and Meth. in Phys. Research* A, 523, 217–222.

Yoneyama, A., Takeda, T., Tsuchiya, Y., Wu, J., Lwin, T. T., & Hyodo, K. (2004b). Large-area phase-contrast X-ray imaging system using a two-crystal X-ray interferometer—development of an interference-pattern-based feedback positioning system. *AIP Conference Proceedings,* 705, 1299–1302.

Yoneyama, A., Takeda, T., Tsuchiya, Y., Wu, J., Lwin, T. T., Hyodo, K., & Hirai, Y. (2005). High-energy phase-contrast X-ray imaging using a two-crystal X-ray interferometer. *J. Synchrotron Rad.*, 12, 534–536.

Yoneyama, A., Amino, N., Mori, M., Kudoh, M., Takeda, T., Hyodo, K., & Hirai, Y. (2006). Non-invasive and time-resolved observation of tumors implanted in living mice by using phase-contrast X-ray computed tomography. *Jpn. J. Appl. Phys.*, 45, 1864–1868.

Yoneyama, A., Wu, J., Hyodo, K., & Takeda, T. (2008). Quantitative comparison of imaging performance of X-ray interferometric imaging and diffraction enhanced imaging. *Med. Phys.*, 35, 4724–4734.

Yoneyama, A., Takeda, T., Yamazaki, T., Hyodo, K., & Ueda, K. (2010). High-energy diffraction-enhanced X-ray imaging, *AIP Conference Proceedings*, 1234, 477–480.

Permissions

All chapters in this book were first published in ABE, by InTech Open; hereby published with permission under the Creative Commons Attribution License or equivalent. Every chapter published in this book has been scrutinized by our experts. Their significance has been extensively debated. The topics covered herein carry significant findings which will fuel the growth of the discipline. They may even be implemented as practical applications or may be referred to as a beginning point for another development.

The contributors of this book come from diverse backgrounds, making this book a truly international effort. This book will bring forth new frontiers with its revolutionizing research information and detailed analysis of the nascent developments around the world.

We would like to thank all the contributing authors for lending their expertise to make the book truly unique. They have played a crucial role in the development of this book. Without their invaluable contributions this book wouldn't have been possible. They have made vital efforts to compile up to date information on the varied aspects of this subject to make this book a valuable addition to the collection of many professionals and students.

This book was conceptualized with the vision of imparting up-to-date information and advanced data in this field. To ensure the same, a matchless editorial board was set up. Every individual on the board went through rigorous rounds of assessment to prove their worth. After which they invested a large part of their time researching and compiling the most relevant data for our readers.

The editorial board has been involved in producing this book since its inception. They have spent rigorous hours researching and exploring the diverse topics which have resulted in the successful publishing of this book. They have passed on their knowledge of decades through this book. To expedite this challenging task, the publisher supported the team at every step. A small team of assistant editors was also appointed to further simplify the editing procedure and attain best results for the readers.

Apart from the editorial board, the designing team has also invested a significant amount of their time in understanding the subject and creating the most relevant covers. They scrutinized every image to scout for the most suitable representation of the subject and create an appropriate cover for the book.

The publishing team has been an ardent support to the editorial, designing and production team. Their endless efforts to recruit the best for this project, has resulted in the accomplishment of this book. They are a veteran in the field of academics and their pool of knowledge is as vast as their experience in printing. Their expertise and guidance has proved useful at every step. Their uncompromising quality standards have made this book an exceptional effort. Their encouragement from time to time has been an inspiration for everyone.

The publisher and the editorial board hope that this book will prove to be a valuable piece of knowledge for researchers, students, practitioners and scholars across the globe.

List of Contributors

Manuel G. Forero
Cardiff University, United Kingdom

Alicia Hidalgo
University of Birmingham, United Kingdom

Dongxiao Zhu
University of New Orleans, New Orleans, U.S.A
Research Institute for Children, Children's Hospital, New Orleans, U.S.A.

Lipi R. Acharya
University of New Orleans, New Orleans, U.S.A

Lidia Vilca-Quispe, Alejandro Castilla-Loeza, Juan José Alvarado-Gil and Patricia Quintana-Owen
Centro de Investigación y de Estudios Avanzados del IPN, Unidad Mérida Mérida, Yucatán, México

Gregor Kijanka, Robert Burger, Ivan K. Dimov, Rima Padovani, Karen Lawler, Richard O'Kennedy and Jens Ducrée
Biomedical Diagnostics Institute - Dublin City University, Ireland

Javier Sanz-Valero, Rocio Guardiola-Wanden-Berghe and Carmina Wanden-Berghe
University Miguel Hernández, University of Alicante, University CEU Cardenal Herrera, Spain

Alexandros Karagiannis and Philip Constantinou
National Technical University of Athens, School of Electrical and Computer Engineering, Mobile Radio Communication Laboratory

Demosthenes Vouyioukas
University of the Aegean, Department of Information and Communication Systems Engineering, Greece

Craig Jin
School of Electrical and Information Engineering, The University of Sydney, Sydney NSW, Australia

Virginia Best, Gaven Lin and Simon Carlile
School of Medical Sciences and Bosch Institute, The University of Sydney, Sydney NSW, Australia

Dhananjay Singh
Future Internet Team, Division of Fusion and Convergence of Mathematical Sciences, National Institute for mathematical Sciences (NIMS), Daejeon, South Korea

Pilar Del Valle García, Ignacio Martínez Ruiz, Javier Escayola Calvo, Jesús Daniel Trigo Vilaseca and José García Moros
Aragon Institute for Engineering Research (I3A), University of Zaragoza (UZ), Zaragoza, Spain

Tetyana Torchynska
ESFM - National Polytechnic Institute, México D. F., México

Yuri Vorobiev
CINVESTAV-IPN, Unidad Querétaro, Querétaro, QRO., México

Mette Ebbesen
University of Aarhus, Denmark

Zhaopeng Fan, Gong Zhang and Simon Liao
University of Winnipeg, Canada

Akio Yoneyama
Advanced Research Laboratory, Hitachi Ltd., Japan

Shigehito Yamada
Congenital Anomaly Research Center, Kyoto University, Japan

Tohoru Takeda
Allied Health Sciences, Kitasato University, Japan

Index

www.ingramcontent.com/pod-product-compliance
Lightning Source LLC
LaVergne TN
LVHW081019210926
848485LV00004B/902